10

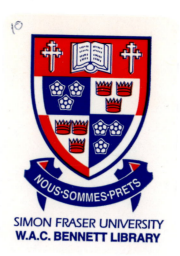

SIMON FRASER UNIVERSITY
W.A.C. BENNETT LIBRARY

Gender, Health and Healing

Gender, Health and Healing presents a whole range of issues which are brought together and connected to emerging concerns in contemporary life such as the new genetics and transformations in biomedical knowledge and practices. It offers a challenging assessment of gender relations and embodied practices across the public/private divide, using health and healing as paradigmatic examples.

This thought-provoking volume lies at the intersection of gender studies, the sociology of health and healing, health policy, the critical analysis of scientific knowledge and the current debates around the body, health and emotions. Bringing together new and leading scholars in the field, it provides a unique, critical overview of contemporary debates in health care for an interdisciplinary readership.

Gillian Bendelow, **Mick Carpenter**, **Caroline Vautier** and **Simon Williams** are all members of the Centre for Research in Health, Medicine and Society, University of Warwick.

Gender, Health and Healing

The public/private divide

Edited by
Gillian Bendelow, Mick Carpenter,
Caroline Vautier, Simon Williams

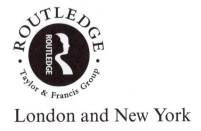

London and New York

First published 2002
by Routledge
11 New Fetter Lane, London EC4P 4EE

Simultaneously published in the USA and Canada
by Routledge
29 West 35th Street, New York, NY 10001

Routledge is an imprint of the Taylor & Francis Group

Typeset in Times New Roman by RefineCatch Limited, Bungay, Suffolk
Printed and bound in Great Britain by
Biddles Ltd, Guildford and King's Lynn

British Library Cataloguing in Publication Data
A catalogue record for this book is available from the British Library

Library of Congress Cataloging in Publication Data
A catalog record for this book has been requested

ISBN 0–415–23574–X (pbk)
ISBN 0–415–23573–1 (hbk)

Contents

Contributors

Priscilla Alderson is Professor of Childhood Studies at the Social Science Research Unit, Institute of Education, University of London.

Gillian Bendelow is Senior Lecturer in the Department of Sociology, University of Warwick.

Lynda Birke is a feminist biologist and a freelance writer in North Wales, formerly of the Centre for the Study of Women and Gender, University of Warwick.

Geraldine Brady is an ESRC-funded PhD student in the Department of Sociology, University of Warwick.

Joan Busfield is Professor of Sociology at the University of Essex.

Mick Carpenter is co-Director of the Centre for Research in Health Medicine and Society and Reader in the Department of Sociology, University of Warwick.

Celia Davies is Professor of Health Care at the Open University, Milton Keynes.

Lesley Doyal is Professor of Health and Social Care at the University of Bristol.

Renée C. Fox is Annenberg Professor Emerita of the Social Sciences in the Department of Sociology and a Fellow of the Center for Bioethics at the University of Pennsylvania, also a Research Associate at the Queen Elizabeth House at the University of Oxford.

Joan Haran is an ESRC-funded PhD student in the Department of Sociology, University of Warwick

Gillian Lewando Hundt is Professor of Social Studies and Medicine at the University of Warwick.

Anne Murcott is Professor Emerita at South Bank University, London.

Virginia Olesen is Professor Emerita of Sociology, University of California, San Francisco, USA.

Hilary Rose is Visiting Research Professor of Sociology at City University, London and joint Professor of Physics, Gresham College London.

Ursula Sharma recently retired from the University of Derby where she held the post of Professor of Comparative Sociology.

Meg Stacey is Professor Emerita in the Department of Sociology, University of Warwick.

Caroline Vautier is an ESRC-funded PhD student in the Department of Sociology, University of Warwick.

Simon J. Williams is a Warwick Research Fellow and Reader in the Department of Sociology, University of Warwick, and co-Director of the Centre for Research in Health Medicine and Society.

Acknowledgements

The Conference and the production of this book have been collective efforts of considerable proportions, but we should like to make special mention of the following.

The idea of a *festschrift* for Meg Stacey was initially suggested by Priscilla Alderson at a London Medical Sociology meeting. Simon Williams took the initiative and laid the groundwork to make the conference happen through the newly emerging Centre for Health Medicine and Society, aided by co-director Mick Carpenter and Caroline Vautier. The Warwick conference was also made possible by the untiring efforts of Geraldine Brady and Becky Elford. Thanks are also due to Frances Jones and other members of the secretarial staff in the Departments of Sociology and of Social Policy and Social Work and for financial support from the Medical Sociology Group of the British Sociological Association and the University of Warwick.

Sadly, this collection was unable to encompass the contributions of everyone who took part in the conference, and we offer our deep apologies to all those we were unable to include. Other people would have liked to take part but were unable to do so, some of whom are mentioned in the volume.

Meg, herself, would like to acknowledge the continued support of Jennifer Lorch throughout the whole process. Special mention should be made of the tremendous amount of input to the editorial work made by both Meg and Jennifer, for which the members of the team are very grateful.

Finally, we wish to thank Edwina Welham, Michelle Bacca and Routledge for their patience and support in helping us to realise this ambitious volume. We hope the final result does everyone justice.

GILLIAN BENDELOW
MICK CARPENTER
CAROLINE VAUTIER
SIMON WILLIAMS

Introduction: Overcoming divisions

Reflections on tradition, change and critical continuity

Gillian Bendelow, Mick Carpenter,
Caroline Vautier and Simon Williams

This volume arose from a *festschrift* held to celebrate the life and work of Meg Stacey that was organised by the Centre for Research in Health, Medicine and Society at Warwick, of which Meg is a founder member, and which has evolved in the university where she taught for many years and has continued working as *emerita* professor. The conference was held in April 1999, was hugely successful, and many of those who took part – including ourselves – will remember it for years to come as a remarkable event that was intellectually challenging, convivial and comradely.

Some of the spirit of that conference, we hope, permeates the book itself, although this is not just an attempt to reproduce it in the cold light of print. That would be impossible; and in any case we decided from the outset not to produce the kind of 'presentation tome' that primarily celebrates and reminisces about a person. Rather, what we seek to do is represent the vital *tradition* of analysis that Meg's work represents as one of the animating forces of contemporary sociology and social policy. In a world which seems in headlong rush down 'modernising' freeways of all kinds, the notion of 'tradition' might be seen as cautious, unreflective and conservative, to be discarded in favour of 'the new' and the speedier. However, what we mean by tradition is not unreflective acceptance, but a sense of *critical continuity*. It can be argued that what has characterised all types of sociological theorising since its emergence as an intellectual creation of nineteenth-century European social formations has been an ambivalence towards 'the modern' without which it could not have entered the world (Bauman 1997). This complex parent–child relationship is still working itself out in contemporary analysis, because profound changes continue to take place, the solid is still 'melting into the air' and the aim of social analysis (the only ultimate justification, surely, for devoting so much of society's surplus resources to it) is to help us to understand so that we can *choose* rather than simply be swept along or even trampled underfoot by social change.

The theme of this book, like the conference from which it originated, and on which all authors were asked to 'reflect', was the public/private divide in relation to gender, health and healing. The purpose of this title was to focus contributors' attention on the dichotomy between the two spheres that emerged with modern industrial capitalist societies and which, despite the various attempts to transcend it, remains a prominent feature today, whether societies are characterised variously as post-industrial, late- or postmodern. Whereas 'malestream' sociology and social policy had primarily expressed its critical ambivalence or opposition towards unequal social arrangements in the public sphere, the worlds of market work and formal politics, feminist criticism and social thought not only 'added' gender inequality into the equation, but also drew attention to the taken-for-granted divide between these public spheres and those of the family, domestic relations and daily life, which had in the process become subordinated. This insight raised intellectual, political and moral agendas. At the intellectual level, as Meg Stacey wittily pointed out, there was a need to explain the origins of the 'two Adams': not just the public subordination associated with Adam Smith's formal division of labour, but also the private one associated with Adam and Eve's informal division of care (Stacey 1981). Both were seen as socially created. However, this was associated with a political agenda of transformation, not just separately within the two spheres, but also the power relations between them. There was a widening of the political and moral agendas which was represented most clearly in the feminist rallying cry that 'the personal is political'. This has certainly resonated through all the fields of contemporary critical sociology, social policy and cultural studies, and its influence is now all the greater for the fact that it is no longer formally asserted but has become part of the customary analytical narrative.

Within this shift in social and political consciousness, and highly germane to the current book, is the part that health has played in contemporary critical feminist analysis. At first sight the lines of division between the public and private divides seem clear enough. One of the key important and continuing issues has been the extent to which health work should be produced 'differently' from the rest of the capitalist division of labour as a form of 'professional autonomy', and whether the state rather than the market should act as regulator and distributor of professional care. We can also 'add in women' by showing that within the public sphere there is a clear if changing gendered division of labour in which men usually come out on top, though sometimes different men – doctors, politicians, managers and even nurses. We can then rightly point out that this focus on the public division of labour must also take account of the fact that most care takes place within the 'private' informal sphere which people do for themselves, or is done for them by others, and which typically is seen as primarily the responsibility of women. However, we then have to go one step further to show how the public and private *intersect*. Health work spans both the public and private spheres, and professional interventions can be seen as attempts to mobilise knowledge and power in order to restructure the private sphere (the core principle around which Meg's textbook (Stacey 1988) is organised). Indeed, one of the key insights of feminist sociology and social policy has been a focus on medicalisation as a process of control over the body, contingent and always open to challenge, as one of the central props of patriarchal relations and of power relations generally within modern societies. What this has done is to bring into focus the embodied nature of the social and the human nature of the embodied. By picturing 'our bodies' as 'ourselves' the feminist health movement sought to counter the imposition of mechanistic principles of biomedical science from above in order to assert 'popular' lay control from below (Boston Women's Health Collective 1979). Thus although this was primarily asserted for women, it had universal implications. This insight has become one of the commonplaces of analysis now, but in the process its origin is not always fairly attributed. The current explosion of interest in the 'sociology of the body', for example, is often seen as having derived from a male French thinker, Michel Foucault. While not denying his importance, the danger is that the contribution of the feminist health movement will not be recognised and also that, as a result, analysis will become distorted in certain ways. While some of the ways in which feminism of the 1960s and 1970s polarised the biological and the social in the 'sex' and 'gender' distinction can now be regarded as problematic (see, for example, Oakley 1972), at least the excesses of latter-day social constructionism were avoided. Above all the concern to outline the relationship between bodily and personal identity in a holistic way raised ethical and humanistic concerns that have often tended to get lost or to be regarded as irrelevant in the wordplay of the 'linguistic turn'.

The purpose of the current collection therefore is to take stock, to celebrate and consolidate the traditions of analysis which Meg pioneered alongside others, but also to show how these remain vitally relevant to contemporary concerns. We hope that this has been achieved in two ways. First, the contributors are a mix of authors, many of whom have worked and collaborated with Meg on these issues over many years, but they also include representatives of the emergent generation of researchers. In this respect, the book seeks to overcome yet another potential divide, the importance of which should not be overlooked: that of the generations. Meg herself, as a member of the Second World War generation, has at times challenged the notion that second-wave feminism of the 1960s emerged because the original feminist impulse of a first wave had become exhausted, and because it overlooked the feminists of the nineteenth century (and earlier). Rather, the struggle for gender justice and a more caring world where women's issues become everyone's concerns is a continuous process, in which nobody starts from scratch. In the contemporary era postmodern forms of analysis have repaid the compliment by suggesting that the intellectual and political agendas of second-wave feminism have now become problematic or even passé. This too, can be regarded as representing something of a generation break, and this book, while recognising the tensions, seeks to keep open the dialogue by asserting the existence of critical continuity between the various 'waves', rather than focusing one-sidedly on the disjunctures between them. And, to maintain the thematic links of this discussion with Meg's own work, this emphasis on both tradition *and* change was the core theme of her more general sociological research on the town of Banbury in the post-1945 era (Stacey 1960; Stacey *et al.* 1975).

Second, the essays in the book address urgent theoretical, political and ethical concerns, as both the need for social relevance and an emphasis on the *applied* aspects of sociological analysis are strong features of Meg's example to us as both an academic and activist. In other words, sociology should help to improve the world, not just analyse it. This collection therefore seeks to transcend the artificial divisions between social theory and social policy which have particularly emerged for specific historical and cultural reasons in the English-speaking world. In addressing these applied issues, the volume seeks to make a critical appraisal of biomedical science and practice, its impact on gendered inequality and society generally. Taking their lead from Meg, the aim of these essays is not just to criticise science or scientists or reject medicine or health professions; but, through asking hard questions, to establish a dialogue in which there can be meaningful conversations between lay and professional concerns and understandings. In this respect the sociology and social policy of health and healing provide bridges between the two worlds and sets of discourses that confront scientists and professionals with the social implications of their theories and interventions, and thereby help to empower public choices and the exercise of democratic control.

There is no doubt that one of modernity's greatest achievements, involving real gains for many people, has been in the sphere of health and health care. In developed capitalist societies people generally live longer, and they enjoy a standard of health provision that is unique in human history, one also that is still not to be found in much of the rest of the world today, for example in developing or post-communist countries. Perhaps women have gained most from this, if increased life expectancy is seen as the yardstick. Yet although the patient according to the objective signs may be doing better, she or he is often feeling worse, the paradox being that it is women particularly who have mounted critical assaults on the citadels of contemporary science and medicine. The 'and yet . . .' is where, in diverse ways, all the contributors to this book commence, taking up these central themes of ambivalence towards modernity's achievements in relation medicine and health, focusing particularly on their gendered features, but using this as a launching pad for analysis of more universal concerns.

A number of other books, both new and established, address specific issues relating to gender, medicine and health on such issues as professions and the health care division of labour, patriarchal implications of reproductive technologies, gender inequalities of health, gender and mental illness (for example, Martin 1987; Stacey 1993; Riska and Weger 1993; Witz 1992; Doyal 1995; Sabo and Gordon 1995; Busfield 1996; Annandale and Hunt 2000). To our knowledge, this current volume is unique in bringing together this whole range of issues, connecting them also to new emerging concerns such as the new genetics and the problematic transformations in biomedical knowledge and practices occurring under late modern capitalism. Its assessment of gender relations and embodied practices across the public/private divide draws upon and uses health and healing as paradigmatic examples located within these broader tensions and transitions. The contributors maintain a consistent emphasis throughout on critical debates and key developments, and their efforts have produced an exciting volume that lies at the intersection of gender studies, the sociology of health and healing, health policy, the critical analysis of scientific knowledge and current debates around the body, health and emotions. There could, in our view, be no better way than this of celebrating Meg's life and work.

In order to achieve coherence, but avoiding the imposition of a rigid structure, the collection has been organised into three sections around themes which Meg has consistently addressed; these are given contemporary relevance by the contributors to the current volume, focusing on key debates and developments. Meg's work has always been 'realist' in the sense that the sociology of health and illness has been seen as a central element in the development of a sociology sensitive to the fact that the biological provides the irreducible framework within which social life takes place (Stacey 1988). In this regard, her work has also featured the analysis of human reproduction as a core social activity, and the way that struggles for control over it involving professional and scientific interventions have impacted in both positive and problematic ways on the embodied lives of women and men (Stacey 1993). Part 1, 'Biology "revisited" and human reproduction', refocuses attention on the knotty problem of how to envisage the biological within the social sciences in general and feminisms in particular, without slipping into the reductionist or dualistic traps of the past or the excessively constructionist errors and blind alleys of the present. In this regard the cracking of the human genetic code with the associated efforts to develop genetic therapies and the accelerating development of reproductive technology raise significant issues for analysis and policy.

Chapter 1, by Simon Williams, tackles head-on the 'problem' of biology, both inside and outside feminist scholarship, and attempts to rethink these issues avoiding reductionism, dualism and constructionism alike through principles of irreducibility and emergence: a complex intertwining, in effect, of biological and social processes which takes us well beyond either/or debates. Far from legitimating existing social inequalities, moreover, biology provides the kernel for a radical critique of social oppression, both past and present. It is not therefore, from this viewpoint, a question of choosing between biology or society, but of rethinking this relationship – and the former dichotomies it entails – in new, mutually informing terms. Developments such as the new genetics, the disability debate and other life-political agenda make this an urgent priority at the turn of the century.

Building upon these issues, Lynda Birke (Chapter 2) considers how people in Western cultures perceive the insides of their bodies in particular ways, by drawing upon some key ideas in anatomy and physiology and the kinds of representations these offer. She analyses how students of biology 'learn to see' the body's inner mysteries and focuses particular attention on how scientific diagrams convey images of the body machine, of the body's inner spaces, or of the body as servomechanism. There are implications here too, in terms of social divisions such as gender, particularly in how scientific diagrams are read. There are also, of course, implications for how we come to understand our bodies (in terms of passivity or agency, for example), and hence, for our experiences of health and disease as well as for medical practice. And finally, again, there are implications for social theory, which has tended to marginalise 'the biological', thus further contributing to notions of the physiological body as fixed or passive.

Human reproduction now enters the highly charged and contested terrain of the new genetics and new reproductive technologies, including the cultural imaging of the gene and the moral and ethical dilemmas of reproductive 'choices'. In Chapter 3 Hilary Rose takes as her starting point the historically troubled relationship between 'genetics' and 'eugenics', which have often been equated. Although this was marked and transparent in relation to Nazi pseudo-science and the social practice of the death camps, she argues that it also featured as a significant feature of 'progressive' political ideologies such as British Fabian socialism and Swedish social democracy. The relationship remains a troubled one, in that eugenic tendencies still lie behind the apparently socially neutral face that the 'new genetics' now presents to the world in the wake of the postwar discovery of the double helix and the recent mapping of the human genome. The new genetics/new reproduction theme is then taken in a somewhat different direction by Joan Haran (Chapter 4), who shows how analysis of feminist science fiction can help generate a cultural critique of some of the most troubling aspects of these developments.

Another central contribution of Meg's was the notion of health practices as both formal and informal forms of work, spanning the whole division of labour, including carers and patients themselves. The implications of this were theoretically and politically profound as it cut professionals down to size, showed that informal carers were not necessarily always motivated by love, and made patients active producers of their own health: ideas that undercut the then emergent but now rampant health policy emphasis on 'consumers' (Stacey 1976). It is therefore highly appropriate that the second key thematic, 'Gender (in)equality and (emotional) division of labour', builds upon this tradition of analysis of the gendered relations of health care and the role of emotional dynamics in relations of health work. The first three chapters in this section address health work in diverse ways. Celia Davies (Chapter 5) takes off from Stacey's insights into the elite status, closed culture and autonomy of medicine, and the observation that regulation does not and cannot work in the same way for other professions in the health care division of labour. It then goes on to consider the tensions which have arisen between nurses and midwives in the unified regulatory structure that was put in place in the early 1980s, arguing that this can be seen in the light of two historically distinct forms of gendered regulatory subordination. Giving these themes an empirically international insight, and widening our horizons beyond a Euro/US-centric focus, Gillian Lewando Hundt (Chapter 6) reflects how unpaid health work in the form of informed and selective choices about packages of maternity care has been a constant theme throughout her thirty years of research with marginalised Negev Bedouin women.

Taking a highly original approach to the social history of death and dying, whilst echoing the earlier cries of tradition and change, Anne Murcott's research (Chapter 7) on the division of labour in death work in Banbury revisits those earlier 'locality' studies (she herself was part of the research team), bringing an evocatively poignant note to those earlier recurrent themes of inequality and division of labour.

The last two chapters in Part 2 focus more directly on emotion: Joan Busfield (Chapter 8), on the gendering of mental health, works through two main issues. First, there is the increasing attention paid to the less severe mental disorders where women tend to be over-represented as patients. Issues explored here include the way in which disorders, which often start with a more masculine identity, quite frequently end up as more feminised mental disorders. Second, we have the feminisation of the mental health labour force and the role of women as carers for those with mental health problems. Finally, Gillian Bendelow and Geraldine Brady (Chapter 9) use examples drawn from empirical studies of children's beliefs about health and illness, focusing in particular on children with a diagnosis of attention deficit/hyperactive disorder, to explore the relative influence of children's and parents' voices, and the salience of emotion work and emotion management across the public/private, paid/unpaid, formal/informal health care divides.

The third and final part of the book attempts to follows Meg's initiative in seeking to link issues of theory to urgent questions of policy in relation to the broader and more immediate social changes affecting the health system. Thus 'Health care in transition: ferment and change?' provides a critical up-dating and assessment of various 'paradigmatic challenges' and 'shifts' occurring in the health policy arena at the turn of the twentieth century; developments which underpin many of the foregoing arguments and the push towards a more 'women-friendly' and 'gender-sensitive' pluralism in health care policy and provision. To this end, in Chapter 10 Lesley Doyal brings a global perspective to bear on gendered patterns of health, and particularly on the policy implications of current trends. It distinguishes between strategies for 'equality' and for 'equity', and the complex dilemmas that might arise from these. It invites debate by suggesting that we should strive for equity, rather than equality, the outcome of this might still at the end of the day be gender differences in health which leave men with higher mortality rates and a lower life expectancy than women. In addition, the need to address women's morbidity, which is typically worse than men's, might have costs as well as benefits for men, and it therefore should not always be assumed that a 'non-zero-sum game' operates in relation to equalising health chances between men and women.

Priscilla Alderson (Chapter 11) raises the thorny issue of informed consent as a problematic area of medical practice, signifying a range of changes such as growing uncertainty in medical practice, the emergence of rationing, and new conceptualisations of relations between practitioners and users based on a consumerist view of citizenship. In particular, she explores these in relation to children as health users who are embedded in a network of relationships between professionals, institutions, parents and the state. Recent critical cases have generally illustrated both the dilemmas posed by uncertain medicine and children's and parents' responsibility in relation to informed consent. In turn, these illustrate the ways in which issues such as informed consent are inevitably complicated by the wider sets of social and power relations in which users are enmeshed.

'Alternative' forms of healing were issues that Meg Stacey focused on before many others sought to account for their growing popularity, and in Chapter 12 Ursula Sharma examines the extent of the change of attitude of the biomedical establishment in a number of Western countries to complementary and alternative medicines (CAMs). In Britain, while certain CAMs are being provided on the NHS to some patients under a variety of institutional arrangements, there is very little reciprocal impact on medical education and training. She argues that there are a number of practical problems in developing a genuinely integrated health care system, problems which relate to both forms of knowledge and forms of practice, and asks whether there can indeed be any integration into medicine without biomedical dominance. Widening the issues for debate still further, Fox's classic chapter develops Roy Porter's conclusion in *The Greatest Benefit to Mankind* (1998) that the 'medical history of humanity' is in a state of anomie despite and in some ways because of its diagnostic, therapeutic and preventative advances. The chapter goes several steps further than does Porter in interpreting what he calls the 'disorientation' of medicine. It explores various forms of epistemological uncertainty with which medicine is grappling at the end of the twentieth century, and deals with the meta-significance of the emergence and continuing development of bioethics during the past three decades.

Finally, providing an appropriately wide overview to end this part, Virginia Olesen argues in Chapter 14 that the sociology of health and illness has, in its brief history, struggled to understand micro–macro tensions in social life. These struggles will take on new fervour and meaning as society and the discipline enter the new millennium in the bureaucratised West with significant alterations in large-scale health structures and contextualised relationships of care seekers and providers. A new repertoire of conceptualisations, she argues, will be required in these struggles; conceptualisations which will find their roots in contemporary feminist thought and practice.

The book ends appropriately with concluding reflections on future agendas by Meg Stacey herself. She argues forcefully that underpinning all the diverse issues addressed in the volume is a call to engage critically in a series of (bio)ethical, theoretical and political debates. She insists that the ultimate aim of our research and analysis must be to help to mitigate intended, unintended and unnecessary human suffering associated with gendered inequality and ill health and with patriarchal forms of health intervention, both now and in the future, as an urgent agenda for the twenty-first century.

References

Annandale, E. and Hunt, K. (2000) *Gender Inequalities in Health*, London: Macmillan.

Bauman, Z. (1997) *Postmodernity and its Discontents*, Cambridge: Polity Press.

Boston Women's Health Collective (1973) *Our Bodies, Ourselves*, New York: Simon and Schuster.

Busfield, J. (1996) *Men, Women and Madness: Understanding Gender and Mental Disorder*, London: Macmillan.

Doyal, L. (1995) *What Makes Women Sick? Gender and the Political Economy of Health*, London: Macmillan.

Martin, E. (1987) *The Woman in the Body*, Milton Keynes, Bucks: Open University Press.

Oakley, A. (1972) *Sex, Gender and Society*, London: Temple Smith.

Porter, R. (1998) *The Greatest Benefit to Mankind: A Medical History of Humanity*, New York: W.W. Norton.

Riska, E. and Wegar, K. (eds) (1993) *Gender, Work and Medicine: Women and the Medical Division of Labour*, London: Sage.

Rose, H. (1994) *Love, Power and Knowledge: Towards a Feminist Transformation of the Sciences*, Cambridge: Polity Press.

Sabo, D. and Gordon, D. (1995) *Men's Heath and Illness: Gender Power and the Body*, London: Sage.

Stacey, M. (1960), *Tradition and Change: A Study of Banbury*, Oxford: Oxford University Press.

—— (ed.) (1976) *The Sociology of the NHS*, Sociological Review Monograph 22, University of Keele.

—— (1981) 'The division of labour revisited, or overcoming the two Adams', in P. Abrams, R. Deem, J. Finch and P. Rock (eds), *Development or Diversity: British Sociology 1950–1980*, London: Allen and Unwin.

—— (1988) *The Sociology of Health and Healing*, London: Allen and Unwin

—— (1993) *Changing Human Reproduction: Social Science Perspectives*, London: Sage.

—— Batstone, E., Bell, C. and Murcott, A. (1975) *Power, Persistence and Change: A Second Study of Banbury*, London: Routledge and Kegan Paul.

Witz, A. (1992) *Professions and Patriarchy*, London: Routledge.

Part I

Biology 'revisited' and human reproduction

Old problems, new dilemmas?

1 Corporeal reflections on the biological

Reductionism, constructionism and beyond

Simon J. Williams*

Introduction

It is perhaps only the bold or foolhardy, in an era of floating signs and signifiers, who dares to resurrect the thorny question of biology. From Darwinian evolutionary theory, on the one hand, to the perils of eugenics and the pitfalls of socio-biology, on the other, the question of biology if not the spectre of biologism has been an implicit if not explicit theme: a foil, in effect, for the sociological imagination itself. The 'repressed' however, as Freudians are keen to remind us, has a habit of returning, for better or worse. Certainly it is possible to detect signs of this reappearance. New ways of understanding science and its relationship to culture, alternative ways of philosophically ordering scientific knowledge, together with newly influential movements – from ecology to animal rights – have combined in recent years, as Benton (1991) suggests, to compel or facilitate new ways of thinking about biology and the human sciences.[1] To this we may add the recent upsurge of interest in the body and emotions, both inside and outside the academy. The body, it seems, is everywhere and nowhere today: a victim, like the sociology of emotions, of its own success perhaps (Wouters 1992: 248). Here, on this contested corporeal terrain, claims and counter-claims as to what precisely the body is (or is not) abound, the push for more integrated modes of theorising themselves at a relatively early stage of development.

In this chapter I take a closer look at these corporeal issues and the deeper ontological and epistemological questions they raise, taking feminist scholarship as a paradigmatic example. The aim in doing so is to provide a series of thoughts and reflections on the biological which avoid the pitfalls of (biological) reductionism and (social) constructionism alike. It is not, I shall argue, drawing on a variety of recent work in support of my claims, a question of choosing between *either* biology *or* society, but of *re-envisioning* this

* I would like to thank my colleagues on the editorial team who have read and commented on earlier drafts of this chapter. Thanks also to Lynda Birke for her perceptive comments and valuable insights into these biological matters, within and beyond this chapter.

very relationship – and the former dichotomies it entails – in new (emergent, irreducible) ways which go beyond these existing terms of debate, without leaving out what is important to them in the process. In these and other respects, I hope, the chapter marks in spirit, if not content, Meg Stacey's (1988) own non-determinist approach to the 'biological base'. How then has the biological fared in these debates to date, and where do we go from here? It is to these and other related questions that I now turn.

The dilemma of biology: a 'corporeal' feminism?

Feminisms, in many ways, provide a paradigmatic expression of the tensions and dilemmas of recourse to the 'biological' body, both in theory and practice (Birke 1999): something, according to writers such as Spelman (1988), which has bordered on the 'somatophobic'. All too often, it seems, the link made between women and their bodies has been used against them as a means of curtailing their own freedom like that of 'others' (that is, blacks, lesbians, children, the disabled) (Spelman 1988; Birke 1995). In challenging such 'biological determinism', Spelman argues, the body has remained under-theorised; feminists pointing instead towards broader social, cultural and political determinants of women's oppression in Western patriarchal society. This charge, made well over a decade ago now, may seem somewhat dated, particularly in the light of recent feminist scholarship. It does none the less contain more than a germ of truth, particularly in relation to the biological. Theorising the body may now be a central feminist preoccupation – some would doubtless claim it has never been otherwise – yet the nature and status of biology, qualifications apart, remains somewhat 'problematic' in many of these discussions and debates to date.

One response to this corporeal dilemma, as Birke (1995, 1999) notes in relation to past feminist theories of biology and the body, has been to claim that women are 'biologically disadvantaged' relative to men. From this perspective, social reform can only achieve so much, leaving the rectification of remaining inequalities to increases in 'control' over nature (i.e. biology) itself. Firestone (1970), for example, in *The Dialectic of Sex* provides a clear expression of these concerns, including the 'liberatory' potential of science for women. The answer to women's subordination, from this perspective, lay in future technological control over the 'tyranny' of their reproductive biology. The 'specificity' of the reproductive body, in other words, had to be 'overcome' if sexual equality was to be achieved (Birke 1995).

An alternative position has been to suggest that women should not aspire to be 'like men' at all. Rather, women should celebrate and affirm their bodies, including the capacity to recreate and nurture, care and love – a 'biophilic' position, that is to say – *vis-à-vis* the selfish, 'necrophilic' or 'gynophobic' nature or traits of men (Daly 1978). *Essential* sexual difference should, therefore, for theorists of this persuasion, be retained rather than overcome through scientific intervention (Birke 1995). Hovering somewhere in between these two strands of essentialism lies the work of feminist writers who, in their differing ways, highlight how women, as potential or actual reproducers, experience oppression (Birke 1995). O'Brien (1981, 1989), for example, sees women's oppression as originating in the male discovery of their role in paternity. Physiology is 'fate' for men, she suggests, paternity itself an 'alienated' experience, based on abstract knowledge rather than the 'unity of knowing and doing, of consciousness and creativity, of temporality and continuity' which comes through the very process of giving birth (O'Brien 1989: 14). Whilst this statement implies a biological determinism of sorts, it is in fact, as Birke (1995) comments, deeply rooted in material and cultural processes of patriarchal oppression for writers such as O'Brien. Unity with 'nature' (itself a contested or problematic term) therefore becomes a desirable future state of affairs from this viewpoint (Birke 1995).

Rich (1976), in a similar (albeit more radical) vein, asks women to reconsider their so-called 'problematic' relationships to their bodies and to female biology (Birke 1995). Rather than simply perpetuate dominant (masculinist) views, women must instead, Rich argues, learn to 'repossess' their bodies:

> In arguing that we have by no means yet explored or understood our biological grounding, the miracle and paradox of the female body and its spiritual and political meanings, I am really asking whether women cannot begin, at last, to *think through the body, to connect what has been so cruelly disorganised – our great mental capacities, hardly used; our highly developed tactile sense; our genius for close observation; our complicated, pain-enduring, multi-pleasured physicality*.
>
> (Rich 1976: 284; emphasis added)

Whilst these responses to women's corporeal specificity are often taken to exhaust the 'sexual equality versus sexual difference debate', they are, as Gatens (1992) notes, ultimately caught up in one and the same paradigm, which understands the body as a biologically 'given' entity and assumes rather than transcends a mind/body, nature/culture dualism. The sex/gender distinction in particular, a central issue within feminisms of the 1970s and early 1980s – see, for example, Oakley (1972) among others – failed to question how society constructs the 'natural body' itself.[2]

Recognition of this important fact has led recent feminist scholarship to an alternative view of the body and power; one which highlights the discursive construction of 'sex' itself, thereby challenging the dualistic manner in which sexual difference has been articulated to date. Instead of seeing 'sex' as a biological phenomenon and gender as a cultural category, these thinkers are concerned to undermine the dichotomy altogether. Within the corpus of Judith Butler's (1993) work, for example, materiality itself becomes an 'effect of power', indeed as power's most 'productive effect'. Once 'sex' is understood in its 'normativity', she claims, the 'materiality of the body will not be thinkable apart from the materialisation of that regulatory norm' (ibid.: 2).

Seen in these terms 'sex' is not simply what one has, or what one is, rather it is one of the regulatory and reiterative norms by which one becomes 'viable' at all. At stake in such a reformulation, for Butler, are five key propositions. First, a recasting, in Foucauldian terms, of body matters and the matter of bodies as a dynamic effect of power, and the regulatory norms that govern their materialisation and signification. Second, the understanding of 'performativity' as a reiterative power of discourse to (re-)produce the very phenomena that it regulates and constrains. Third, the construal of 'sex' as no longer a 'bodily given' upon which gender constructs are artificially imposed, but instead a 'cultural norm' which governs the materialisation of bodies. Fourth, a rethinking of the process by which a bodily norm is assumed, appropriated or adopted as one in which the very subject, the 'speaking I', is constituted by virtue of having gone through the process of assuming a 'sex'. Finally, a linking of the assumption of 'sex' with the question of 'identification', and the discursive means by which the 'heterosexual imperative' enables certain 'sexed' identification whilst foreclosing and/or disavowing others (ibid.: 2–3).[3]

The (mythical) 'pre-social' body, from this viewpoint, is rejected in favour of a discursive body, a body which is bound up in the 'order' of desire, power and signification. Related to this, as alluded to above, is an acknowledgment (and/or celebration) of 'difference': one in which culture rather than biology 'marks' bodies and creates the specific conditions in which they live and recreate themselves (Grosz 1994). The emphasis here, broadly speaking, is 'deconstructive'; a position which seeks to 'destabilise', 'challenge', 'subvert', 'reverse', 'overturn' ossified conceptual forms in favour of more plural, fluid or 'leaky' positions (see also Barrett and Phillips 1992; Shildrick 1997; Battersby 1998).

Problems remain none the less with both these positions (i.e. essentialism and constructionism). Biology, in the former case, whether celebrated or bemoaned, remains essentially fixed or determinative, save the 'transformatory' (*qua* liberatory) potential of technology itself. Constructionism, on the other hand, takes us in precisely the opposite direction through a problematic series of conflationary moves. To the extent that biology figures at all here, it becomes yet another form of discourse (i.e. 'written in/out' of the picture): a 'reductionist' one at that. The body that 'performs' moreover, as Grosz reminds us, must nevertheless '*abide between performances*, existing over and above the sum total of its performances' (1995: 212, my emphasis). Sexuality, in this sense, is more than simply a position in social space (Turner 1995). There is little attempt here, by writers such as Butler, to understand the physicality of the body, or its material decline and decay across the lifecourse (Turner 1995, 1996). 'Like many women', as Birke (1995: 2) rightly comments, 'I have trouble thinking about theories of social construction that ignore or play down my bodily pain and bleeding, or that ignore the way that desire (however constructed) finds expression through my material body.' The upshot of these and related embodied matters, is that discursive (i.e.

performative and citational) approaches to the body of this kind, at one and the same time, remain both promising and problematic.

What we have here, to put it in slightly different terms, is a conflation of the epistemological with the ontological – that is, the 'epistemic' fallacy' (Bhaskar 1989) in which *what* we know and *how* we know it is confused with what there *is* to know. Like the biological itself, moreover, the social is *reduced* to language (i.e. the subtle play of signs and symbols): a form of 'discourse determinism' (Turner 1995) based on an inversion rather than overcoming of the problems of essentialism (Sayer 1997).[4] This, in turn, suggests that the socially *constructed* and the socially *constituted* world cannot simply or unproblematically be equated: the former, *qua* discourse, merely one aspect of the latter (perhaps the most obvious one at that).[5] Biology does not, it is clear, have to be 'written out' of existence in this way, or any other way for that matter; nor, however, does it have to be seen as 'determinative' (Birke 1995, 1999). In raising these issues and putting matters this way, I have perhaps set myself a somewhat easy or straw target: a caricature, in effect, of a far more complex, subtle and sophisticated series of arguments and debates. There is, I concede, some truth in this. A number of other more promising positions, both inside and outside feminist scholarship itself, are indeed now beginning to emerge with which to 'rethink' the biological in other non-reductionist or non-conflationary ways (Birke 1999; Rose and Rose 2000a; Rose 1997; Benton 1991). What then do these theories constitute, and where do we go from here? It is to these very questions, and the embodied agendas they call forth, that I now turn.

Where do we go from here? Five key issues

Duality and dualism, ontology and epistemology

The first issue to tackle here, head on, concerns the knotty problem of dualism itself. Do we, given their dubious Western history, need dichotomies? If so, how best might they be pressed into service? This is hotly contested terrain, upon which much debate, both past and present, has turned. It may, however, as a preliminary contribution to these debates, be useful to distinguish here between dual*ity* and dual*ism*.[6] As the process of Cartesian duality suggests, it is only through an act of conscious reflection (i.e. *Cogito ergo sum*) that the split between mind and body is effected. This duality, to be sure, represents a stage in the development of 'human consciousness', but is nevertheless, as we know only too well, founded upon a series of problematic assumptions about mind/body relations which have served neither women nor, ultimately, men (Seidler 1994), well. This stage of development (i.e. duality), in turn, leads to its own illusory appearance, namely the problem of dualism. As a doctrine, dualism turns duality into an 'ism': one in which the mind/body split appears somehow 'natural', rational and unconditioned. Moreover, it also spawns a number of other unfortunate, unhelpful dualisms such as nature/culture, reason/emotion, public/private, together with the associated ideological baggage and hierarchical orderings this involves. The critique of dualism, as a critique of the illusions of duality, and the critique of duality as a critique of a certain stage of development of human conscious, must therefore look forwards rather than backwards, to a 'third' stage of development, which is 'prepared for' as it were by the previous stage(s).

It is dualism, within this particular framework at least, which is most to blame for the problems of Western culture to date – that is, the turning of duality into an 'ism', and the hierarchical prioritisation of one binary term over the other. Duality indeed in some respects is inescapable: non-dualists themselves pitched against their dualist counterparts. Duality it follows, qua *analytic* device, may still have something useful to offer here (as a preliminary point of departure at least), enabling us to examine, through principles of interplay, irreducibility and emergence, the complex intertwining of biological and social processes, conceived in spatio-temporal terms. The body itself, from this point of view, is at one and the same time both biological and social, material and cultural, shaping and being shaped by on-going social-cultural relations or liaisons, yet irreducible to any one domain or discourse none the less: a 'threshold' or 'borderline' concept, in Grosz's (1994: 23) terms, that hovers 'perilously and undecidably at the pivotal point of binary pairs'. In the face of social constructionism therefore, 'the body's tangibility, its matter, its (quasi) nature may be invoked; but, in opposition to essentialism, biologism and naturalism, it is the body as cultural product that must be stressed (ibid.: 24). This, I hasten to add, is merely one way forward (promising or otherwise), of which there are many. Numerous competing conceptualisations, moreover, as Benton (1991: 18) reminds us, are also be found within the biological themselves, including 'several well-articulated alternatives to reductionist materialism available for use as philosophical means in the attempt to re-think the biology/society relationship'.

Underlying these points, as touched on earlier, is a series of deeper ontological and epistemological issues, including the so-called 'epistemic fallacy' and the confusion of having *something* important to say with the having of *everything* important to say on the matter (Craib 1995). Rose (1997) for example, in his insightful account of biology, freedom and determinism, puts the matter well. We live, he argues, in *one* world, but with *many* ways of knowing it. A 'material world', in formal terms, which is an 'ontological unity, but which we approach with epistemological diversity' (ibid.: 304). Different scientific disciplines therefore, from the social to the sub-atomic sciences, deal with different levels of organisation of matter, levels which themselves, in some respects, are 'confused':

> In part they are *ontological*, and relate to scale and complexity, in which successive levels are nested one within another . . . each level appears as a holon – integrating levels below it, but merely a subset of the level above it. In this sense, levels are fundamentally irreducible . . . However, to

some extent – and this is where the confusion enters – the levels are *epistemological*, relating to different ways of knowing the world, each in turn the contingent product of its own discipline's history. The relation-ship between such epistemological levels . . . is best described in the *metaphor of translation* . . . problems arise when one attempts to apply concepts and terms applicable at one level to phenomena on another level . . . the power of metaphor is such that we always run the danger of confusing it with reality.

(Rose 1997: 304–5, my emphasis)

The argument at this point, to summarise, is one premised on an acknow-ledgement of epistemological and ontological distinctions and an acceptance of principles of interplay, irreducibility and emergence: issues, I suggest, which point the way out of former reductionist and constructionist traps alike and the blind alleys to which they lead.

Enabling biology: an 'unfinished' matter?

These points, in turn, prepare the ground a second key proposition; namely that biology, far from being a mere constant or given, constraint or determin-ing factor, is itself a relatively open, pliable or unfinished matter, one com-pleted and depleted by society so to speak. This, of course, is not to deny various biological limits or constraints – a man cannot (yet), for example, give birth to a child, and we do not have wings to fly (without mechanical aid) – but simply to point towards various degrees of freedom rather than determin-ism. It also, moreover, as the very prerequisite or precondition of social and cultural relations – without our biological capacities and endowments noth-ing, social or otherwise, is possible – disposes us, in myriad ways, towards society, displaying what Wentworth and Yardley (1994) appositely refer to, in the context of emotions, as a 'deep sociality'. The so-called 'natural' proper-ties of human bodies, in this respect – themselves a product of both biological and social processes involved in evolution – are inseparable from the cultural practices and achievements of humans (Shilling 1993: 105).[7] Even in those cases where the biological is 'mediated' in almost every respect, however, this does not mean, as Archer (1995: 288) (echoing Sayer 1992) emphasises, that the 'mediated is not biological nor that the physical is epiphenomenal': a point which again reinforces the limits of a wholly constructionist viewpoint. To refer to the body as a 'post-biological social entity' or a 'pre-social bio-logical entity' remains therefore, given its *simultaneous* biological and social nature and the complex intertwining this entails, equally problematic or mistaken (Shilling 1993: 105).

Elias's (1991a) processual account of emotions, for example, provides one potentially promising illustration of these issues; one which articulates key elements of his more general *Symbol Theory* (Elias 1991b) in which biological and social processes are more or less successfully brought together.[8] Three key hypotheses, in particular, are ventured here by Elias in taking these issues forward. The first of these concerns the fact that human beings, as a species, represent something of an evolutionary 'breakthrough'. Here Elias draws attention to the fact that the ability to steer conduct with the help of learned knowledge, itself a product of biological evolutionary processes, accords human beings a distinct advantage over all other species whose behaviour, in contrast, is largely governed by instincts. Indeed, it is this dominance of learned over unlearned characteristics in humans which, he emphasises, provides a *biological framework for social developments.*

Elias's second hypothesis concerns the fact that human beings not only can but must learn far more than any other species, as a consequence of the 'civilising process' (cf. Elias [1939a] 1978, [1939b] 1982) and the maturation of the child to an adult: itself a process in which that achieved over the course of many centuries is passed through within the short span of each and every individual's lifetime. Here again, Elias points out how a child's learning of a language, for example, is made possible by the interweaving of two processes: a biological process of maturation and a social process of learning. Indeed, it is through this biological ability to understand and transmit symbols via language that social developments and transformations can occur independently of further evolutionary change – what Elias (1991b) refers to as 'symbol emancipation'. 'The biological dominance gained by learned forms of steering experience and conduct over unlearned forms of conduct', Elias (1991a: 115) states, 'links irreversible evolution with reversible development.'

Finally, Elias's third, perhaps most important, hypothesis is that no emotion is ever an entirely unlearned, genetically fixed reaction pattern. Rather, like human languages more generally, human emotions result from a merger of an unlearned and a learned process. In this respect, whilst humans share certain reaction patterns, such as the fight–flight reaction, with non-human species, there are also marked differences in that humans are capable of far greater diversification in accordance with different situations and antecedent experiences. It is on this basis that Elias is able to demonstrate how biological and social processes mesh in the human experience and communication of emotion (i.e. unlearned emotional impulses are always related to a person's learned self-regulation, including learned social control of emotions).

These processes and the 'balances' they involve are fleshed out further by Elias through the fascinating, rich and complex example of the face. The unique character of the face, he argues, serves as an important reminder of the singularity of human beings: one has to be human in order to read the signals of human faces properly. In this respect, the capacity for both giving and perceiving facial signals has an 'innate – that is to say species-specific – *plastic* core which in every particular case is *capable of being re-modelled through learning in varying degrees*' (1991a: 122, my emphasis). Thus whilst a baby's smile is more or less wholly innate, as human beings grow older its innateness is greatly weakened and becomes instead much more *malleable* in relation to antecedent as well as immediate experiences. As such, the adult smile can be used to convey a subtle variety of feelings and shades of meaning ranging from happiness to pride, and from hesitancy to insincerity. In each particular case, however, Elias insists, the same processes manifest themselves, namely, 'a learned and deliberate steering of conduct merges with an unlearned form of steering one's face muscles' (ibid.: 123).

The strength of Elias's position, as this brief exposition suggests, lies in the more or less successful demonstration that 'going beyond' the biological within sociology does not have to mean leaving it out altogether: a non-reductionist, unfinished, enabling formulation as itself the precondition of social relations and our profound dependence upon them. Emotions, from this perspective, *qua* irreducible human compounds, are 'one of the indicators that human beings are by nature constituted for life in the company of others, for life in society' (ibid.: 125).[9]

Negation and transcendence: biology as critique?

A third crucial factor to bring out here, given the dubious ideological claims of the past, is that far from legitimating existing social practices and arrangements, recourse to the biological may itself serve as a profound critique of them; practices, that is to say, without permanent foundation in the body. What is remarkable about the species of human beings, as Shilling remarks, is not the 'few biological differences that exist between them, but their *shared* capacities for action' (1993: 108, original emphasis). 'We share the same biology', as the lyrics of a popular Sting song ('The Russians love their children too') put it, 'regardless of ideology'. In other words, there is more, biologically speaking, which unites than divides us, childbearing capacities notwithstanding. It is social practices, therefore, which distort or exaggerate, negate or transform this (common) biological base, including the 'amplification' of so-called 'natural' difference (see also Birke 1999, 1986; Fausto-Sterling 2000, 1992).

Connell (1983, 1987), for example, points the way here through a strong, non-reductionist formulation of these issues: one which stresses the active role of social praxis in what he takes to be the negation and transcendence or transformation of our reproductive biology. Reproductive biology, Connell (1987: 79) claims, is 'socially dealt with' in the historical process we call gender, a history that negates its biological as well as its social materials. Social categories (*qua* negation) and practice (*qua* transcendence or transformation), from this perspective, give new meanings to bodies which – herein lies the crucial point – cannot be justified with reference to their biological constitution (Shilling 1993: 107). Indeed, if these differences are natural, Connell asks, then why do they need to be marked so heavily? Social practices, in other words, are:

> not reflecting natural differences with these diacritical marks of gender. They are weaving a structure of symbol and interpretation around them,

and very often vastly exaggerating or distorting them . . . Social emphasis on difference negates natural similarity . . . an effect that is necessary precisely *because the biological logic*, and the inert practice that responds to it, *cannot sustain the gender categories.*

(Connell 1987: 81, original emphasis)

This, in turn, underscores the more general point that the body, in and through these modes of practical transcendence, is 'carried forward' into the next transaction, so to speak, through a process of symbolic and material incorporation: a 'presence, indeed a ferment, in the order of things constituted by more complex social processes' (ibid.: 82). The social definition of men as power holders, for instance, is translated:

not only into mental body-images and fantasies, but into muscle tension, posture, the feel and texture of the body. This is one of the many ways in which the power of men becomes 'naturalized', i.e. seen as part of the order of nature. It is very important in allowing belief in the superiority of men, and the oppressive practices that flow from it, to be sustained by men who in other respects have very little power.

(Ibid.: 85)

The body, in short, reinforcing the above points and propositions, is 'never outside history', whilst history, likewise, is 'never free from bodily presence and effects on the body'; an incorporative logic in which complex processes of interplay occur (ibid.: 87).

Another promising formulation of these issues, from a feminist standpoint, is provided by Grosz (1994) who, in her insightful book *Volatile Bodies*, provides a series of corporeal reflections on the matter of 'sexed bodies'. It is through the complex intertwining and interchanging of writing and bodies, Grosz stresses – bodies as 'blank or already encoded surfaces of inscription' – that the 'sexed' body emerges. The sexed body cannot, that is to say, be understood in terms of a fixed, ahistorical biology, although it must clearly contain a biological dimension. Instead, biology must itself, in keeping with the general thrust of this chapter, be reconceptualised as an:

open materiality, a set of (possibly infinite) tendencies and potentialities which may be developed, yet whose development will necessarily hinder or induce other developments and trajectories . . . The kind of model I have in mind here is not simply then a model of an imposition of inscription on a blank slate, a blank page with no 'texture' or resistance of its own . . . a more appropriate model for this kind of body writing is not the writing of the blank page . . . but *a model of etching, a model which needs to take into account the specificities of the materials being thus transcribed and their concrete effects on the kind of text produced.*

(Grosz 1994: 191, original emphasis)

To these attempts to grapple with the so-called 'knot of natural difference' (Connell 1987) and the critiques contained therein, we may add the important point that biological factors themselves, of course, provide an instructive index or point of commentary upon existing social practices and arrangements through the recalcitrant language of disease and disorder – or perhaps, to put it more sociologically, the health and illness of the embodied agent. From Engel's ([1845] 1987) damning documentation of the capitalist contortions and distortions of proletarian bodies within the factories and mines of nineteenth-century England – and the many lives unnecessarily sacrificed therein – to other more recent evidence of the widening gap between wealth and health (Townsend *et al.* 1988; Wilkinson 1996; Shaw *et al.* 1999), the 'afflictions of inequality', quite literally, speak volumes.

Freund (1990, 1998), for example, highlights an important part of the contemporary picture here, incorporating both the sociology of emotions and the sociology of health along the way, through the expressive body and the broader questions of power and status, domination and control this raises. Differing modes of emotional being, Freund argues, are in effect differing ways of feeling empowered or disempowered, feelings very much linked to people's material and social conditions of existence. Having one's feelings ignored or treated as irrational – what Hochschild (1983) terms the absence of 'status shields' to protect the self – is analogous to having one's perceptions invalidated. Less powerful people, it is claimed, face a 'structurally inbuilt handicap' in managing social and emotional information which may, in turn, contribute to 'dramaturgical stress' (cf. Goffman 1959), existential fear or ontological insecurity (cf. Laing 1965), and neuro-physiological perturbations of various sorts (for example, endocrinological disorder, hypertension and so on). Emotional being, social agency and structural context therefore interpenetrate. It is this relationship, Freund suggests, which comes to be physically and emotionally embodied in many different ways.

In particular, Freund argues, social relationships may engender a form of what he terms 'schizokinesis' in which a split arises between what is consciously shown and experienced and what occurs somatically. As continued emotional and other kinds of distress alter physiological reactivity, neuro-hormonally related functions such as blood pressure may markedly increase in response to the stressor, yet not be consciously experienced as such.[10] Here Freund poses two extremely pertinent sociological questions: first, just how 'deep' can the social construction of feelings go? Second, can emotion work (cf. Hochschild 1983) eliminate the responses of an 'unconsciously knowing body'? The implications of his argument seem to suggest that society affects physiological reactivity deep within the recesses of the human body although, as the notion of schizokinesis implies, the mind, consciously at least, may be unaware of the body's knowing response. As Freund (1990: 470) states:

> One's positions, and the roles that accompany them in various systems of social hierarchy, shape the conditions in which one lives. This position

influences access to resources. It may also determine the forms of emotion-social control to which one is subject as well as the severity of the impact these controls have on the person ... Such as process may mean internalising the emotional definitions that others impose on what we are or 'should be'. The physiological aspects of such processes are of interest to those studying emotions. However, these physical aspects may also be seen as examples of ways in which controls are sedimented and fixed in the psycho-soma of the person. Physiological aspects of social activity can also act as a form of feedback that colours the tone of existence. This feedback can *indirectly* serve social control functions. For instance, conditions that create depression ... construct an emotional mode of being where motivation to resist is blunted.

The argument here, as the above quotation suggests, is for a subtle and sophisticated form of 'socialised' or 'pliable' biology which, in an important sense, expresses the deleterious consequences of inequality in a bodily manner; one that accords emotional modes of being a central role in linking the health and illness of the existentially embodied social agent with wider structures of power and domination, civilisation and control. Far from providing a legitimation of existing social practices and (hierarchical) arrangements therefore, biology, to repeat, may provide an important rebuke or critique of them, given the distortions and transformations, amplifications and negations they entail and embody.

Being and becoming: 'going with the flow'?

From the previous three premises concerning epistemology and ontology, the unfinished matter of biology, and issues of negation and transcendence, a fourth and equally crucial issue emerges: that of being and becoming. Biology, it is clear, is a pulsing, moving lifeforce, not an innate, fixed or static entity. Reductionism, in this sense, rests on series of distortions which effectively place in a straitjacket, both literally and metaphorically, our understanding of biology in these latter, more open, mobile, dynamic terms. Rose (1997) again provides a key point of reference here, sketching out, in the process so to speak, the *autopoetic* principles of our lifelines and the complex trajectories this entails – that is to say, the dynamic or processual capacity of all life forms to build, maintain and preserve themselves within an ever-changing environment. To put these principles back at the core of our thinking on the biological, Rose stresses, helps counter the 'gene's-eye' view of the world which has come to dominate much popular and scientific deliberation and debate over the past two decades, including the advent of evolutionary psychology (Rose and Rose 2000a).[11] Our lives, from this viewpoint, form a

developmental trajectory, or lifeline ... This trajectory is not determined by our genes, nor partitioned into neatly dichotomous categories called nature and nurture. Rather it is an autopoetic process, shaped by the interplay of specificity and plasticity . . . This autopoetic interplay is in a sense captured by that old paradox of the Xeno – the arrow shot at a target, which at any instant of time must be both somewhere and in transit to somewhere else. Reductionism ignores the paradox and freezes life at a moment of time. In attempting to capture its *being* it loses its *becoming*, turning processes into reified objects. This is why reductionism always ends by impaling itself on a mythical dichotomy of materialist determinism and non-materialist free-will. Autopoiesis, self-construction, resolves these paradoxes.

(Rose 1997: 306)

To these issues of being and becoming we may add a broader series of (feminist) reflections and debates on issues of corporeal fluidity and flow, 'sexed' or otherwise. From the cultural imaging of the immune system (Haraway 1991; Martin 1994, 2000) to the post-structuralist metaphysics of fluidity and flow, dominant Western (*qua* masculine) notions of 'containment' and the autonomous 'bounded' self are now being critically questioned and rethought. The emphasis here, as writers such as Irigaray (1991) and Cixous (1991) suggest, is on a *process* metaphysic which thinks 'being as fluid', and which privileges the 'living, moving, pulsing, over the inert dead matter of the Cartesian world view' (Young 1990: 193). Movement and energy, from this viewpoint, are ontologically prior to 'containment' or 'thingness': views with a Nietzschean and Bergsonian, amongst others, pedigree (Battersby 1998). Thinking in these more 'fluid' or 'leaky' terms, it is argued – ways, to repeat, in tune with the rhythms of biological and emotional processes themselves – provides the basis of moving beyond the deconstruction of boundaries, to the reconstruction of former (Aristotelean) notions of (fixed) 'essences', (permanent) 'substances' and (unchanging) 'being' (Battersby 1998). (See also Shildrick 1997; Spivak 1989, 1990; Deleuze and Guattari ([1980] 1988, [1972] 1984); and Fox 1999).[12] The so-called 'new sciences', for writers such as Haraway (1991) and Battersby (1998), provide some promising leads here, from chaos theory with its dissipative systems, to the rhythmic repetitions of sound and music: topological models for imaging an embodied (fleshy) self 'birthed' out of movement and relationality, potentialities and flow (Battersby 1998: 57–60). Bodies, in short, 'irreducible' to any one domain or discourse, are processual rather than fixed, incorporating flows, both literal and metaphoric, which expose the limits of reductionism in myriad ways: issues captured in the paradox of being and becoming.

Reasonable emotions in an '(un)reasonable' world: towards a 'passionate' sociology?

Here we arrive at a fifth and final point that underpins much of this chapter: the importance of emotions to our knowledge of the world and our place within it, including a fundamental rethinking of reason itself in other less 'unreasonable', self 'contained' terms. The opposition between reason and emotion, as a variety of classical and contemporary commentators have pointed out, is in fact far less durable than belief in the opposition itself, masking as much as it reveals about the precise nature of this relationship, both past and present (Barbalet 1998; Williams 2001). Emotion, for instance, *qua* embodied modes of being and becoming, knowing and relating to the world, are crucial to all aspects of our lives, from the supposedly dispassionate, detached, value-neutral observations of scientific inquiry (Jaggar 1989; Rose 1994), to the affective basis of effective decision making (Damasio 1995) and the intersubjective, intercorporeal nature of communicative understanding within the lifeworld (Crossley 1998). Rather than repressing emotion in Western epistemology, therefore, it is necessary fundamentally to:

> rethink the relation between knowledge and emotion and construct conceptual models that demonstrate the *mutually constitutive* rather than oppositional relation between reason and emotion. Far from precluding the possibility of reliable knowledge, emotion as well as value must be shown as necessary to such knowledge ... the ideal of dispassionate enquiry is an impossible dream but a dream nonetheless or perhaps a myth that has exerted enormous influence on Western epistemology. Like all myths, it is a form of ideology that fulfils certain social and political functions.
>
> (Jaggar 1989: 157)

Not only would this serve to breathe new emotional life into conventional (Kantian) ethical paradigms – particularly in the light of developments such as the new genetics (Conrad and Gabe 1999) and the bioethical tensions and dilemmas they place upon existing frameworks (Shildrick 1997) – it may also serve to promote a more full-bodied, 'passionate' sociology in general; one which takes the embodiment of its practitioners, as well as those it seeks to study, seriously. This, moreover, would entail or necessitate a similar shift within existing specialisms such as the sociology *of* the body and the sociology *of* emotions, both of which (intentionally or not) imply a more or less detached, disembodied set of sociological reflections on these matters. A passionate sociology, as Game and Metcalfe put it:

> celebrates an *immersion in life, a compassionate involvement with the world and with others* ... An engaged or passionate sociology involves *a sensual, full-bodied approach to knowing and to practices of knowledge* such as reading, writing, teaching ... passion, social life and sociology only exist in the in-between, in specific, moving social *relations*.
>
> (Game and Metcalfe 1996: 5, my emphasis)

In these and other respects, it may be ventured, the challenges within and beyond sociology may not simply be reconfigured or re-envisaged, but also re-embodied in less 'unreasonable' terms: a guide both to life and living in ways which expose the limits of dominant Western rationalist viewpoints and the (bio)ethical dilemmas to which they give rise.

Concluding remarks

Let me take this opportunity to sum up what precisely I am and am not saying here. Biology, I have argued, for understandable reasons perhaps, has in large part been neglected if not dismissed in favour of sociocultural processes and the matters, or perhaps the non-material matters, to which they speak. A variety of forces, both inside and outside the academy, however, are compelling or facilitating a revisiting or rethinking of the biological: a 'return of the repressed' perhaps, but one, echoing Benton, we should (albeit cautiously) welcome rather than lament. Feminisms, in this respect, provide a clear illustration of what is at stake here, including some promising new ways forward, embryonic or otherwise (Birke 1999; Grosz 1994). An eclectic series of points or propositions, in keeping with these trends, have therefore been put forward, some no doubt more fruitful than others. In these and other ways the call, echoing Stacey (1988) in spirit if not content, has indeed been to acknowledge the 'biological base' and to give the biological its due, in a non-reductionist manner: one which enables us to move beyond the either/or logic (i.e. the Scylla and Charybdis) of biology versus society.

Key issues here, as we have seen, concern duality and dualism, epistemology and ontology; the 'unfinished' matter of biology; processes of negation or distortion, transcendence or transformation; the dynamics of being and becoming; and finally, in keeping with the intertwining of biological and social processes, an emphasis on emotions, *qua* embodied ways of knowing and relating to the world, themselves no longer the 'scandal' of Western thought and practice – an incorporative viewpoint which includes the 'passionate' vocation of sociology itself (cf. Game and Metcalfe 1996). These propositions, to be sure, are in no way exhaustive. Nor do the eclectic theoretical positions they draw upon necessarily sit easily or compatibly together. My aim, instead, has simply been to approach these issues from a variety of viewpoints which, each in its different way perhaps, help us to think through the non-reductive possibilities of bringing the biological 'back in' – exposing a series of former errors or misconceptions along the way. Much work, none the less, remains to be done here, itself a source of challenge and opportunity. These very issues, as noted above, are presaged in critical new ways through developments such as the new genetics (Conrad and Gabe 1999), the challenges and dilemmas of (bio)ethics (Shildrick 1997; Frank 2000), and the rise of evolutionary psychology (Rose and Rose 2000a).

One final issue, perhaps, within all this remains to be (explicitly) addressed here: the question of 'risks'. Are there, for instance, risks in reopening the biology/society debate? If so, what are they, who benefits, and in what ways? On the one hand, in not fully taking up the challenge, we run the risk of perpetuating existing either/or type debates concerning the biological and the social. Going beyond the biological, to repeat, does not mean leaving it out altogether; nor, however, does recourse to the biological imply an inescapable or ineluctable slide into the quagmire or murky depths of reductionism, essentialism or determinism. We can no longer, in other words, afford to 'write' the biological more or less out of existence, to 'interpret it away', or to deny it a place in our theorising.

On the other hand, the risk in taking up this challenge, particularly for those of a strongly constructionist persuasion, is that some ground may indeed have to be conceded here, forcing a rethinking or revision of our own preferred theories about the world and our place within it, including the disciplinary (if not imperialist) claims this entails (Craib 1997; Strong 1979). Doing so, moreover, requires an acknowledgement of the paradoxical fact – obvious for some, unpalatable for others – that it is precisely our biological capacity for thought, language and tool use, amongst other things, which enables the very denial or explaining away, in a (self-serving) sociological fashion, of the biological body itself: a constructionist ruse or conceit to be sure, which in turn betrays a deeper undercurrent of 'sociologism' (i.e. the temptation to explain everything in sociological terms) that, potentially at least, knows no bounds (Craib 1988). This, however, in keeping with the general thrust of the chapter, turns out to be no real risk at all, given the limits of (biological) reductionism and (social) constructionism alike, and the need to go beyond the biological without leaving it out altogether. A more 'balanced' viewpoint may therefore, in effect, emerge here through a bringing of the biological back in, placing minds in bodies, bodies in society and society in the body in the process.

The matter of bodies, to conclude, matters: a biological as well as a social matter which our theorising about the world, and our place within it, must both incorporate and respect in newly enmattered ways.

Notes

1 A distinction between the 'biological' as a material, animating life-force, and 'biology' as a disciplinary way of knowing, ordering and understanding this matter, may be drawn here at the outset, although I do not adhere to it rigorously in this particular chapter. See also the following discussion of ontological and epistemological issues under the first of the five key ways forward proposed in this chapter.

2 As Fausto-Sterling's (2000) *Sexing the Body* makes abundantly clear, moreover – drawing upon biological evidence in support of her case – 'two sexes' do not exist in any simple, straightforward fashion. See also Birke (1999, 1986) and Kaplan and Rogers (1990).

3 For an illuminating comparison and contrast of Butler and Bourdieu, and their respective merits for feminist theory, see Lovell (2000).

4 Sayer (1997) in fact goes further here, arguing, in the face of anti-essentialism, for

a 'moderate', non-deterministic essentialism (*vis-à-vis* a strong, deterministic essentialism); something which, he claims, is necessary for a social science with critical or emancipatory potential.

5 This distinction was first introduced, in the context of a realist critique of the social construction of emotions, by Greenwood (1994). See also Craib (1988) for a further critique of the collapsing of the social into the liguistic, alongside the dangers or limits of 'sociologism' in general.

6 I would like to acknowledge here a series of very useful debates with Robert Fine on these and associated matters.

7 Mention of Mauss's ([1934] 1973) notion of body techniques and Bourdieu's (1984, 1990) appropriation of the habitus and bodily hexis is also important here. There is, Mauss proclaims, no such thing as a 'natural' way for the adult. Rather, every society has its own corporeal habits, movements and customs. Body techniques identified in one society or historical period therefore may have no equivalent in another. See Williams and Bendelow (1998) for a fuller discussion of these and related issues. See also Ingold's (2000) dissussion of the Maussian paradigm case of walking; something, Ingold argues, which cannot simply be explained as an evolved, innately developing skill, independently of the circumstances and contexts within which indivuals learn and develop within and across their lifetimes/lines.

8 For other biologically informed accounts of emotions within sociology, see Wentworth and Ryan (1994), B.S. Turner (1996), J.H. Turner (2000), Burkitt (1997), Lyon (1998) and Williams (2001). See also Hirst and Wolley (1982) for a more general discussion of social relations and human attributes.

9 Elias's own position here, it should be noted, is not immune from criticism. Post-symbol emancipation, for example, as Shilling (1993) points out, the biological constitution of human action tends to recede from Elias's view in favour of the civilising process (that is, the socialisation, rationalisation and individualisation of bodies). There is also, as Lynda Birke rightly comments (personal communication), a problematic distinction drawn by Elias (amongst others) between learning humans and instinctual animals. See, for example, Birke (1994) on this more general point and its implications within and beyond feminism.

10 Lynch (1977) reaches similar conclusions in his book *The Broken Heart: The Medical Consequences of Loneliness*, where he presents compelling evidence of the links between cardiovascular disease and emotionally distressing life events. See also Lynch (1985) and Brown and Harris (1978, 1989) for further research on the relationship between life events and illness, and Wilkinson (1996) on issues of income distribution, social cohesion and the psychosocial pathways to disease, the emotional dimensions of which are theorised in Williams (1998).

11 The claims of evolutionary psychology, as contributors to Rose and Rose's (2000a) co-edited volume convincingly demonstrate, are for the most part not merely 'mistaken, but culturally pernicious' (Rose and Rose 2000b: 3).

12 Respect for the integrity of some sort of borders or boundaries, however, as Lynda Birke has pointed out to me (personal communication), may none the less be important to the maintenance of fundamental human as well as animal rights, and the political struggles contained therein. The Deleuzo-Guattarian (1984, 1988) deterritorialisation (or dissolution) of the body (without-organs) and the nomadic forms of becoming it entails, for example, may be achieved at too great a cost for the furtherance of women's own particular interests (Grosz 1994; Battersby 1998). See also Sayer (1997), cited in note 4 above, concerning the importance of a 'non-deterministic essentialism' in relation to the maintenance and defence of basic human rights and needs.

References

Archer M.S. (1995) *Realist Social Theory: A Morphogenetic Approach*, Cambridge: Cambridge University Press.

Barbalet, J. (1998) *Emotion, Social Theory and Social Structure*, Cambridge: Cambridge University Press.

Barrett, M. and Phillips, A. (1992) *Destabilizing Theory: Contemporary Feminist Debates*, Cambridge: Polity Press.

Battersby, C. (1998) *The Phenomenal Woman: Feminist Metaphysics and the Patterns of Identity*, Cambridge: Polity Press.

Benton, T. (1991) 'Biology and social science: why the return of the repressed should be given a (cautious) welcome', *Sociology* 25 (1): 1–29.

Bhaskar, R. (1989) *Reclaiming Reality*, London: Verso.

Birke, L. (1986) *Women, Feminism and Biology: The Feminist Challenge*, Brighton, Sussex: Wheatsheaf.

—— (1994) *Feminism, Animals and Science: The Naming of the Shrew*, Buckingham: Open University Press.

—— (1995) *Our Bodies, Ourselves? Feminism, Biology and the Body*, Working Paper, Centre for the Study of Women and Gender, University of Warwick.

—— (1999) *Feminism and the Biological Body*, Edinburgh: Edinburgh University Press.

Bourdieu, P. (1984) *Distinction: A Social Critique of the Judgement of Taste*, London: Routledge.

—— (1990) *The Logic of Practice*, Cambridge: Polity Press.

Brown, G.W. and Harris, T.O. (1978) *The Social Origins of Depression*, London: Tavistock.

—— and —— (eds) (1989) *Life Events and Illness*, London: Hyman Unwin.

Burkitt, I. (1997) 'Social relationships and emotions', *Sociology* 31 (1): 37–55.

Butler, J. (1993) *Body Matters: The Discursive Limits of 'Sex'*, London: Routledge.

Cixous, H. (1991) 'The laugh of Medussa', in S. Gunew (ed.), *Feminist Knowledge: A Reader*, London: Routledge.

Connell, R.W. (1983) *Which Way is Up?*, Sydney and London: George Allen and Unwin.

—— (1987) *Gender and Power: Society, the Person and Sexual Politics*, Cambridge: Polity Press.

Conrad, P. and Gabe, J. (eds) (1999) 'Sociological perspectives on the new genetics', *Sociology of Health and Illness* (Special Issue) 21 (5).

Craib, I. (1988) *Psychoanalysis and Social Theory: The Limits of Sociology*, London: Harvester Wheatsheaf.

—— (1995) 'Some comment on the sociology of emotions', *Sociology*, 29 (1): 151–8.

—— (1997) 'Social constructionism as social psychosis', *Sociology* 31 (1): 1–15.

Crossley, N. (1998) 'Emotion and communicative action: Habermas, linguistic philosophy and existentialism', in G. Bendelow and S.J. Williams (eds), *Emotions in Social Life: Critcal Themes and Contemporary Issues*, London: Routledge.

Daly, M. (1978) *Gyn/ecology: The Metaethics of Radical Feminism*, Boston, MA: Beacon Press.

Damasio, D. (1995) *Descartes' Error*, New York: Putnam.

Deleuze, G. and Guattari, F. ([1972] 1984) *Anti-Oedipus: Capitalism and Schizophrenia*

I, trans. R. Hurley, M. Seem and H.R. Lane, preface by M. Foucault, London: Athlone Press.

—— and —— ([1980] 1988) *A Thousand Plateaus: Capitalism and Schizophrenia II*, trans. B. Mussumi, London: Athlone Press.

Elias, N. ([1939a] 1978) *The Civilizing Process*, vol I: *The History of Manners*, Oxford: Basil Blackwell.

—— ([1939b] 1982) *The Civilizing Process*, vol II: *State Formations and Civilization*, Oxford: Basil Blackwell.

—— (1991a) 'On human beings and their emotions: a process-sociological essay', in M. Featherstone, M. Hepworth and B. Turner (eds), *The Body: Social Process and Cultural Theory*, London: Sage.

—— (1991b) *The Symbol Theory*, London: Sage.

Engels, F. ([1845] 1987) *The Conditions of the Working Class in England*, Harmondsworth, Middx: Penguin.

Fausto-Sterling, A. (1992) *Myths About Gender: Biological Theories About Men and Women*, 2nd (rev.) edn, New York: Basic Books.

—— (2000) *Sexing the Body*, New York: Basic Books.

Firestone, S. (1970) *The Dialectic of Sex: The Case for Feminist Revolution*, London: Women's Press.

Fox, N.J. (1999) *Beyond Health: Postmodernism and Embodiment*, London: Free Association Books.

Frank, A.W. (2000) 'Review essay: social bioethics and the critique of autonomy', *Health* 4 (3): 378–94.

Freund, P.E.S. (1990) 'The expressive body: a common ground for the sociology of emotions and health and illness', *Sociology of Health and Illness* 12 (4): 452–77.

—— (1998) 'Social performances and their discontents: reflections on the biosocial psychology of role-playing', in G. Bendelow and S.J. Williams (eds), *Emotions in Social Life: Critical Themes and Contemporary Issues*, London: Routledge.

Game, A. and Metcalfe, A. (1996) *Passionate Sociology*, London: Sage.

Gatens, M. (1992) 'Power, bodies and difference', in M. Barrett and A. Phillips (eds), *Destabilizing Theory: Contemporary Feminist Debates*, Cambridge: Polity Press.

Goffman, E. (1959) *The Presentation of Everyday Life*, New York: Doubleday Anchor.

Greenwood, J.D. (1994) *Realism, Identity and Emotion: Reclaiming Social Psychology*, London: Sage.

Grosz, E. (1994) *Volatile Bodies: Toward a Corporeal Feminism*, Bloomington and Indianapolis: Indiana University Press.

—— (1995) *Space, Time and Perversion*, London: Routledge.

Haraway, D. (1991) *Simians, Cyborgs and Women*, London: Free Association Books.

Hirst, P. and Wolley, P. (1982) *Social Relations and Human Attributes*, London and New York: Tavistock.

Hochschild, A.R. (1983) *The Managed Heart: The Commercialisation of Human Feeling*, Berkeley, CA: University of California Press.

Ingold, T. (2000) 'Evolving skills', in H. Rose and S. Rose (eds), *Alas Poor Darwin: Arguments Against Evolutionary Psychology*, London: Jonathan Cape.

Irigaray, L. (1991) 'The sex which is not one', in S. Gunew (ed.), *Feminist Knowledge: A Reader*, London: Routledge.

Jaggar, A. (1989) 'Love and knowledge: emotion in feminist epistemology', in

S. Bordo and A. Jaggar (eds), *Gender/Body/Knowledge: Feminist Reconstructions of Being and Knowing*, New Brunswick, NJ, and London: Rutgers University Press.

Kaplan, G. and Rogers, L. (1990) 'The definition of male and female: biological reductionism and the sanctions of normality', in S. Gunew (ed.), *Feminist Knowledge: Critique and Construct*, London: Routledge.

Laing, R.D. (1965) *The Divided Self*, Harmondsworth, Middx: Penguin.

Lovell, T. (2000) 'Thinking feminism with and against Bourdieu', *Feminist Theory* 1 (1): 11–32.

Lynch, J. (1977) *The Broken Heart: The Medical Consequences of Loneliness*, New York: Basic Books.

—— (1985) *The Language of the Heart: The Human Body in Dialogue*, New York: Basic Books.

Lyon, M. (1998) 'The limitations of cultural constructionism in the study of emotions', in G. Bendelow and S.J. Williams (eds), *Emotions in Social Life: Critical Themes and Contemporary Issues*, London: Routledge.

Martin, E. (1994) *Flexible Bodies*, Boston, MA: Beacon Press.

—— (2000) 'Flexible bodies: science and the new culture of health in the US', in S.J. Williams, J. Gabe and M. Calnan (eds), *Health, Medicine and Society: Key Theories, Future Agendas*, London: Routledge.

Mauss, M. ([1934] 1973) 'Techniques of the body', *Economy and Society* 2: 70–88.

Oakley, A. (1972) *Sex, Gender and Society*, Aldershot, Hants.: Gower.

O'Brien, Mary (1981) *The Politics of Reproduction*, London: Routledge and Kegan Paul.

—— (1989) *Reproducing the World*, Boulder, CO: Westview Press.

Rich, A. (1976) *Of Woman Born*, London: Virago.

Rose, H. (1994) *Love, Power and Knowledge: Towards a Feminist Transformation of Science*, Cambridge: Polity Press.

—— and Rose, S. (eds) (2000a) *Alas Poor Darwin: Arguments Against Evolutionary Psychology*, London: Jonathan Cape.

—— and —— (2000b) 'Introduction', in H. Rose and S. Rose (eds), *Alas Poor Darwin: Arguments Against Evolutionary Psychology*, London: Jonathan Cape.

Rose, S. (1997) *Lifelines: Biology, Freedom, Determinism*, Harmondsworth, Middx: Penguin.

Sayer, A. (1992) *Method in Social Science: A Realist Approach*, 2nd edn, London: Routledge.

—— (1997) 'Essentialism, social constructionism and beyond', *Sociological Review* 45 (3): 453–87.

Seidler, V. (1994) *Unreasonable Men*, London: Routledge.

Shaw, M., Dorling, D., Gordon, D. and Davey Smith, G. (1999) *The Widening Gap: Health Inequalities in Britain*, Bristol: Policy Press.

Shildrick, M. (1997) *Leaky Bodies and Boundaries: Feminism, Postmodernism and (Bio)Ethics*, London: Routledge.

Shilling, C. (1993) *The Body and Social Theory*, London: Sage.

Spelman, E. (1988) *Inessential Woman: Problems of Exclusion in Feminist Thought*, Boston, MA: Beacon Books.

Spivak, G.C. (1989) 'In a word', interview with Ellen Rooney, *Differences* 1 (2): 124–56.

—— 1990: *The Post-colonial Critic: Interviews, Strategies, Dialogues*, ed. S. Harasym, London: Routledge.

Stacey, M. (1988) *The Sociology of Health and Healing*, London: Routledge.

Strong, P. (1979) 'Sociological imperialism and the profession of medicine: a critical examination of the thesis of medical imperialism', *Social Science and Medicine* 13A: 199–215.

Townsend, P., Davidson, N. and Whitehead, M. (1988) *Inequalities in Health: The Black Report and the Health Divide*, Harmondworth, Middx: Penguin.

Turner, B.S. (1995) *Medical Power and Social Knowledge*, 2nd edn, London: Sage.

—— (1996) *Body and Society*, 2nd edn, London: Sage.

Turner, J.H. (1996) 'The evolution of emotions in humans: a Darwinian–Durkheimian analysis', *Journal for the Theory of Social Behaviour* 26 (1): 1–33.

—— (2000) *On the Origins of Human Emotions*, Stanford, CA: Stanford University Press.

Wentworth, W.M. and Ryan, J. (1994) 'Introduction', in W.M. Wentworth and J. Ryan (eds), *Social Perspectives on Emotion*, Greenwich, CT, and London: JAI Press.

——, —— and Yardley, D. (1994) 'Deep sociality: a bioevolutionary perspective on the sociology of emotions', in W.M. Wentworth and J. Ryan (eds), *Social Perspectives on Emotion*, Greenwich, CT, and London: JAI Press.

Wilkinson, R.G. (1996) *Unhealthy Societies: The Afflictions of Inequality*, London: Routledge.

Williams, S.J. (1998) ' "Capitalising" on emotions? Rethinking the inequalities debate', *Sociology* 32 (1): 121–39.

—— (2001) *Emotion and Social Theory*, London: Sage.

—— and Bendelow, G. (1998) *The Lived Body: Sociological Themes, Embodied Issues*, London: Routledge.

Wouters, C. (1992) 'On status competition and emotion management: study of emotion as a new field', *Theory, Culture and Society* 9: 229–52.

Young, I. (1990) *Throwing Like a Girl and Other Essays in Feminist Philosophy and Social Theory*, Bloomington and Indianapolis: Indiana University Press.

2 Anchoring the head

The disappearing (biological) body

Lynda Birke

Introduction

> My body and I have never been friends . . . I tend to think of my body as
> something to anchor my head, the place where the really important stuff is
> going on.
>
> (Bray 1994)

The body is highly fashionable in the academy. But, like the body invoked in
Bray's short story, it has largely been a place to anchor the head – an entity
apart from the 'I' that does the theorising about it. Its materiality is something we generally take for granted (unless we get sick); indeed, its materiality
is so taken for granted in the new theorising that it seems not to exist except as
surface – an endlessly malleable surface on to which culture writes (Ferguson
1997).

In writing and teaching about feminism and the body, I have searched in
vain for the presence of the biological body below the surface – our interior
bits and pieces, our inner processes. To locate those, I have to turn (back) to
the narratives of biomedicine, for there seem to be no other ways of speaking
about our innards in our technoscientific culture. Perhaps that is one reason
why biological bodies are conspicuously absent from much of the new social
theory (see Birke 1999).

Focusing on the body as surface extends another sociological preoccupation with ideas of social construction (of gender or sexuality, for example).
Underlying this is a rejection of any notion that human behaviour is biologically determined. With that I must agree; determinism implies that
change is difficult. But that does not mean that biological processes are irrelevant to our conceptualisation of the body. All it means is that some concepts
in biology are more useful than others to our theorising and politics.

Like many women, I have trouble in thinking about theories of social
construction that ignore my bodily pain and bleeding, or that ignore the
suffering of people in war or torture (see Scarry 1985). The emphasis in 'body
theory' on the body's surface presents problems, too, in relation to illness.
Arthur Frank (1996) has noted, for example, how odd the idea of body as

surface is to someone suffering from cancer; illness, for Frank, means living the body, experiencing it through a 'shifting synthesis of this perpetually spiralling dialectic of flesh, inscription and intention' (ibid.: 58). You cannot live *in* an empty surface.

In this chapter, I want to look at some of the ways in which we have come to think about the 'biological body'; inevitably, these ideas draw heavily on biomedicine. My own training in the biological sciences also provides source material for questions: How did I come to think in those ways? What do these modes of thought imply for how we think about the biological body? For feminism? Or for illness and health? An undercurrent to all this is my insistence that we have to find ways of thinking about the body that disavow determinism, yet acknowledge the material entity we call the body – along with its pains, its bleeding, its suffering.[1]

My immediate focus is on scientific diagrams as representations of the ways in which we think 'things happen' inside. I shall draw out two themes: that of the body as encapsulating inner space, and that of the body as a tightly controlled set of systems. Each of these connects, I shall argue, to themes in sociological theorising about the body, even if 'the biological' is played down in that theorising. The metaphor of 'space', for instance, is implicit in the theoretical preoccupation with the body as surface; for if cultural inscription on the surface is all there is to bodies, then there can be nothing inside *but* space. Similarly, the theme of control finds echo in concepts of bodily control in/through the social order. These two strands intertwine most closely through our experiences of illness and the related practices of biomedicine.

Picturing inside

> The Female Body is made of transparent plastic and lights up when you plug it in. You press a button to illuminate the different systems . . . each Female Body contains a female brain. Handy. Makes things work.
>
> (Atwood 1994: 90–2)

To imagine our insides, we in Western culture usually invoke images drawn from science. Not for us the ebbs and flows of earlier humoral doctrines (Duden 1993); rather, we tend to think in terms of machine metaphors. Similarly, most of us recognise the line drawing of (say) a uterus, and can promptly add the labels. Indeed, we tend to do so uncritically, to forget what we have learned in other disciplines of the academy about deconstructing images:[2] anatomical diagrams seem somehow so far removed from that world.

In thinking about the biological body, it is inevitable that I too draw on those biomedical representations. I am a child of that technoscientific culture; I have also been trained in biology – thoroughly immersed in the narratives and concepts of biomedicine. In doing so, I learned about bodily controls, how the internal state is maintained. I also, of course, learned the tacit assumptions of science; among other things, I learned 'how to see' specific pictures down a microscope, for example (see Keller 1996). I was also immersed in the conceptual dismemberment of the body as it is portrayed through reductionist rhetoric: the animal bodies of my training were merely walking machines, assemblages of moving parts.[3]

Here, I explore briefly one aspect – diagrams – of my own journey through scientific training, and what they taught me about 'how bodies work' (Birke 1999). Such scientific images are, however, widely available within the culture and roughly familiar to most of us, whatever our training. Take, for example, the plastic model of a woman described in Margaret Atwood's short story. As a child, I had one of these 'Visible Woman' models; you could paint the organs and reassemble them. The reproductive system, naturally, came in two types – pregnant or not.

What can one learn from models such as these? Perhaps not surprisingly, I did learn something about anatomy from my Visible Woman. But I also learned some other, less overt, lessons, too; I learned, for instance, how squashed up the intestines become in late pregnancy. No wonder I avoided pregnancy ever after. Even less overtly, I learned to conceptualise the inner organs as coexisting within an inner space – a theme I want to pick up here. The metaphor of 'inner space', I suggest, is a powerful one in the diagrams of Western biomedicine. It is perpetuated – often quite implicitly – through the kinds of images and diagrams that biomedicine uses to get its ideas across to generations of students. What then are the implications for how we view our bodies and for health care?

Inner spaces

It is, perhaps, rather less uncomfortable to look at the diagrammatic drawings of modern textbooks than the carefully detailed and shaded drawings of Vesalius' sixteenth-century anatomies.[4] Like viewing film clips of open heart surgery, his detailed drawings are rather too vivid in their portrayal of anatomical structures. Abstracted diagrams don't so easily remind us of our literal flesh.

Abstraction in scientific illustration developed over the centuries. Early illustrations attempted to represent through shading the literal shape of internal organs and their location in the body. Gradually, however, these details fell away, until the highly abstracted and stylised form of illustration, with which we are now familiar, emerged (Laqueur 1990).

Modern scientific illustrations of the body are highly stylised: organs appear as outlines, taken out of the context of a body. They simply appear on the page as sets of lines. Sometimes, they are so abstracted they no longer bear much relationship to the living organism: a rough oval, for instance, might serve to symbolise the body plan of a 'typical vertebrate'. Details are lost in the process of abstraction – not only of the organ(s) themselves but also of their context; the organ/body thus becomes free-floating. The body is typically presented as if sectioned longitudinally; the front is removed so that we can 'see in' to the outlined organs. Now, the only details that might be added are notations that indicate that what we are seeing is a *scientific* text; these notations might include mathematical symbols, arrows, graphs, tables superimposed on or juxtaposed to the diagrammatic organ.[5]

Where representations of 'real' bodies appear in medical textbooks, it is often as illustrations (photographs, for instance) of pathologies; a photo might appear to show, say, a person with thyroid dysfunction. Or an outline of a human body might accompany an inset graph to demonstrate the location of a specific function – perhaps a graph showing the electrical changes of the heart superimposed on an outline of a human thorax. But these are the exceptions. In general, the shape of the human body disappears completely in scientific illustration, to be replaced by graphs and diagrams of finer details such as histology.

Learning to interpret these diagrams is a crucial part of 'learning to see' as a scientist-in-training. Like students confronted with a microscope slide for the first time (Keller 1996), you have to learn *how* to read a scientific diagram, to understand what and how it represents. And what it represents is no longer the specific tissue that might appear under a microscope; rather, the diagram stands for a generalised cell/tissue, just as diagrammatic human bodies are supposed to represent a generalised human.

Yet what is a generalised human? Abstraction enables the illustrator to omit details, in effect to censor what goes into the image. And it is at this point that *how* we read the images becomes most salient. A few diagrams do attempt to show some part of the body outline. But this outline, especially in older textbooks, is usually one of a man – European and young adult, at that. Even in more recent texts, which might include the use of colour printing, beige (to represent 'white' skin) appears more often than any other colour in representations of the scientifically portrayed body (see Birke 1999). And bodies other than the young adult male are rarely shown; significantly, the exceptions are either younger bodies (to illustrate growth and changes at puberty, for example), or bodies showing pathologies (obesity in certain endocrine disturbances, say). The generalised human body of the scientific diagram is thus rather less than fully representative.

Not surprisingly, diagrammatic abstraction conveys other gendered meanings. In diagrams, the 'female reproductive tract', for example, is usually shown from the front (at least in elementary textbooks). The uterus can then be drawn as a triangle, with Fallopian tubes either side. Below are lines representing the vagina. What is missing here are details that are seen as scientifically irrelevant to the narrative of reproduction: typically, neither the clitoris nor the lubricating glands appear in these highly stylised and abstracted diagrams. The clitoris is removed by the longitudinal section, which has erased everything situated in front of the uterus.

Diagrams representing a sideways section should in theory be more anatomically inclusive; after all, this should 'cut' through the whole of the external genitals. But no. The clitoris is usually missing (Moore and Clarke 1995).[6] Analysing medical texts, Moore and Clarke note how the labelling of the clitoris was actively removed from the 1948 edition of *Gray's Anatomy*, and repeated in several other texts through the 1950s and 1960s.

Despite the detailed labelling that inevitably was included in feminist books about women's bodies (such as *Our Bodies, Ourselves*: Boston Women's Health Collective 1973), clitoral erasure continues. Recent medical texts, Moore and Clarke found, still ignore or downplay the clitoris, and emphasise the narrative of reproduction. Vaginas exist for penises, and lubrication exists for heterosexual intercourse in these accounts. Abstraction – in the diagrams and in the accompanying text – clearly has implications for women. We are divorced from our bodies; even those parts that give us pleasure disappear or have no names.

Abstraction must be interpreted; viewers/readers must do work to fill in the gaps, to give the image meaning. (And in the case of the missing clitoris, the gender of the viewer/reader becomes highly significant.) But the meaning as constructed in medical diagrams is not arbitrary. We are not supposed, as viewers, to see the thoracic cavity as, say, a cooking pot (as medieval doctors sometimes did: Pouchelle 1990). Rather, we are to read it as scientific, as mathematical, as abstract.

Abstractions contribute, moreover, to a conception of the inner body as *space*. We are so used to seeing lots of space on the page around the diagrammatic organs that space becomes part of the imagined body's interior.[7] Organs appear almost free-floating within these spaces. This impression is augmented when we see televised or film images of the inner body; we can witness surgical procedures, for instance, or we can undergo a 'voyage' via fibreoptic tubes. Here, in that watery world, we travel along our inner passageways; we move along through what seem like oceanic spaces.

Inner space is further invoked through cyberspace if we explore webpages showing anatomical details – the images of the Visible Human Project is one example (Cartwright 1998). We can, we learn from the webpages, 'fly around the thighs' of the Visible Woman:[8] space and sexuality evoked both at once. For even more abstraction, we can visit the Stanford Visible Female – the cryopreserved pelvis of a young woman. Not the rest of her body, mind you – just her pelvis, so reinforcing the concept of woman as reproductive organs. Images of male scientists cutting up the lump of frozen female flesh disturbed me when I found the site. But so too did the highly abstracted coloured models that resulted from digitised sections of her pelvis. Apart from the sexual overtones of the accompanying text ('entering posteriorly', for example), the models are eerily disembodied, totally devoid of context (see Birke 1999: 77). Abstraction indeed.

Now I am not suggesting that more realist representations are somehow freer of interpretative possibilities (the gallows in the background of one of the more vivid of Vesalius' sixteenth-century drawings reminds us of that).

Nor am I suggesting that we should avoid diagrams: simplified diagrams help to get the message across to students where more complex details would obscure. My point, rather, is to emphasise that the abstractions and their necessary ommissions help to determine how we, the readers, *read* the images. It is at that point that hidden assumptions – of gender and race, for example – become particularly significant.

Learning to 'see' the inner body in terms of spaces, as the generalised cell or the generalised torso, makes it much easier to do a cut-and-paste with different organs. Just as I could easily move plastic organs around in my childhood model, so we can (re)move the organ from the corpse on to paper or into the even greater abstractions of cyberspace. The body thus becomes a set of replaceable parts – as indeed it is within the rhetoric of biomedicine. Transplant surgery is a clear example; there, organs have meaning only as bits of machinery. Thus the heart is 'only a pump', easily interchangeable even with the heart of another species (Birke and Michael 1998; Williams and Bendelow 1998).

Such reductionism does not always match up to how people live their bodies, however. On the contrary, studies of people facing transplant surgery have noted the contradictions, as people must try to make sense of the reductionist rhetoric alongside other cultural images (such as the heart as the seat of the emotions: Sharp 1995). Pregnant women, too, must deal with the contradictory narratives of 'their' baby ('seen' through ultrasound imagery, for instance, and thus extrapolated from its context: Petchesky 1987), and their experiencing of the foetus in relation to themselves (Mitchell and Georges 1997). We may learn to read scientific diagrams in particular ways, to learn that these lines and spaces represent 'the' 'universal' body. But it is much harder to learn to connect these to *our* lived bodies, in all their differences; these are erased by abstraction.

Living machines

Alongside the spaces of anatomical diagrams is the rhetoric of the body as machine – another metaphor far removed from the lived experiences of bodies. While this notion has a long history, it developed particularly (and unsurprisingly) in the wake of the Industrial Revolution (Kremer 1990). In the second half of the twentieth century, it gained new momentum in association with cybernetics: the body as a set of interlocking and cybernetically controlled systems was born. It was this body that I found throughout my undergraduate training – the 'living control systems' of my textbooks.

The accompanying diagrams were (and are) highly stylised and abstract, a set of interconnecting lines indicating feedback and control. These are entirely abstracted from the living organism; there are no animals – or bodies – here, only machines and systems, represented by boxes and interconnecting lines: feedback, comparator, input, output. The empty space of the anatomical diagram becomes further consolidated; even the organs now disappear within the rectangular images. This is far removed from the glistening flesh exposed to view by the camera or in Vesalius' anatomical illustrations.

Learning 'how bodies work' was, for me, a fascinating experience: that animal bodies function so marvellously was (and is) a never-ending source of wonder. Yet the learning was also violating, for what had begun in my life with an awe and delight at the complexities of living animals was slowly being translated into horror at their (literal) dismemberment in the teaching labs. The linear diagrams of systems theory took further that process of abstraction, and helped to gloss over the horror: it is harder to think of whole animals (and their suffering) when you are confronted with a systems diagram.

Analogies abound in portraying the inner body and play a useful role in helping us to understand it. But they also structure our understanding in particular ways. Earlier in the twentieth century, analogies for the human body were largely mechanical. The 'factory' metaphor predominated, for example (and, indeed, can still be found in textbooks). These stories typically portray the body's workings as a factory (with the proviso that the factory can itself move: see Bayliss 1966: 1), with implications of (gendered) hierarchy, management and control.[9] We are so familiar with these mechanical devices that comprise our inner bodies that they occasion little surprise. Representing the heart as 'merely a pump' allows us to gloss over the many cultural meanings attached to the heart, which in turn facilitates our acceptance of techniques such as heart transplants (Radley 1996).

Yet the body-machine, as it was imagined by scientists a century ago, was rather inefficient. How much more efficient it could become, they dreamed, with the help of electricity some time in the future:

> The digestive organs and the organs of assimilation which are the boiler plant, have an efficiency much lower than a steam boiler plant. The fact is that the old machine consumes too much vital energy in preparing the fuel (food) for assimilation ... [but electrical energy no doubt] will be utilised as an assistant to the natural forces of the body.
>
> (Foree Bain 1910; cited in Marvin 1988: 142)

Perhaps not quite in the way that Bain forecast, we do indeed use electricity now to extend our bodies' capacities. One part of the heritage of systems theory applied to the body is an emphasis on information flow. Information, whether in the form of genetic material in DNA or as electrical traces in the nervous system, flows through our bodies (thus connecting to other forms of electronic information).[10]

These developments have led to major shifts in how we perceive the functioning of the human body, particularly in how we understand the electrical nature of nerve action. Integrated circuits and information flow rely on pathways of information; within the body, a major conduit of such 'information' is the nervous system and its electrical flow. Our bodies and their illnesses, moreover, become exteriorised by means of those conduits; we can be connected up to machines for various purposes, from diagnosis to dialysis. It is, moreover, now quite easy to envisage ourselves as inexorably plugged into feedback circuits, to understand ourselves as cyborgs; we become boundaryless, part of a global integrated circuit (see Haraway 1991; Tomas 1996).

Body metaphors and social theory

I began this chapter by remarking that recent theorising about the body in sociology and feminism has tended to ignore inner, biological, processes. That in turn rests on their taken-for-grantedness. I can assume my body will get on with its business while I write – and if not, then I had better get it mended. But what is taken for granted is a steady state: too much disturbance of that state and I would be unable to function at the keyboard. That in turn implies fixity, a lack of change; I can ignore my body because I assume that 'its business' is to maintain my bodily order. In this section, I want to turn from the metaphors of biomedicine back to the social theory and its underlying assumptions about the body, to ask questions about the relationship between the two. Control, for example, is a theme that links both the biomedical and the sociological narratives.

As I have noted, the controlled and thus unchanging body lies at the heart of physiology (so to speak); in physiology classrooms, students learn about the maintenance of bodily control systems through homeostasis. Too much change and the systems go out of control. Now homeostasis is indeed crucial; in general, my body temperature remains around 37° Celsius. But that emphasis on maintenance can become normalising. Bodies that deviate from controls thus become deviant, pathologies. The taken-for-grantedness of the body rests on a prototype – predictably, of the adult, male body. So, if my becoming-menopausal body goes into apparent temperature swings then it must be, in some sense, deviant[11] by comparison to that mythically predictable norm.

Similarly, much recent work about the body draws on ideas of control (and, relatedly, power) within the social order; so how do these link to the biomedical models I have been discussing? There are two broad themes on which I draw. One approach within sociology is to emphasise social control *over* the body; another is to emphasise the willed control of the body within society, by which we learn how to 'live in' our bodies within a particular culture (Williams and Bendelow 1998).

Foucault's work (e.g. Foucault 1973), for instance, has been particularly influential as an example of control through the social order. He put particular emphasis on the power of discourse to effect social control, and thus to exert disciplinary power. Discourses of femininity and thinness, for example, act to discipline us into seeking to achieve a leaner body (Bordo 1993). Medical discourses are crucially part of that disciplining, Foucault argues, serving to create or maintain control, to create 'docile bodies' – a control which has been escalating with the rise of medical power since the eighteenth century.

Armstrong (1993), following Foucault, describes how disease was re-mapped during the twentieth century, from the inner organs of the body into the social spaces between people. Tuberculosis, for example, became seen increasingly as a social disease, indicating poor living conditions rather than a disease of the individual body. These changes helped to extend the medical gaze; thus, when we become aware of our body in illness, our experiencing of the body is controlled through encounters with doctors, the structure of the hospital, and by the visualisation technologies that determine the diagnosis, as well as our expectations of technological medical practices.

An alternative way of conceptualising bodies and control is through a focus on control over the body through its functioning within society; that is, we learn to use our bodies (to control them) in particular ways in particular societies. Bourdieu's work on body 'habitus' is significant here (Bourdieu 1984).[12] We learn to comport ourselves, to exert control over our bodies, in particular ways – through participation in particular sports, for example, or through the kind of food that we eat. Here, the implications for health have to do with the consequences of that comportment, in terms of the effects of diet for example.

Both themes have been important in directing attention to how 'bodies' are constructed in Western culture, and have contributed greatly to the recent resurgence of interest in this theme. But neither, it seems to me, really addresses the *biological* body. Approaches such as Foucault's render the body passive; his insistence on the power of discourse and disciplinary power allows biological, material, bodies to drop out of theorising altogether, as several critics have pointed out (e.g. Shilling 1993; Williams and Bendelow 1998). Bourdieu's approach seems, by contrast, to acknowledge the material-ity of the body in the behaviour of that body. Yet it too ignores the inner body; rather, its focus is the disposition of the physical body in its social world rather than inner workings. The latter seem always to remain within the purview of biomedicine, removed from sociological theory.

It is, however, in the biological body and the maintenance of its health that the two approaches of social theory meet, I would argue. What we eat is a matter of constant surveillance: health promotion campaigns advocate that we eat less fat if we want to stay healthy, for example. But what we choose to eat is also part of our bodily habitus (cf. Bourdieu and control of the body). We control it; yet our bodily systems also control it, and through what we eat we are connected to our outside world.

'Control' is a motif running through biomedical narratives of 'how the body works'. Control was a significant organising principle for the physiology of my training, and has become incorporated into the way most of us view the body's inner processes, as I have already noted. Our understandings, through exposure to biomedical ideas, of how bodies work and operate within society cannot be separated from that theme; it is a two-way traffic, and the biomedical models and social theory go hand-in-hand. Control, however, is now becoming incorporated into newer models that emphasise flexibility.

Metaphors of bodily inner control were developed in the context of war; they grew alongside ideas about social control and were deeply entwined with them (see Birke 1999). In her analysis of changes in the way that immunity has been conceptualised and represented, Emily Martin (1994) noted a major shift from the machine metaphor (which emphasised the fortress-body, under siege from marauding micro-organisms) to the metaphor of a dispersed immune system, relying on information flow, and always ready to respond and change – the flexible body, as she termed it.

If, however, such narratives of information flow imply a loose fluidity, they persist alongside narratives of regulated and tightly controlled systems. Both inform how we think about the body. As Martin notes, many lay people now draw on discourses of the body as something which can be immunologically 'tuned up', acting upon information; yet we simultaneously use discourses of the body-machine – we want to 'fix' things that don't work properly, and often speak of health in terms of self-control (Crawford 1993).

Martin's work on concepts of the immunological body demonstrates how lay understandings of bodily function shift alongside scientific models, incorporating many new elements. Lay perceptions of immunology have changed, Martin suggests, in the wake of AIDS; where once the immune system was perceived as a set of strategic defences, that image has now been (partly) superseded by a narrative of a system that can be 'tuned up', to become more 'flexible'.

Control, flexibility and space are thus distinct – if overlapping – narratives within biomedical accounts of how the body works. Fluidity and flexibility may indeed be significant themes in emerging narratives of, say, the immune system (Martin 1994; also see Grosz 1994); yet they coexist with the theme of control. Together, these entwined themes help to structure our perceptions of our inner biology. What, though, are the consequences of them for our experiences of health and disease? In the first place, they are reductionist, combining to create a story of the body's insides as a set of parts (whether those are organs free-floating in inner space or a set of abstracted processes we have learned to call control systems). The reductionist practices of medicine are then justified; perhaps nowhere is this more obvious than in the case of transplant surgery.

The narratives of systems theory, in particular, help to structure how we think about bodily experience. They are, for example, normalising, contributing to a perception that 'other' ways of being in the body are pathological, just because they do not represent a tightly controlled system – whether because of age, illness or disability, for example.

How we draw on these narratives are, however, changing. Emily Martin's account of discursive shifts in talking about immune function is one example.

The experience of pregnancy provides another; Barbara Duden (1993) has argued, for example, that the embryo/foetus is increasingly seen as a cybernetic state, a repository of an abstraction called 'life'. This shift in turn helps to engender a shift of focus away from the necessity of women's bodies and towards the separate entity of the foetus – a shift which is of great concern to women.

The biomedical models of 'how the body works' and the narratives of social theory are inevitably deeply interconnected; it is not surprising that we can trace the theme of bodily control as a reflection of industrial machinery. But what is less obvious is how the emergence of new forms of power/control themselves affect bodily function, rather than the representations by which we understand that function. Following Foucault, we can map the ways in which power operates throughout the different institutions of our society; we can explore the ways that 'the body' becomes relocated into social spaces (as Foucault described for diseases in the twentieth century). But what about the material processes *of* that body?

Given that we are now quite used to thinking in terms of control systems, let me take these as an example. Bodily systems are controlled from within, to maintain homeostasis. These systems, in turn, connect to an outside world. We could perhaps think of these as a set of interlocking systems. Now, within this rhetoric, if we are subject to control(s) within the wider society (whether in the sense of Foucault or of Bourdieu), then it is not only the entity called the deportment of the body that is subject to control, but also the systems within it. Yet we know almost nothing about how living in a particular society affects those internal processes.

We can perhaps identify some differences; women tend to experience the menopause differently in different cultures, for example (Lock 1993). Perhaps this is 'just' cultural; perhaps it also reflects cultural impacts upon the material processes of the body: we cannot tell. My point, however, is that we rarely think in terms of how living the body within society (the subject of so much recent theorising) impacts upon that body's internal processes. And one reason why we don't think in such terms is the predominant assumption of taken-for-grantedness, the steady state of the normalising body.

Focusing on the body as a surface on which culture inscribes itself, as recent theory has often done, ensures that the inner processes of the material body disappear. They are rendered unintelligible by the insistent voice of social construction. Important though that voice has been (to feminist politics, for example), it separates itself from the material body; that body then becomes fixed, pre-social. Such a theoretical position then colludes with the narratives of biomedicine to create a story of biological bodies as somehow unchanging, controlled. But bodies are not biologically unchanging – even the 'gold standard' young adult male body does not remain the same.

We know little about how living in culture affects our bodies, partly because we do not ask (or at least we don't ask below the surface). Just as sociology and feminism have tended to avoid confronting biology, so biomedicine tends to avoid thinking sociologically (or about feminism!). Apart from the territorial disputes of academic disciplines, the failure to bridge the gap comes partly from entrenched reductionism, which ensures that we lose sight of the context within which biological processes operate. So, for example, we are bombarded with the language of 'the gene', encouraging us to view genes as influencing, say, the kinds of sexual behaviour we show as adults. But much more rare is the approach that asks about how the gene's context (a particular body, living in a particular society) itself affects how the gene operates.

As biomedicine places more and more emphasis on reductionist language (and specifically on genetics), so this process of forgetting becomes more entrenched. Forgetting context also – and importantly – obscures the *agency* of the organism (or of a specific body). In its development, an embryo/foetus is not simply the outcome of a genetic blueprint; rather its development involves active and dynamic processes of becoming. Whole animals, too, are much more than sets of parts; they are creators of their own worlds.

In this chapter, I have sketched out some themes threading through scientific representations of the body, focusing particularly on space, control and flexibility. These narratives inevitably influence how we perceive our bodies and how we come to understand our health and our bodily disease(s). They have also influenced social/feminist theory precisely *because* they are so profoundly reductionist and determinist. But avoiding thinking about 'the biological' does not solve any problems. On the contrary, it merely reinforces the determinist message by sleight of hand, as the taken-for-granted body – like the anchor for the head in the quote opening this chapter – is a fixed one. But there are other narratives, even within the sphere of biomedicine; discourses insisting on agency provide one example of approaches which might serve our theory better (as well as being, I would argue, more accurate descriptions of biology[13]). Dialogue across the disciplinary divide would serve us well.

Notes

1 The call to integrate social theory with recent insights from biological theory – and to do so in ways that resist genetic determinism – has been made by a number of authors. See, for example, Benton 1991; Williams and Bendelow 1998.
2 I was struck forcibly by how differently we perceive 'scientific' images while co-teaching a course on 'Feminism and the body' at the University of Warwick (with Terry Lovell). Students were much more likely to view these images as simply 'fact'.
3 It is a conceptual dismemberment (*sic*) paralleling and drawing on the literal dismemberment of the corpse in the dissecting room (Romanyshyn 1989), and of the multitudes of animal bodies used for dissection. Animal physiology books in my undergraduate training frequently spoke of animals' bodies *as* machines, so reinforcing the reductionist and mechanistic message.
4 Andreas Vesalius' drawings are well known in the history of anatomy. His *De Humani Corporis Fabrica* (On the Fabric of the Human Body) was first published in 1543. The book included very finely executed drawings, based on his

observations of dissected corpses (often obtained from the gallows). His work departed from traditional styles of scholarly teaching in that, unlike his predecessors, he did not read from classical texts but insisted on cutting into corpses himself (see Schiebinger 1993)

5 Bruno Latour (1987) emphasises the significance of such graphs and other output of machines (which he calls inscription devices) in laboratory practice. These help to persuade the reader of the truth of the claims; it is the graphs and diagrams which help to make the claims *scientific*, and to give them scientific authority.

6 Its absence – even from many feminist texts (Moore and Clarke 1995) – has been dubbed 'critical clitoridectomy' (Bennett 1993: 242).

7 Artists designing part of an exhibition on the body in London ('Science for life'; formerly at the Wellcome Trust building, now moved to the Manchester Museum) were thus surprised at how tightly packed the internal organs are; they had anticipated that organs float around in an inner space of the body (D. Janson-Smith, personal communication).

8 The Visible Woman and the Visible Man are sets of scanned images derived from cryopreserved bodies, and available on the Internet (http//:www.nlm.nih.gov/research/visible/visible_human.html; accessed June 2001). The project was set up by the US National Institutes of Health.

9 It is significant that Walter Bradford Cannon, who introduced the term homeostasis to physiology, wrote about extending the concept to society: homeostasis to maintain social order (Cannon 1932).

I do not wish to imply here that gender is relevant only in terms of the social relations of the factory metaphor. Rather, gender relations are often built into the design of technology (Wajcman 1991), so that any machines used as analogies for the body are likely to be gendered from the start.

10 'Information' is transmitted as pulses of electrical charge, called action potentials, which travel along nerve fibres. For a history of work on the biology of nerve conduction, and the social context of that work, see Trumpler 1997.

11 Emily Martin (1987) noted the negative narrative of the menopause in biomedical literature, which typically portrays the menopause as 'deficiency'. Also see Lock (1993). Interestingly, there is growing debate about the possibility of a 'male menopause'; one wonders whether that will have the same negative connotations?

12 Bourdieu emphasised that our bodies bear the imprint of living in particular societies (and thus of divisions within those, such as social class and gender). The result is the habitus, an acquired way of being in and using the body. For feminist critique of Bourdieu's analysis, see Lovell 2000.

13 See Steven Rose (1997) for a sustained analysis of such alternative frameworks to the prevailing deterministic ones. These alternatives emphasise the ways that order (in, say, the emergence of particular structures in embryonic development) emerges in nature from previous structures. What alters the path of development is how different parts interact: this is not a deterministic process (see also Goodwin 1994). To challenge determinism, we need to emphasise these and similar stories which insist on agency and dynamic process in nature.

References

Armstrong, D. (1993) 'From clinical gaze to regime of total health', in A. Beattie, M. Gott, L. Jones and M. Sidell (eds), *Health and Wellbeing: A Reader*, Milton Keynes, Bucks.: Open University, and London: Macmillan.

Atwood, Margaret (1994) 'The female body', in P. Foster (ed.), *Minding the Body: Women Writers on Body and Soul*, New York: Anchor Press.

Bain, Foree (1901) 'Looking Forward', *Western Electrician* (Chicago), 5 January.

Bayliss, L.E. (1966) *Living Control Systems*, London: English Universities Press.

Bennett, P. (1993) 'Critical clitoridectomy: female sexual imagery and feminist psychoanalytic theory', *Signs* 18: 235–59.

Benton, T. (1991) 'Biology and social science: why the return of the repressed should be given a (cautious) welcome', *Sociology* 25: 1–29.

Birke, L. (1999) *Feminism and the Biological Body*, Edinburgh: Edinburgh University Press.

—— and Michael, M. (1998) 'The heart of the matter: animal bodies, ethics and species boundaries', *Society and Animals* 6: 245–62.

Bordo, S. (1993) *Unbearable Weight: Feminism, Western Culture and the Body*, Berkeley, CA: University of California Press.

Boston Women's Health Collective (1973) *Our Bodies, Ourselves*, New York: Simon and Schuster.

Bourdieu, P. (1984) *Distinction: A Social Critique of the Judgement of Taste*, London: Routledge.

Bray, Rosemary (1994) 'First stirrings', in P. Foster (ed.), *Minding the Body: Women Writers on Body and Soul*, New York: Doubleday.

Cannon, W.B. (1932) *The Wisdom of the Body*, New York: W.W. Norton.

Cartwright, Lisa (1998) 'A cultural anatomy of the Visible Human project', in P. Treichler, L. Cartwright and C. Penley (eds), *The Visible Woman: Imaging Technologies, Gender and Science*, New York: New York University Press.

Crawford, R. (1993) 'A cultural account of "health": control, release and the social body', in Alan Beattie, Marjorie Gott, Linda Jones and Moyra Sidell (eds), *Health and Wellbeing: A Reader*, London: Macmillan, and Buckingham: Open University Press.

Duden, B. (1993) *Disembodying Women: Perspectives on Pregnancy and the Unborn*, Cambridge, MA: Harvard University Press.

Ferguson, H. (1997) 'Me and my shadows: on the accumulation of body-images in western society. Part Two: The corporeal forms of modernity', *Body and Society* 3: 1–31.

Foucault, M. (1973) *The Birth of the Clinic*, London: Tavistock.

Frank, Arthur (1996) 'Reconciliatory alchemy: bodies, narratives and power', *Body and Society* 2: 53–71.

Goodwin, Brian (1994) *How the Leopard Changed its Spots*, London: Phoenix.

Grosz, Elizabeth (1994) *Volatile Bodies: Toward a Corporal Feminism*, Bloomington, IN: Indiana University Press.

Haraway, D. (1991) *Simians, Cyborgs and Women*, London: Free Association Books.

Keller, E.F. (1995) *Refiguring Life: Metaphors of Twentieth-century Biology*, New York: University of Columbia Press.

—— (1996) 'The biological gaze', in G. Robertson, M. Mash, L. Tickner, J. Bird, B. Curtis and T. Putnam (eds), *FutureNatural: Nature/Science/Culture*, London: Routledge.

Kremer, Richard L. (1990) *The Thermodynamics of Life and Experimental Physiology, 1779–1880*, New York and London: Garland Publishing.

Laqueur, T. (1990) *Making Sex: Body and Gender from the Greeks to Freud*, Cambridge, MA: Harvard University Press.

Latour, B. (1987) *Science in Action*, Buckingham: Open University Press.

Lock, Margaret (1993) *Encounters with Aging: Mythologies of Menopause in Japan and North America*, Berkeley, CA: University of California Press.

Lovell, T. (2000) 'Thinking feminism with and against Bourdieu', *Feminist Theory* 1 (1): 11–32.

Martin, Emily (1987) *The Woman in the Body*, Milton Keynes, Bucks.: Open University Press.

—— (1994) *Flexible Bodies: Tracking Immunity in American Culture from the Days of Polio to the Age of AIDS*, Boston, MA: Beacon Press.

Marvin, Carolyn (1988) *When Old Technologies Were New: Thinking about Electric Communication in the Late Nineteenth Century*, Oxford: Oxford University Press.

Mitchell, Lisa M. and Georges, Eugenia (1997) 'Cross-cultural cyborgs: Greek and Canadian women's discourse on fetal ultrasound', *Feminist Studies* 23: 373–401.

Moore, L.J. and Clarke, A.E. (1995) 'Clitoral conventions and transgressions: graphic representations in anatomy texts, c1900–1991', *Feminist Studies* 21: 255–301.

Petchesky, Rosalind (1987) 'Fetal images: the power of visual culture in the politics of reproduction', *Feminist Studies* 13: 263–92.

Pouchelle, M.-C., (1990) *The Body and Surgery in the Middle Ages*, New Brunswick, NJ: Rutgers University Press.

Radley, Alan (1995) 'The elusory body and social constructionist theory', *Body and Society* 1: 3–23.

—— (1996) 'The critical moment: time, information and medical expertise in the experience of patients receiving coronary bypass surgery', in S.J. Williams and M. Calnan (eds), *Modern Medicine: Lay Perspectives and Experiences*, London: UCL Press.

Romanyshyn, R.D. (1989) *Technology as Symptom and Dream*, London: Routledge,.

Rose, Steven (1997) *Lifelines: Biology, Freedom, Determinism*, Harmondsworth, Middx: Penguin.

Scarry, E. (1985) *The Body in Pain*, Oxford: Oxford University Press.

Schiebinger, L. (1993) *Nature's Body: Sexual Politics and the Making of Modern Science*, Boston, MA: Beacon Press.

Sharp, Lesley (1995) 'Organ transplantation as a transformative experience: anthropological insights into the restructuring of the self', *Medical Anthropology Quarterly* 9: 357–89.

Shilling, C. (1993) *The Body and Social Theory*, London: Sage.

Tomas, David (1996) 'Feedback and cybernetics: reimaging the body in the age of cybernetics', in M. Featherstone and R. Burrows (eds), *Cyberspace/Cyberbodies/Cyberpunk: Cultures of Technological Embodiment*, London: Sage.

Trumpler, M. (1997) 'Converging images: techniques of intervention and forms of representation of sodium-channel proteins in nerve-cell membranes', *Journal of the History of Biology* 30: 55–89.

Wajcman, J. (1991) *Feminism Confronts Technology*, Cambridge: Polity Press.

Williams, S. and Bendelow, G. (1998) *The Lived Body: Sociological Themes, Embodied Issues*, London: Routledge.

3 Building genethics from below

Hilary Rose

Eugenics and social policy

As in the aftermath of war the horror of the Nazi period was fully grasped, the concept of eugenics became suffused with moral revulsion. Such was the grip of this intense revulsion that to say that some policy or practice is eugenic is to demonise it. Thus for solid historical reasons the disability movement is committed to maintaining this revulsion, even though, as they gradually admit the materiality of the body into their social constructionist model of disability, the movement is likely to find itself in that hard territory of whether all potential lives are worth living and who is to judge. But for the discourse and practice of social policy this demonisation has created huge problems, for at the height of the eugenics movement, roughly the interwar period, key theorists of the welfare state, such as the Swedish Myrdals and the British Beveridge and Titmuss, took eugenics to be an integral aspect of social policy. Quite soon in Britain but, for reasons I shall try to sketch out briefly, rather more slowly in Scandinavia, the word eugenics became unusable and with singularly little intellectual courage social policy failed to reflect on its own history as actively shaping eugenic policies. This silence about the discipline's past does not help us now as we try to think about how to cope with the new genetics.

Something of the cultural price of silence over social policy's outworn domain assumptions is reflected in the story of the Swedish moral panic of the 1990s stirred up by an article in the leading newspaper, *Dagens Nyett*, over the 'discovery' that Sweden had been compulsorily sterilising feeble-minded women until the mid 1970s. Yet this was no 'discovery' for it was no secret that this was Scandinavian state policy; indeed, leftists and reformers had successfully campaigned against it during those self same 1970s. Dropping the policy was thus part of a much wider move from a confident patriarchal statism to a more individual approach to welfare energised by the new women's movement. What was new in the 1990s was that this was the occasion when the wider Swedish public and the political classes explicitly confronted their eugenicist past. By contrast Britain has never confronted the eugenic aspect of the long history of the institutional sexual segregation of the feeble-minded – even though this policy was vigorously proposed by the Eugenic Society as the most acceptable form of eugenic control. Both Swedish surgical intervention and British sexual segregation served the same end of controlling the reproduction of the unfit and both faded away during the 1970s.

Thus state eugenics extended (although rarely using the demonised 'E' word after 1945) until the 1970s as integral to the basic assumptions of the welfare state. Improving the national stock, with all that connotation of good husbandry, was initially based on the science of eugenics with a mixture of clinicians and geneticists/eugenicists at the helm. This commitment to enhancing the life chances and social wellbeing of all the nation's people led to a clear-eyed recognition that this could weaken natural selection. Put plainly, weak, incapable babies would no longer die naturally; instead, with support of the new welfare state, they would live and would demand a disproportionate share of welfare. Logically, without some form of unnatural selection, the nation state would have to carry a burden greater than its level of economic wealth could bear. Such theorising brings evolutionary theory into the active management of human populations, for eugenics is unquestionably unnatural selection. However, as the concept of eugenics means the wellborn it is, unlike evolutionary theory proper, profoundly linked to an interventionist notion of human improvement and progress.

The move from state to consumer eugenics

In the state interventionist past genetics – which then proudly called itself eugenics – primarily focused on which women are 'fit' to mother; outside assisted conception, the focus is on which embryos are 'fit' to survive. The prime means by which the fitness of embryos to survive is assessed is through DNA analysis and 'informed choice'. In this chapter this shift of focus is spoken of as the move from state to consumer eugenics. Thus I leave for others those important issues of genetic testing for both employment and insurance. None the less, given the increasing marketisation of welfare and the move to the flexible and less-protected labour market currently taking place within Europe, it seems to me imperative that we look at the best of over fourteen US state attempts to regulate testing so as to prevent the development of a 'genetic underclass' in a hyper-marketised context. At state level policy makers have been quick to move to anticipate the risk that genetic tests would add even more people to the current 42.5 million Americans without medical insurance. Even in the context of universal National Health Service provision it is depressing news that the UK government will permit the insurance industry to ask if tests for Huntington's disease have been performed. Certain uninsurability now enters as a further consideration and burden for the at-risk person's informed choice. But it is as a feminist sociologist that I want to pull into visibility the historical changes and continuities between who gets to decide, using what kinds of discourse, who or what is 'fit'. For those who want to reconcile the claims of women's reproductive freedom with the promises and risks offered by the new genetics there are few simple solutions.

This new fusion between genetic testing and the new reproductive technologies forms one of the most powerful sites of moral anxiety about the limits to biomedical intervention: it deeply affects our cultural ideas about who we are. Thus the new DNA testing has radically changed the nature of risk assessment for severe inherited disease but has also opened up a Pandora's box in terms of fears and enthusiasms for 'designer babies'. With the advent (birth is too simple a word) of Dolly the sheep, *Brave New World* threatens to become reality for humans. No longer a science fiction narrative so remote as to be only a matter for dinner table debate, it becomes an actual possibility in the everyday world. This is not to say that the moral anxiety cannot be appropriated and turned into a profitable entertainment. The judicious mixture of pleasurable titillation and social reassurance at work in the science fiction film *Gattaca* is exemplary. Here the usual boy-gets-girl Hollywood narrative is set in a future world, *Gattaca* (a name composed from the four letters of DNA sequences), in which all the elite have been genetically engineered; the normals, meanwhile, are cast in the position of an underclass. The plot provides social reassurance through the figure of the young hero as a mere normal and hence destined to be an intellectual and physical inferior (needless to say because of his mother's foolish naturalistic longings), who none the less sets himself to pass for a genetically engineered superior. *Gattaca* thus works on two levels: first, to mobilise pleasurable anxiety about the unnaturalness of a genetically manipulated future and, second, to give conservative reassurance that, given sufficient and heroic determination, the normal man will still triumph. Because *Gattaca* is a truly appallingly made film it has not had the influence of, say, *Brave New World*, which put such speculations strongly on to the cultural map. Instead it has been the dystopic speculations by the leading US molecular biologist Lee Silver which have sustained these fears and enthusiasms. His book *Remaking Eden* has in many ways become today's cultural equivalent of *Brave New World.* Where *Brave New World* posited a powerful state as its taken-for-granted context, Silver assumes the context of an hyper-marketised society. Thus his argument is the epitome of consumer eugenicism; his thinking is located within a distinctively US context with its current adverts seeking to purchase for $40,000 the gametes of high IQ, 175 cm tall, Ivy League women. (Which out of this *mélange* of characteristics are believed to be transmissable through genetics is intriguing.) From this location Silver argues that it is inevitable that well-off people, given the technical possibility of genetically engineering their offsprings' appearance and behaviour, will do so.

This new possibility, in which intending parents get to choose the eye colour, height, intelligence, looks and so on, is part of a new consumer culture without limits. If you want it, can pay for it and someone can provide it, then, whatever that 'it' is, it is yours. In Silver's future scenario a revitalised economic liberalism enthrones the consumer as king or – even – queen. Of course there will be some moral discourse questioning the desirability of letting the market into parenthood, but the ethicists within such a context are themselves weakened by their subscription to the thesis of the importance of the market as the chief arbiter of our futures. Thus while tasteless, absurd, even impossible, the dream of the perfect baby takes its place alongside other consumer fantasies: of the perfect house, suit, job, garden, partner, drink and so on. The epitome of this unrestrained consumerism is as usual the US, and it is important not to dismiss or undermine the institutional structures of social solidarity still evident in European countries which, though weakened, still serve as a constraint against the marketisation of everyday life.

The Nash family and consumer eugenics?

In recent days the case of Lisa and Jack Nash and their now two children has served as a microcosm of current genetic testing/eugenic anxieties. Have the well-heeled Nashes opened the door to the commodification of children, the eugenicism of the consumer society, or are they more mundanely and humanly an expression of parental love muddling its ethical way through biotechnologically advanced times? Here I want to extend this analysis of the Nashes by looking not only at the story as it is told to us by the media, but at the mixed and varying responses reported in the media.

On 4 October 2000 the headlines of the broadsheet newspaper the *Guardian* were: 'Test-tube child designed in US as cell transplant donor'. While the story was in every newspaper, I here use the *Guardian* as a left of centre paper which followed the debates closely. The account reported the case of Lisa and Jack Nash, parents of Molly, a six-year-old with the fatal inherited disorder Fanconi anaemia, who had learnt that her best chance of therapy was a cell transplant from an unaffected sibling. The parents, who wanted a second but unaffected child, had decided to seek pre-implantation genetic diagnosis to select an unaffected embryo – but also one well-matched to Molly. Thus the second baby was both to be free from Molly's life-threatening genetic condition and also to provide a potential life-saving cell transplant resource to its sibling. Lisa Nash had to undergo four IVF cycles to produce the twelve embryos to test and select one matching both criteria. The resulting baby, Adam, is free from the disorder and blood from the umbilical cord (thus a non-invasive procedure) has been used to treat his sister. So far it is too soon to say whether the treatment has worked.

Few commentators have seen the actions of the Nash family and their clinicians as straightforwardly unethical unless the entire procedure is ruled out by religious conviction. Secular-minded others have drawn on the Kantian imperative that people should be treated as ends not means to argue that the new baby Adam has been treated unethically: he has been treated as a means, not as an end in himself (see, for example, the letter from D.S King in the *Guardian*, 5 October 2000). But this abstract imperative remains rather a long way from most people's decision to parent. Scrupulously examining any longings to have a child that you or I may have experienced is a confusing task. What did it mean that I wanted to have a baby? Where did that longing come from? Alongside the distinctly remote evolutionary view that such longings are necessary for the continuity of the species, recent anthropological work studying the decisions to parent made by young couples, whether married or living together, shows that it is social expectation on the part of family and friends which chiefly and more immediately influences why they chose to have a baby (Edwards 2000). Their social circle assumes that the reason the couple chose to live together is a statement of their wish to have a family. Thus the casual questioning about 'when are you going to have a baby' is translated into a steady pressure to conform to expectation. For those of us who are parents it is a little uncomfortable to reflect that deciding against having children may reflect a more worked-out position than mere social compliance. But for all too many bioethicists the tendency is to turn to abstract philosophy, not least to principalism, rather than either to the distal explanations of evolutionary theory or to the messiness of proximal explanation rooted in the everyday world.

However, there is an uncomfortable awareness that the Nash case, with all its genetic testing and embryo selection for what is widely seen as a benign outcome, simultaneously opens the door to 'designer babies'. In Britain the press has actively acknowledged and fostered widespread sympathy for the Nashes as parents who carry severe genetic risk. What is spoken of as a 'let the parents decide' position is curiously seen by commentators such as science writer James Meek (*Guardian*, 5 October) as supporting Lee Silver and his argument that all rich would-be parents in a high-tech market society would opt for genetically engineered infants. Both Silver and Meek following him thus ignore the invasive IVF procedures to be undergone by only one of the partners; instead, they assume that women would freely choose to enter such invasive procedures simply to enhance their child. A recent article from a member of the Human Fertilisation and Embryology Authority pointed out just how invasive and uncertain IVF still is. With one move the male scientist and the male science writer had equated Lisa Nash's courage and physical endurance with Jack Nash's important but supporting role. In this language, undifferentiated by gender, the Nashes become not two people but one homogenised entity – the parents. Silver and Meek fail to recognise that in a loving partnership, such an invasive procedure and risk to one may well be only tolerable to either or both if there is deep moral agreement that this risk is necessary to avert a huge and evident danger.

In the everyday world, where parents cope with their own and their would-be children's actual or potentially flawed bodies and the limits of reproductive and genetic medicine, not the world of the andro-centric science fantasists, positive enhancement through genetic engineering looks risky both ethically and practically. In the present state of know-how, enhancing a child's physical and mental endowment comes more directly from its access to life chances in historical context. Thus beautiful teeth are today the birthright of any child from a well-off US family, but it has been wealth and dental technology which has brought about this enhancement, not genetics. Meanwhile the fantasy of genetic enhancement threatens to weaken our cultural confidence that our societies can manage the new genetic technologies.

Building genethics from below

Thus I want to distinguish between the ideologically constructed and homogenised 'parents' of the andro-centric fantasists and contrast these parents not only with the Nashes but with the social research studies of the social world of genetic testing. One recently reported 10-year study carried out by the anthropologist Rayna Rapp and her colleagues has been studying New York women in all their diversity, confronting genetic risk together in negotiation with their genetic clinicians, their counsellors, their partners and their families. Rapp argues that these women are moral innovators. They are successfully negotiating the complex and historically new moral problems thrown up by the new genetics. It is interesting to find the US geneticist and leading figure in the Council for Social Responsibility in Genetics, Paul Billings (1994), who is an outspoken opponent of consumer eugenics, echoing the view that such painful ethical matters are best decided by the people confronting the difficulty. He says of the Nash case: 'this could theoretically commodify children, but on the other hand there is no evidence that children who are conceived this way are loved any less'. He goes on: 'There is a danger we are making a mountain out of a personal tragedy. I don't think people are going to rush to IVF treatments which are an alienating and expensive procedure.'

This view of genethics as best 'bricolaged from below', by directly affected women, their partners and their families, is in some tension with conventional approaches to new social, cultural and ethical problems generated by advances in genetics. First, genethics from below questions the cultural hegemony of mainstream bioethics. The expert in this ethics-from-below perspective becomes not the moral philosopher, the religious leader or the leading biomedical researcher but women and their partners confronting entirely new moral and material risks produced by genetics and reproduction in everyday life.

Such individual women, supported by their partners, families and friends, have to make their decisions within a macro-context; and although so far I have spoken negatively of the pressures stemming from a hyper-marketised society on the practices of prenatal genetic testing and selection, here I want to turn to the macro changes that have taken place not least in the practice of eugenics over the course of the twentieth century.

The recovery of the history of state eugenics

For the second half of the twentieth century the Nazi episode has stood as the historical embodiment of state eugenics in all its violent horror. Indeed, for much of that time eugenics became synonymous with the Nazi practice of compulsory sterilisation and the seemingly inexorable path to the death camps, with some modest acknowledgement given to US eugenic practices. Although many, even most, contemporary geneticists hate to be reminded of it, genetics was both the scientific and institutional child of eugenics. Nowhere was this connection made more sharply than in the case of the Nazi race science. The critical histories of genetics and biomedicine, produced by a post-1968 generation of scholars (cf. Muller Hill 1988; Weindling 1989), pointed to the distasteful evidence that the directors of leading laboratories in the immediate postwar period had also been directors during the Nazi period and deeply implicated in Nazi eugenic practices. In Britain, Darwin's cousin Galton founded the discipline of eugenics and occupied its first chair at University College London; subsequently this department was to become a leading department of genetics. Both J.B.S. Haldane, a co-theorist of the modern synthesis in the 1930s, and the currently hugely successful popular-iser of genetics, Steve Jones, have held chairs there. Similarly the famous US Cold Spring Harbor laboratory was the home of first eugenics then of Jim Watson of DNA fame. The story can be endlessly repeated.

For many years following the Second World War the eugenic practices of other countries were allowed to pass more or less unremarked. Even in the case of the US it was difficult to gather statistics on compulsory sterilisation for this was primarily a state activity. In consequence it has taken historians a tremendous effort to make visible just how widespread the practice was. But historians of eugenics have always had to work knowing that few contemporary fellow citizens want them to discover this particular aspect of our past. It has been much more politically comfortable to demonise the Nazis and ignore our own histories. Thus for today's intellectuals it is still uncomfortable to recall the huge enthusiasm for eugenics in most industrial countries – socialist well as capitalist – energetically supported by socially progressive scientists and social thinkers. It would be true to say that in the early twentieth century, barring Catholic intellectuals, eugenics commanded the support of most EuroAmerican intellectuals including feminists, reformers and Marxists as well as racists and reactionaries (Pickens 1968; Weeks 1981; Kevles 1985).

The nineteenth-century theory of evolution, with its central notions of fitness, natural and unnatural selection, was crucial in this: it played into how nations, particularly as 'race', conceived of themselves. Nations as race both stood in competition with one another and had to be managed internally so as to minimise the production of the unfit. Darwinism, and even more potently Social Darwinism, thus became a hugely influential cultural current that could be mobilised around a range of political projects and take a multiplicity of forms. The Nordic countries saw compulsory sterilisation as integral to the formation and management of the social democratic welfare state, sterilising those who were 'unfit' to parent, thus reducing the potential burden on the state and enabling it to provide universal high-quality welfare. That Britain progressed little farther than a policy of custodial care and sexual segregation for mentally impaired women and men was less personally violent but it amounted to the same denial of what we now see as a basic human right – the right to a family life. It was only the advent of the Nazi mass extermination of the mentally impaired and sick in the hospitals and the mass exterminations in the death camps which silenced such dangerous enthusiasms for racial improvement. These eugenicist histories and enthusiasms have been, if not actually hidden, at least distinctly underplayed in national cultural self-accounting, leaving the Nazi episode to stand out as a singular horror story rather than as the monstrous epitome of a broad current. Consequently the critique of 'state eugenics' is almost always set against the Nazi horror rather than this much more pervasive state eugenicism which lies uneasily, only half silenced, within culture and history. As repressed rather than confronted, such histories have returned slowly and with shame.

Thus for many years the Nordic experience was rendered invisible even though it was practised up to 1976. It was only during the very last years of the twentieth century that the Swedish government apologised to and compensated those women whose ability to bear children had been taken away from them, typically on the grounds that they were unfit to mother. One of the specific features of Nordic sterilisation programmes is that they were primarily directed against women, sometimes in 90 per cent of all cases. Whatever role 'unfit' men might have to play in reproducing the 'unfit' was set to one side by the biomedical professional discourse and practice. Other states, including the Nazi, were sexually equal in sterilisation practices. Nordic biomedical science in the service of the welfare state had special skills: it saw itself as entirely able to judge that these women should be sterilised because they were 'unfit in mother' in two distinct senses, to breed and to care. The centrality of children in the Nordic welfare state and culture (so unlike the British variant) meant that the deemed 'unfitness' to provide adequate maternal care sustained sterilisation long after human genetics supplied any legitimacy that feeble-mindedness (above all in the form of Down's syndrome) was inherited. (The key chromosome work concerning Down's syndrome was done in the 1950s; sterilisation went on until the mid 1970s.)

Eugenicist enthusiasms died hard. In Britain the distinguished biologist Peter Medawar, in his 1958 Reith lectures, expressed his concern that the welfare state was permitting too many unfit children to live whom nature would have selected out. The wellbeing of the national stock depended on an acceptable version of eugenics. Such thinking gave ideological support for birth control and pro-abortion policies and made an extraordinary alliance with feminist ideology. (In the 1960s these were distinctive strands; earlier in the century numbers of feminists, *pace* Marie Stopes, feminist founder of the birth control clinics, were passionate eugenicists.) The 1967 UK legislation on abortion, which was greeted with joy by the embryonic women's movement, is written in eugenicist language quite shocking to the contemporary ear. It has taken more than 30 years to develop a practice of abortion more or less on demand on the ground.

Even in 1968, that year of revolutionary hope, eugenic enthusiasm was still openly expressed:

> There should be tattooed on the forehead of every young person a sym-
> bol showing possession of the sickle cell gene or whatever other similar
> gene. . . . It is my opinion that legislation along this line, compulsory
> testing for defective gene before marriage, and some form of semi-public
> display of this possession, should be adopted.
>
> (Linus Pauling, quoted in Kay 1993: 276)

What is painful is that the author of this appalling statement was not some bizarre figure from the racist right, but a hero of the anti-war and alternative health movements, none other than Nobel prize-winning biologist Linus Pauling.

The Janus face of clinical genetics

It was against this history of eugenics genetics that the clinical speciality now called medical or clinical genetics had to reconstruct itself in the postwar years. Partly it was about changing names, rebranding the profession in today's advertising language, but also hugely about developing – in the light of Nuremberg and subsequently Helsinki – ideas of patients' informed consent. Counselling, spending time with patients to make sure that co-operation was freely given, became the hallmark of the best clinical practice. The non-directive nature of the genetic clinic stands in sharp contrast to other clinical specialties. In the antenatal clinic, women have long been expected to comply with medical guidance to follow life-style regimes, give blood and urine samples to be tested all for the good of the baby. Indeed, here and elsewhere in medicine 'compliance' is a routinely discussed problem. Occasionally welfare benefits have been linked to participation to ensure compliance. But while this non-directive approach to patients was developing, clinical geneticists had to make their case to the state for support. To this resource-granting or -denying the argument radically changes, and the profession now speaks in distinctly eugenic language about reduction in the births of impaired infants and thence about savings to the public purse. This Janus-like stance implicitly assumes that the informed decisions of individual patients and the needs of the state will conveniently coincide. More recently, Phillip Kitcher has adopted the same Janus-like position, indeed describing it as Utopian eugenics.

Remembering that the original Utopia was 'nowhere', the more sceptically minded might well note that this double agenda simply produces invisible norms which set the 'acceptable number' of genetically impaired infants to be born. Indeed, UK clinical geneticists, aware of these pressures, report the invisible norms which indicate the acceptable number of Down's syndrome babies to be born in their patch. To meet the invisible norm satisfies the double demands of Janus – first, that the pregnant woman is enabled to make an informed choice and, second, that the state's burden of genetically impaired is minimised. Given the current cultural struggle being waged by people with Down's and their allies to insist that theirs is life worth living, it is reasonable to anticipate that Kitcher's eugenic Utopia is more accurately viewed as Panglossian (all is for the best in the best . . .). Meanwhile, discovering how such invisible norms are negotiated, established and then renegotiated is a research task yet to be carried out. What only can be clear is that as new responses – whether social (support for learning-disabled people) or biomedical therapeutics (as in, say, PKU, phenylketonuria) – are available then the definition of an unlivable life is likely to change in both clinical and public perception.

Pointing to the statistic that genetic impairment constitutes only some 3 per cent of all impairment may weaken the cost-benefit effectiveness of the claims of clinical genetics to save public resources, but the ideology of eugenicism still echoes in which some 'right hands' (Fox Keller 1992) decide which 'impaired' foetuses need to have maternal decisions made about their survival (Hubbard and Henifin 1984). It might seem straightforward, at least for lay people outside the genetic or the prenatal clinic, to see the value of pre-natal tests which permit the identification of genetically transmitted conditions associated with terrible pain and premature death, and thus offer the possibility of terminating the pregnancy. However valued and however secure women and their partners are in their choices, dealing with this knowledge has a human cost. Over the past 20 years research has systematically indicated that the decision to have an abortion as the result of prenatal diagnostic testing is associated with high levels of personal distress even where supported with appropriate levels of counselling. This high level of distress stands in marked contrast with the much lower levels felt by women who find themselves pregnant and choose an abortion because they have decided they do not wish to mother a potential child. The point is not that women who want to mother necessarily want to reverse the informed choice which led them to elect an abortion after genetic testing, simply that the personal costs associated with living with genetic testing are high.

Scarcely surprisingly, the movement of disabled people is deeply suspicious about the proliferation of genetic testing and sees it as inherently eugenic (Shakespeare 1995). Learning-disabled people have been at the forefront of these confrontations. In a culture which has for so long taken for granted that a woman would not want to give birth to a child with Down's syndrome and would see amniocentesis or chorionic villus sampling (CVS) as helpful, these challenges are both disturbing and long overdue. Defending women's reproductive freedom while refusing to subscribe to an automatic categorisation of the life of a person with Down's as not worth living is not easy. When this debate takes place with learning-disabled people arguing their rights to life itself, the old certainties begin to yield.

Understanding the speed of technical change that this Janus-like profession must presently contend with is crucial. As Dorothy Nelkin and Lawrence Tancredi document in *Dangerous Diagnostics* (1995), the new genetics has proliferated tests but few therapies. Indeed diagnostic technology is integral to the development of the field, both in the sense of the technics of production of the knowledge and in a more directly commercial sense. While the Human Genome Project was launched to promises of gene therapy, and thus secured substantial investment from both state and venture capital, the new diagnostics, even without therapies, offers to provide those promised profits. But as leading French molecular biologist Bertrand Jordan recognised, in so far as tests are offered to pregnant women, the only 'medical treatment' that can be proposed is abortion for those foetuses defined as not normal: 'The impact of the genome programme on society as a whole is far from insignificant. The new knowledge thus gained leads to the elimination of embryos through prenatal diagnosis and pregnancy termination' (Jordan 1993: 168).

Arguments within biology

With proliferating genetic diagnostics the meaning and value of the predictive claim comes under sharp questioning from fellow biologists, including leading geneticists and molecular biologists. Over the years, particularly the leading US biologists, such as Jonathan Beckwith, Ruth Hubbard, Sheldon Krimsky and Richard Lewontin, have successfully punctured the self-reported success story of the new genetics. Among the more conspicuous recent examples of such interventions was Lewontin's challenge to the near-absolutist truth claims being made for the DNA 'fingerprinting' (Lewontin 1991). In similar vein, Hubbard, as a feminist biologist deeply involved with the women's health movement, has set out both to demythologise the new genetics and to alert women to the imperialising and mythical claims of the new diagnostics (1984, 1990, 1995). The pressures for genetic testing bear particularly sharply on pregnant women and, despite their ideological claim to certainty and precision, are often rather coarse indicators which offer little other than abortion as a therapeutic response. Within Europe similar waves of technical criticism linked to a profound social distaste for the eugenic past led the German Greens to mount successfully a critique of the European genetic programme which was to be launched under the title 'Predictive Medicine'. Such technical criticisms challenge the crudity of the 'gene for' ideology constantly displayed in press releases from the biology laboratories and amplified in the media. Genes, the critics endlessly argue, do not determine; but their message, even while unquestionably integral to the genetic discourse, is almost drowned out by the deluge of gene-talk.

Critical arguments from within biology have been supported by those from within the social sciences. Economic studies of the costs and benefits of genetic screening programmes can strengthen the state's hand in resisting pressures to misallocate limited public health care resources to such projects. US sociologist Troy Duster contrasts the UK experience in successfully resisting such programmes on the basis of cost-benefit economic analysis. As an African American, Duster has less confidence that state eugenics belongs entirely to the past. His study (1990) documents the replacement of material support for poor African American families by genetic testing programmes, and concludes that genetic testing in this context is best understood as back-door eugenics. As he observes: 'Once again whether this new genetic knowledge is an advantage or a cross depends only partly on how the genes are arranged. It depends as well where one is located in the social order' (Duster 1990: 92).

Risk management of the new risk assessment?

From the inception of the Human Genome Project (HGP) in the 1980s, leading geneticists and molecular biologists have long understood (however much they simultaneously distanced their discipline and themselves from any taint from the topic) that their particular cultural 'bogey' is eugenics. They made sure that around 7 per cent of the total genomic budget, substantial monies by humanities and social research standards, was put into research on the ethical, legal and social 'implications' and/or 'aspects' of genetics. With the HGP came ELSI and ELSA (Ethical Legal and Social Implications [US] and Aspects [Europe]). Optimists could read this as a move to confront serious social and cultural anxieties; sceptics could read this as an attempt to use the social sciences and humanities as hand-maidens whose task was to manage the public perception of the new genetics as positive. The 7 per cent was to be a means of managing risks to genetics as much as risks to the public. I have insufficient space here to detail it, but there is considerable evidence backing both optimists and sceptics.

Today, with a much greater awareness that science and technology generate entirely new and very large risks, above all to nature, there is a much greater consciousness of the need to manage risk. The sociologist Ulrich Beck some while ago called the way we live now the Risk Society. The anxiety around genetic testing is central to this discussion of risk, for what genetic testing does is to change the nature of risk assessment for human beings. In the past the most powerful predictive discourse on morbidity and mortality was epidemiology, the statistical study of the patterns of health and illness in human populations. With this evidence governments in the nineteenth century could be moved to provide sanitation, clean water and eventually, in the twentieth century, clean air. Its interventionist discourse was that of public health, its target the improvement of the health of entire populations. It needed a robustly interventionist state to insist that people comply with its advice. (It is, to say the least, uncomfortable to find that Nazi public health research pioneered work on the tobacco-cancer link.)

However, what genetic testing does is to change the nature of risk assessment from the prediction of the health of populations, or even groups within populations, to that of individuals. It is thus supremely the biomedical discourse, which fits the increasingly individualising discourse of a liberal political economy. Genetic testing thus directs risk primarily towards individuals. Take the second battle to establish the association between smoking and lung cancer: this had its puzzles, for while smoking is statistically dangerous, everyone, especially smokers who were finding it hard to give up, knew people who had smoked heavily for years but died of old age, not cancer. Even then it was obvious that some probably had more constitutional resistance than others; but who was safe and how could one know? Today genetic testing is able to predict for individuals whether in their particular case smoking is extremely dangerous or merely rather unhealthy. Thus the public health struggle against lung cancer is waged on a global level against the machinations of the tobacco industry (and perhaps the tax dependency of governments). At local level it could soon be waged on the predictive reliability of genetic tests for individual risk.

It is by no means clear to me that culturally we are able to deal very effectively with the refinement of risk assessment that genetic testing claims to offer. Numbers of studies of prenatal testing for serious genetic disorders, such as familial cholesterolaemia which, unless the child is homozygote, is relatively clinically manageable, give rise to concern about the psychological effects of genetic knowledge. The mothers of such babies report feeling saddened and fatalistic. Given that treatment for young children with this problem is typically only in terms of managing diet and encouraging exercise, there are good arguments for not testing prenatally but delaying this until the child is old enough to make an informed choice. In the case of genetic disorders – the classic is PKU – where therapeutics need to be started immediately, the argument is different. But here I simply want to emphasise the complexity of genethical thinking. Genetic knowledge has to be situated in intimate context.

It has been the issue of genetic testing for the cruel late-onset disorders such as Huntington's chorea which has taught humility about the value of genetic knowledge. Initially it was thought that those from families at risk would seize on the certainty offered by genetic testing. Some do, some don't, some prefer to live with the general risk, others want to know the exact risk. Observant clinicians working with such families suggest that those who decide not to take a test often have some subtle sense that they are already exhibiting the hints of symptoms associated with the disease. The harsh ethical and practical dilemma for both patient and the clinician is that there is still no effective therapy. The price of certain knowledge in this situation is indeed high.

Genetic testing in the context of a directive medical culture

Despite my analysis of the Janus face of clinical genetics, I want to argue that its non-directive culture by and large serves to protect patients from being prematurely pushed into learning of their own genetic risk status. However, there is good reason to be much more concerned about the spread of genetic testing into the other directive specialties, above all into the antenatal clinics. It is difficult to see how to slow down this process as medicine is being geneticised in its explanation, as both research and any cursory inspection of medical journals reveals. An already identified problem with genetic testing in antenatal clinics is that it claims to give reassurance, to inform a woman that her foetus is 'normal'; yet the very act of testing throws into question the hitherto taken-for-granted 'normality' of the foetus. The test thus raises anxiety which was not there initially. Josephine Green's (1990) survey of the psychological literature on antenatal genetic testing is not by chance called *Calming or harming?*. But even within the context of general practice, where the patient and the clinician often have a long-standing relationship, the increasingly directive culture of general practice is hostile to the non-directive culture required for genetics. This directive culture is embedded increasingly in the statutory requirements for family doctors to try to achieve targets for various measures of biomedical surveillance. Neither, even if the culture can be modified, is it easy on present staffing levels to see where the time for such counselling is to come from. Certainly the current seven-minute consultation per patient in UK general practice does not look to be a psychologically safe starting point.

The societal management of genetic risks assessment

Inevitably the societal management of genetic risk assessment is undergoing rapid change. Here I want to explore the changing contribution of governmental institutions. Because I know it best, I use the UK experience.

The British approach to finding solutions to problems for which the political parties have no predetermined answers is typically to assemble a committee or commission of what are called the 'great and the good'. These committees of eminent people with relevant expertise are supposed to produce disinterested advice that will be acceptable to most acknowledged interests. It is important to note 'acknowledged interests', as while those of science, the arts, the professions and the Church have long been privileged, many interests, not least those of women and other socially weak constituencies, have been silently erased. This process is currently undergoing a considerable change as the management of risk generated by biomedical advance becomes more difficult and requires that hitherto excluded groups are brought in.

The change began with the Warnock Committee in the mid 1980s and its brief to advise on the ethical management of embryological research and *in vitro* fertilisation. It was set up in the wake of the moral anxieties set in train by the birth in 1978 of the first IVF baby, Louise Brown. That the key scientist Robert Edwards had spoken publicly in 1971 of his intention, following the success of John Gurdon with frogs, to produce a human via *in vitro* fertilisation and birth was left out of the discussion. Thus there was advance warning from science but with few influential hearers. The ethical anxieties the British Society for Social Responsibility sought to raise by giving a platform to Edwards were only to be explored *post hoc*. However, the story is a sharp reminder that paying attention to what is happening upstream is potentially much more powerful as a regulatory move than always pursuing events downstream.

The Warnock Committee itself was both a classic example of the old elite approach to the construction of consensus in the face of morally disturbing risk created by biomedical science and also opened the way to a new, more inclusive approach. While the great and the good were in evidence, this was also the first occasion in Britain that such an advisory committee comprised 50 per cent women. Even the Thatcher government, not noted for its sympathy towards women, could see that on this issue of reproduction women and their interests could no longer be safely ignored. Most other European countries with the technical capacity to engage in IVF used not dissimilar committee-like mechanisms, again involving women (even feminists in some, usually Nordic, countries), to establish consensual regulatory mechanisms. This was no fast process: the period between the inception of discussion and the passing of legislation typically was some three to four years. Broadly speaking, European legislation followed substantially a common pattern: embryological research, IVF and other approaches to assisted conception were continued within a now regulated framework.

Not everyone shared this consensus. Much of the feminist movement saw in the birth of this first IVF child the danger that someone other than the woman herself was going to be able to control her reproductive capabilities. Someone other than the woman herself was going to be able to say, first, whether that woman should mother and, second, which foetus should be permitted to come to full term. Unquestionably all the assumptions underpinning Warnock privileged the heterosexual and stable, if not actually married, couple. Although IVF technology was quite limited in its application, the critique was often mounted, as if it was not uncertain, invasive and expensive and that these material barriers in themselves set no limits. IVF and similar forms of assisted conception were powerfully contested by a movement fighting for women's reproductive freedom. Ideologically the movement was right, practically it was wrong. Even today, when IVF and similar technologies are more effective, they are still difficult, and only a minority of would-be mothers entering these programmes take babies home. The uncertainty of the procedures and their invasive and distressing nature ensured that IVF was a measure of last resort. It remains today too much of a craft-based activity, involving high levels of human resources, to offer the possibility of vast markets and corresponding profits.

Genetic diagnostics: a radically different problem

The new human genetics is radically different. This is a highly automated capital-intensive system of production, it mass-produces genetic information and must constantly search for new markets and new outlets. It came into existence initially by huge pump-priming from the state but is now substantially driven by venture capital. As with agricultural applications of biotechnology, there are millionaires to be made from what were formerly public sector scientists. In the accumulation of capital, speedy innovation is of the essence. Thus genetics in its present form presents a huge drive to innovate and impresses its timescale on governments, clinicians and patients alike.

Today the very possibility that genetic profiles can be developed and linked to medical records for ultimately whole populations, as in the case of Iceland and as canvassed for the UK, or as is in place for the entire US military and for all US convicted serious criminals, indicates that big money has entered the picture in a way quite outside the relatively modestly capitalised IVF problematic. Because of this, IVF had 4 years in which to establish an ethical consensus. When immense financial interests are at stake, as with biotechnology and genetically manipulated organisms, the management of risk and satisfying the ethical anxieties surrounding that risk become that much more difficult. The political and cultural task, as the recent WHO advice on legislation suggests, is to go slowly at the speed of society, not that of the biotechnology industry.

The UK's approach to the new genetics began by denying that human genetics produced special problems but was soon moved under the last Conservative government to adopt the suggestion made by the Parliamentary Committee on Science and Technology for a new Human Genetics Commission. Still a young body, this is required by the Labour government to deepen its agenda and widen the range of represented interests. For example, the Commission currently includes a leading figure from the disability movement yet many of the strongest voices within this movement regard genetic testing as inherently eugenic. If genetic testing is to be used at all, it is only to be used when surrounded by robust regulation and by ethically aware professionals and patients. For that matter, the desirable norms of disabled people can be radically different from those of the able-bodied. Thus parents who are themselves genetically deaf and who know from experience that they can successfully bring up a child like themselves to be happy may well think of selecting against a foetus likely to have unimpaired hearing. In consequence admitting such a voice is to include people with potentially very different normative values who have hitherto been deliberately excluded.

A halfway house?

However, given that all the members of the Advisory Commission on Human Genetics are screened and selected, it would be premature to conclude that because it is unquestionably more representative it is the equivalent of a democratically elected body. Thus it would be hard to see the Commission as the practical implementation of Ulrich Beck's ideas concerning the need to develop new social institutions for the democratisation of risk management. The updating of the Commission's form is not unlike a public version of a carefully chosen focus group, a key social research tool in the present government's approach and one much criticised from within and without the social sciences. The question remains whether this halfway house is adequate, or whether the UK government needs to move to new social institutions which are both more transparently democratic and have greater legitimacy and power. Has the halfway house form sufficient legitimacy to effectively advise on the regulation of the immense industrial and financial forces behind the new genetics while paying attention to the messy complex world of the ethics of genetic testing in practice? And how do governments committed to wealth creation and therefore seeking to foster the biotechnology industry receive and act upon such advice? Such questions could be posed even more sharply to numbers of current international bioethics committees whose members are typically either drawn from the great and the good by governments or who are civil servants with a formal brief to cover bioethics. The challenge of genetics is immense. Do such committees have sufficient will and clout to match the situation or do they sometimes feel like a collectivity of mice left with the task of belling the biotechnological cat?

Beyond the halfway house

I am with those who argue that the halfway house is inadequate. To move away from both state and consumer eugenicism requires new social institutions. The task of such new institutions, of consensus fora, citizens' juries and the like, is the socio-technological assessment of both genetic claims and products. Such assessment might entail the rejection of specific technological possibilities and would be unlikely to avoid fierce resistance from vested interests. But such new social institutions do offer the possibility of restoring social trust in the process of technological innovation which is integral to a highly scientific and technological culture. Such trust is massively under siege, not least because of a string of environmental disasters and threats to the environment and to human beings produced by scientific and technological innovation.

Creating new institutions does not itself offer any guarantees of easy consensus. What it does bring is the democratic possibility of conversations between many differently situated people and groups – not least between potential consumers and providers of new technologies. There is some modest evidence that the biotechnology industry is likely to be more open to this than the old secretive traditions of state paternalism. Industry and the Ministry of Agriculture, Fisheries and Food (MAFF) were the joint funders of Dolly, but where industry was willing to talk about the ethics of sheep cloning, MAFF was (as usual) silent. But consumer resistance is also forcing industry to recognise that it must listen. Both in the US and the UK consumer resistance to cystic fibrosis genetic tests is compelling industry to recognise that the market model of the 'consumer' does not fit this world of women and their partners who are thinking about having a baby.[1] Such modest auguries which serve to limit and modify the emergence of consumer eugenics are important to both providers and potential users of genetic tests

In summary, to move on, both out of the old state eugenicism and beyond the emergent consumer eugenicism, requires not only courageous experiment with new social institutions but also the societal acknowledgement of the centrality of women and their partners who, in the process of picking their way through their reproductive choices, are building a genethics from below.

Note

1 Research suggests that social pressure from family and friends on the 'young couple' is much more influential than any version of rational choice theory.

References

Billings, Paul (1994) 'Contribution to an International Seminar on Technology Assessment of Neurogenetics', January, Hamburg University.

Bodmer, Walter and McKie, Robin (1994) *The Book of Man*, New York: Little Brown.

Callon, Michael (1987) 'Society in the making: the study of technology as a tool for sociological analysis', in W. Bijker, T. Highes and T. Pinch (eds), *The Social Construction of Technological Systems*, Cambridge, MA: MIT Press.

Duster, Troy (1990) *Back Door to Eugenics*, New York: Routledge.

Edwards, Jeanette (2000) *Born and Bred*, Oxford: Oxford University Press.

European Science Foundation (1991) *Report on Genome Research*, Strasbourg: ESF.

Fox Keller, Evelyn (1992) 'Nature, nurture and the Human Genome Project', in Daniel Kevles and Leroy Hood (eds), *The Code of Codes: Scientific and Social Issues in the Human Genome Project*, Cambridge, MA: Harvard University Press.

Green, Josephine (1990) *Calming or Harming? A Critical Overview of Psychological Effects of Foetal Diagnosis on Pregnant Women*, vol. 2, London: Galton Institute (Occasional Papers).

Hubbard, Ruth (1984) 'Prenatal diagnosis and eugenic ideology', *Women's Studies International Forum* 8 (6): 567–76.

—— (1995) *Profitable Promises: Essays on Women, Science and Health*, Monroe, ME: Common Courage.

—— and Henefin, Mary Sue (1984) 'Genetic screening of prospective parents and of workers' in James Humber and Robert Almeder (eds), *Biomedical Ethics Reviews*, Clifton, NJ: Humana Press.

—— and Wald, Elijah (1993) *Exploding the Gene Myth*, Boston, MA: Beacon Press.

Irwin, Alan and Wynne, Brian (eds) (1996) *Mis-understanding Science: Making Sense of Science and Technology in Everyday Life*, Cambridge: Cambridge University Press.

Jordan, Bertrand (1993) *Travelling Around the Human Genome*, Paris: Inserm.

Kay, Lily (1993) *The Molecular Vision of Life: Caltech, the Rockefeller Foundation and the Rise of the New Biology*, New York: Oxford University Press.

Kevles, Daniel (1985) *In the Name of Eugenics: Genetics and the Uses of Human Heredity*, New York: Alfred A. Knopf.

—— and Hood, Leroy (eds) *The Code of Codes: Scientific and Social Issues in the Human Genome Project*, Cambridge, MA: Harvard University Press.

King's Fund (1987) *Screening for Foetal and Genetic Abnormality: Consensus Statement*, London: King's Fund Centre.

Kitcher, Phillip (1996) *Biology as Ideology: The Doctrine of DNA*, New York: Harper.

Koshland, Daniel (1989) Editorial, *Science*, 246 (13 October): 189.

Lewontin, R.C. (1991) *Biology as Ideology: The Doctrine of DNA*, New York: Harper.

Luria, Salvador (1989) Letter, *Science*, 246 (17 November): 873.

Meek, James (2000) 'New genetic ethics begins at home', *Guardian*, 4 October.

Muller Hill, Benno (1988) *Murderous Science: Elimination by Scientific Selection of Jews, Gypsies and Others, Germany 1933–45*, Oxford: Clarendon Press.

Nelkin, Dorothy and Tancredi, Lawrence (1994) *Dangerous Diagnostics: The Social Power of Biological Information*, 2nd edn, Chicago: University of Chicago Press.

Petchesky, Rosalind (1985) *Abortion and Woman's Choice: The State, Sexuality and Reproductive Freedom*, Boston, MA: North-Eastern University Press.

Pickens, Donald K. (1968) *Eugenics and the Progressives*, Nashville, TN: Vanderbilt University Press.

Rose, Hilary (1994) *Love, Power and Knowledge: Towards a Feminist Transformation of the Sciences*, Cambridge: Polity Press.

—— and Hanmer, Jalna (1976) 'Women's liberation, reproduction and the technological fix', in D. Leonard Barker and S. Allen (eds), *Sexual Divisions and Society*, London: Tavistock.

—— and Rose, Steven (eds) (1976) *The Radicalisation of Science*, London: Macmillan.

Rose, Steven (1995) 'The rise of neurogenetic determinism', *Nature*, 353 (2 February): 280–1.

Shakespeare, Tom (1995) 'Eugenics by the backdoor? The disability movement's concerns with the new genetics', paper given at the Edinburgh Science Conference, April.

Stacey, Margaret (1969) 'The myth of community studies', *British Journal of Sociology* 20: 134–47.

Stacey, Meg (1992) (ed.) *Changing Human Reproduction: Social Science Perspectives*, London: Sage.

van den Daele, Wolgang (1994) *Technology Assessment as a Political Experiment*, Berlin: Wissenschaftzentrum Berlin für Social Forschung (WZB).

Weeks, Jeffrey (1981) *Sex, Politics and Society*, London: Tavistock.

Weindling, Paul (1989) *Health, Race and German Politics Between National Unification and Nazism, 1870–1945*, Cambridge: Cambridge University Press.

Werskey, Gary (1971) *The Invisible College*, Harmondsworth, Middx: Penguin.

Yoxen, Edward (1983) *The Gene Business: Who Should Control Biotechnology?*, London: Pan Books.

Zipper, Juliette and Sevenhuijsen, Selma (1987) 'Surrogacy: feminist notions of motherhood reconsidered', in M. Stanworth (ed.), *Reproductive Technologies: Gender, Motherhood, and Medicine*, Cambridge: Polity Press.

4   Why turn to speculative fiction?

On reconceiving feminist research for the twenty-first century

Joan Haran

Introduction

> I believe that the abortion issue can never regress to a point where it would be made illegal again. Too many women – and a lot of men – simply wouldn't stand for it.
>
> (Poppema 1996: 233)

> There was Utah, for instance, where the Coalition built its first case that so long as the majority of the state's citizens believed abortion to be murder, the legislature had a mandate. So you got Utah *v.* Doe, making Utah what the Coalition called a prolife state, and then one by one, the other states had fallen into line . . . I did know the text of the Amendment that would land us both in Softjail. It was one of those disarmingly short, simple statements – *No unborn person shall be deprived of life by any person* – and the rights it gave began at fertilization.
>
> (Ferriss 1997: 117–18)

In the United States in 1981, congressional discussions about the origin of human life resulted in a partial victory for 'conservative forces'. According to Hartouni (1997: 34):

> the Senate Judiciary subcommittee concluded, on the basis of the 'evidence' before it, that 'science' had indeed 'demonstrated' the presence of human life at conception. The foetus emerged from these hearings a 'person,' but one without constitutional protection . . . .

The two quotes at the head of this section are extracted from two very different narratives about abortion which respond to the controversial nature of reproductive politics in the United States and to significant shifts in the terrain for debate which have occurred since the 1980s.

Lucy Ferriss's *The Misconceiver*, a dystopian work of speculative fiction (SF), is set in the USA in the third decade of the twenty-first century. In a social and political climate in which women's rights have been sharply curtailed, abortion has been recriminalised and the supply and/or fitting of

IUDs outlawed. Some barrier contraception is available to married couples, on prescription, but the contraceptive pill and the cap are unavailable. IVF procedures have been banned, as has the practice of amniocentesis. Tubal ligation is still legal, but virtually impossible to obtain for white women, although available on demand to black women, as is the contraceptive implant, Norplant.

Poppema's *Why I Am an Abortion Doctor* is the ghost-written auto-biography of a US-based abortion provider, which presents its author's profession as the logical outcome of her personal and political experience of gendered inequality. Brief reference to this life story will provide a counter-point to a more detailed reading of the fictional text. Poppema's narrative is resolutely hopeful and committed to framing the terms of the debate on reproductive rights from a feminist standpoint, and carries the added weight of a feminist empiricist account of the actual practice of abortion which may be contrasted with the bloody rhetoric of the anti-choice coalition.

In this chapter, critical readings of the two narratives will be used to rehearse some key issues related to women's reproductive autonomy. It will show ways in which SF communicates social and cultural complexity through an address to the reader that is formally very different from the analytically distinct categories of abstract social theory, and which resonates with current sociological preoccupations with narrative accounts of subjective experience. The abbreviation SF is used to refer to the multiple literary subgenres abbreviated 'sf', including speculative fiction and science fiction (Haraway 1992: 5). Some thematic links will therefore be made with Poppema's auto-biography[1] (Poppema 1996). This chapter does not present a formal comparison of the two narratives, but the contrasting reader positions available in the two texts are noteworthy. Poppema for the most part presents us with a chronologically sequenced narrative, which seems calculated to eliminate ambiguity, whereas Ferriss requires much more work from the reader in the piecing together of the timeline of her narrative, implicating them (us) much more fully in the meanings created.

This chapter outlines the ways in which critical attention to SF can con-tribute to feminist interdisciplinary research on the social relations of science and technology, before considering the rationale for looking particularly at reproductive technologies. After introducing the key themes of *The Mis-conceiver*, the means by which the text intervenes in feminist 'conversations' about the discursive construction of an adversarial relationship between women and foetuses is considered. This is followed by a discussion of medical and lay practices of abortion which contrasts Poppema's politicised account with the individualised account of the narrator of *The Misconceiver*. Pop-pema's qualifications for intervening in this conversation are unusual. As a university student in the late 1960s she double majored in pre-med and polit-ical science. She was also: 'involved with women's collectives in health-care very early' (early 1970s) (Poppema 1996: 70) and with some other women set up an abortion clinic in 1978 (ibid.: 87). Since 1985 she has run the Aurora

Medical Center in Seattle, providing women's reproductive health services.[2] The chapter concludes with a discussion of the resources that feminist standpoint theory offers to research on reproductive technologies and the ways in which speculative fiction can support the achievement of such a standpoint.

Terminology

The changing discursive field constituted by contested accounts of reproductive technologies has led to a proliferation of terminology which can cause some analytical confusion. The terms reproductive technologies, new reproductive technologies and assisted reproductive technologies all appear in this chapter. Reproductive technologies is used to refer to all enculturated practices of natural-technical knowledge about reproduction, including technoscientific practices (cf. Stanworth 1987a) and the taken-for-granted medical surveillance of women's reproductive bodies. Using this definition, abortion is unequivocally a reproductive technology, whether practised by professionals or by laypersons. New reproductive technologies (NRTs) is deployed in the manner dominant in academic literature of the 1980s and early 1990s to refer to the constellation of technoscientific practices, including IVF, GIFT and other heroic medical-technical conceptive interventions. The term assisted reproductive technologies (ARTs) is used, as has been the case since the late 1990s, to encompass 'low-tech' interventions such as donor insemination and even surrogacy as part of a continuum of social and technical interventions into the 'natural' arena of reproduction.

How can SF contribute to research?

Donna Haraway (1997b: 191) argues:

> An 'ethnographic attitude' can be adopted within any kind of inquiry, including textual analysis. Not limited to a specific discipline, an ethnographic attitude is a mode of practical and theoretical attention, a way of remaining mindful and accountable . . . Textual analysis must articulate with many kinds of sustained scholarly interaction among living people in living situations, historical and contemporary, documentary and *in vivo*. These different studies need each other, and they are all theory-building projects. No one person does all the kinds of work; feminist science studies is a collective undertaking . . . .

Hence there is nothing incongruous about placing textual analysis of a work of fiction alongside empirical research in order to make responsible links between individual feminist research projects that are intended to contribute to the collective undertaking of feminist science studies. Further, critical attention to fictional texts can provide us with theoretical resources that can inform empirical research. Taking seriously the poststructuralist insight that discursive practices shape material reality, a close critical reading of *The Misconceiver* that dramatises the ways in which a particular constellation of discursive practices could conceivably harmfully alter material reality for all women is a valid co-practice with critical attention to the narratives constructed by the 'real life' subjects of reproductive technologies and other medical interventions.

The argument developed in this chapter insists on the need for research on specific reproductive technologies, including, but not limited to, abortion and IVF, to be carried out in the context of a more complex mapping of reproductive choices and with due attention to the subjective bodily integrity and autonomy of all women. The writing and reading of feminist SF is a valuable practice for its contribution to this project, which Haraway calls: 'theory and practice addressed to the social relations of science and technology, including crucially the systems of myths and meanings structuring our imaginations' (Haraway 1991b: 163). It engages its readers emotionally and intellectually, through imaginative identification with the fictional life experiences of protagonists, with Utopian and dystopian alternate (future) histories, and thus the progressive or regressive tendencies and effects of social institutions and practices, particularly those affecting and affected by technology. The address to the reader in speculative fiction not only enables, but invites – or more strongly incites – the reader to engage cognitively and emotionally with subject positions that they do not inhabit in the 'real' world. By identifying with the fictional narrator or with other key protagonists in *The Misconceiver*, an SF novel, we can reorientate our subjective understanding of the social world (of the text or of daily experience).

The Misconceiver speculates about the future of abortion as a medical technology and a social practice precisely in the context of a proliferation of surveilling and interventionist reproductive technologies and the ways in which these are (mis)used to curtail women's subjective autonomy. The emergence of this text may be read as evidence of feminist anxiety about the renewed cultural centrality of contestation around notions of motherhood prompted by the emergence of the NRTs, and public responses to them. This kind of anxiety can be difficult to voice in a research climate which continually insists that the benefits that new technologies offer to some women must not be overlooked; and that it continues to erupt suggests that we need to rethink how we conduct and communicate research.

Why continue to focus on reproduction?

Why is the development of feminist theory and research around human reproduction still an urgent necessity? As Haraway (1997b: 187) asserts:

> Reproduction has been at the centre of scientific, technological, political, personal, religious, gender, familial, class, race and national webs of contestation for at least the past twenty-five years. Like it or not, as if we

were children dealing with adults' hidden secrets, feminists could not avoid relentlessly asking where babies came from. Our answers have repeatedly challenged the reduction of that original and originating question to literalized and universalized women's body parts.

Feminists must continue to repeat that challenge until women are no longer defined primarily in relation to their reproductive capacity; feminism has been only relatively successful in enlarging and complicating the ways in which commonsenses of womanhood are articulated. The complacent view of Patricia Smith (1995: 126) who claims that:

> A reproductive revolution has occurred in this century although the roots of the revolution reach back into the last century and the fruits will be more fully harvested in the next. This revolution is substantially complete and irreversible, and it has profound implications for the traditional role of motherhood

is not warranted with the inauguration of a US President, in the year 2001, who would like to make abortion illegal. As Hartouni (1997: 65) pointed out:

> the radical challenges potentially posed by legalized abortion to trad-itional gender identities and sexual relations were hardly lost on neocon-servatives and their New Right and fundamentalist affiliates, and, over the course of the past decade, have inflamed popular debate while themselves being recast and transformed in the process.

The cultural field of reproduction, with the enormous implications it has for contested notions of gender, sexuality and the public/private divide, is continually shifting as it is contested by different constituencies, so feminists must constantly adjust their analyses and research projects accordingly. An assumption of unidirectional progress is neither sociologically nor politically sustainable.

Despite the work that has been done by a range of theorists, including a strong feminist contribution, to problematise scientific positivism, and teleo-logical narratives more generally, there is still a general tendency, supported by many feminists, including most of the contributors to Stanworth's *Repro-ductive Technologies* (1987a) and, more recently, Dion Farquhar in *The Other Machine* (1996), to assume that recent and prospective developments in NRTs and ARTs will either be beneficial to women or at least not actively harmful. This positive reading is frequently harnessed to research and theoretical projects which are committed to focusing on the ways in which specific tech-nologies are applied and experienced by actual – rather than speculative or theoretical – human subjects. Although there are good epistemological and political reasons for this pragmatic strategy, it does run the risk of capturing only part of the picture.

It can mean that the proposition that the technologies, which medical professionals, laypeople and social theorists represent as filled with potential for expanding choice, also contain the potential to undermine existing, taken-for-granted choices is not taken seriously enough. It is also conceivable that, in this context of researching how social agents negotiate their daily lives, the potential of conservative voices to dominate the debates about what motherhood means following the advent of 'New Reproductive Technologies' is not taken seriously enough by those – feminists and others – who insist on the agency of those non-hegemonic subjects who are fortunate or able enough to negotiate positive reproduction-related outcomes for themselves 'in the chinks of the world machine'.[3]

The Misconceiver

In Lucy Ferriss's *The Misconceiver* (1997) the conservative or reactionary potentials of responses to technology and the social changes they arise from and occasion is imaginatively worked through. The unintended consequences of the new technologies when harnessed to a project of limiting all choices for women, not merely those related to reproduction, are graphically spelled out. Direct links are made between the recriminalisation of abortion and the shift in debates around reproduction enabled by the co-existence of new reproductive technologies and new visualisation technologies.

The story is predicated on a recent history, familiar to many readers of feminist critique: that of the rise of the foetus as public person and the demise of women's reproductive autonomy as its corollary, through the construction of an adversarial relationship between the pregnant woman and the embryo or foetus that she carries (or indeed chooses not to). Petchesky, Haraway, Hartouni and Bordo have each made significant contributions to the understanding of this cultural phenomenon. For example, Susan Bordo (1993: 72) has suggested that there is a legal double standard in the US 'concerning the bodily integrity of pregnant and nonpregnant bodies, the construction of women as foetal incubators, [and] the bestowal of "super-subject" status to the foetus'. Bordo (ibid.) links this double standard with the 'emergence of a father's-rights ideology' which she believes reveals that 'feminist anger and frustration are far from paranoid and anachronistic'. Accounts of the erosion of women's reproductive rights vis-à-vis abortion must be placed side-by-side with accounts of the so-called widening of choice offered by the birth-promoting reproductive technologies and the (limited) availability of surrogacy, to produce a more textured account of the limits of women's reproductive autonomy.

The narrative of *The Misconceiver* takes the form of a self-reflective conversation with an imaginary interlocutor, and charts the narrator's coming-to-terms with her identity as a 'misconceiver': an illegal abortionist. This emotional journey occurs in parallel with physical journeys she takes during the course of the book, and both trajectories enable the reader to consider the fictionalised 'facts' of the case and to comment on the narrator's analysis of what they mean. The overarching message of the novel seems to be that abortion is a woman's choice, but that that choice can only be expressed at the cost of the murder of a foetus. Abortion is therefore conceived of as a necessary evil rather than the legitimate expression of women's bodily autonomy and integrity.

The narrator seems to accept the legitimacy of state control over women's reproductive bodies, but is prepared herself to assist individual women who choose to resist this control. Although, by the end of the novel's consciousness-raising journey, she is eventually able to conceive of taking collective political action to change the terms of the law, she continues to accept the anti-abortionists' discursive equation of abortion with murder.

Although the law that would enshrine the logical outcome of this subsumption of the subjectivity of the 'foetal container' to the 'supersubject' that is the foetus has not yet been re-enacted – 'that old law about natal hierarchy . . . (t)he last frontier. Where you can't save the life of a mother if it means killing the baby' (Ferriss 1997: 28) – the fact that foetal rights discourses have achieved psychic dominance even with individuals whose practice of abortion enables women to reassert control over their own reproductive fate leaves the reader deeply pessimistic. An imaginative leap is required to conceive of more hopeful possibilities, and although the narrator of *The Misconceiver* is unable to make the leap, the discomfort feminists might feel when empathising or resisting empathy with her narrative composure[4] might prompt them (us) to think more radically about possibilities for change.

Published in the US in the late 1990s, *The Misconceiver* emerges from a particular social, political and legal context. In *Understanding the New Politics of Abortion*, Malcolm Goggin (1993: 2) suggests that the 'new' politics of abortion are characterised by: 'right-to-life forces . . . seeking nothing less than a reversal of *Roe*'; the US Supreme Court decision which decriminalised abortion. *Roe* v. *Wade* states that a woman has the right to choose abortion until foetal viability, but that the state's interest outweighs the woman's right after that point. Goggin (ibid.: xi) submits that the *Webster* decision of 3 July 1989 set the stage for this new strategy. In *Webster* v. *Reproductive Health Services*:

> the Supreme Court narrowly upheld a very restrictive anti-choice Missouri statute that prohibited public employees from performing abortions in public facilities, prohibited the use of public facilities to perform abortions, and required doctors to test to see if the foetus could survive outside the womb before performing abortion.

Goggin (ibid.: 7) claims that:

> The essential characteristics of the 'new' politics of abortion [are] – expansion of activities to all levels and branches of government (especially the states); increased levels of public participation for fetal-rights

groups, including an escalation of clinic violence; and pro-choice mobilization and counter-mobilization.

Although the specific 'separation of powers' that applies in the US differs, for example, from that in the UK, there are analogies that may be drawn which may be useful in setting research agendas. For example, activists on either side of the debate in the US have used the contradictions between federal law and state law as a public site on which to stage their contestations, while activists in the UK can make similar use of the contradictions between the law and its differential interpretation and application from one health authority to another. Feminist social research in these areas of contestation could prove particularly fruitful. For example, in *Narratives of Irishness and the Problem of Abortion*, Lisa Smyth points to the 'X Case' in 1992 where activists constructed competing accounts of exactly what composed the national will with regard to the 'pro-life' clause in the Irish Constitution. In her analysis she notes that the legalisation of abortion in the United States was one of the key factors in the emergence of the Pro-Life Amendment Campaign (1979–83): 'given that legalizing abortion had not been on the Irish mainstream political agenda during the 1970s' (Smyth 1998: 65). Thus although the importance of producing situated knowledges and qualitative ethnographic research must not be underestimated, it is crucial to recognise that hegemonic common senses are produced nationally and globally, as well as locally, and must be contested in the same terms.

The Misconceiver and technological innovation

Even the most critical feminist social studies of science and technology can lapse into a kind of positivist technological determinism in which resistance can only be conceptualised as managing the genie that is already out of the bottle. The 'real life' actions of 'pro-life' campaigners and the fictional outcomes of these actions represented in *The Misconceiver* should give us pause for thought. The utopian desire of the pro-life coalition is the total effacement of one specific group of reproductive technologies: those that terminate pregnancy. Comparably totalitarian feminist goals would be anathema, but feminists could consider the possibility of developing more utopian theories and strategies, rather than setting out theoretical, research and political agendas *only* in terms of negotiation and accommodation to existing social conditions and their apparent trajectory.

In *The Misconceiver* virtually the whole gamut of new reproductive and new visualisation technologies:

> those concerned with fertility control . . . more elaborate technologies and screening procedures for monitoring foetal development in the early stages of pregnancy [and] . . . the conceptive technologies, directed to the

promotion of pregnancy through techniques for overcoming or bypass-
ing infertility

(Stanworth 1987a: 10–11)

is explicitly linked by the narrator in the chain of events that leads to the
criminalisation of abortion. This regressive outcome, the text suggests, is
precipitated by the organised response to technological innovations by con-
servatives who have won the rhetorical and representational battle to define
the bodies that matter. Racism, heterosexism and white male economic self-
interest are all portrayed as contributing to a society which defines women
primarily by their ability to reproduce and to service men sexually, and
non-white people as inferior to white.[5]

The power of naming

The narrator dates the coining of the term 'misconception' back to a legal
case focused on a mistake in an infertility clinic that led to 'a Protestant
woman . . . carrying a Tay-Sachs baby'. She compares this to an earlier (real-
life) case in Holland where the mistake was not discovered until after the
baby's birth. In the fictional case the child is aborted because 'The cells in the
mother's uterus, the court essentially maintained, were like Frankenstein's
monster – a misconceived thing, to be corrected only by being destroyed'
(Ferriss 1997: 13). In both the fictional and the 'real-life' case, race plays a
part in defining which children or foetuses are less desirable; Jewish or black
progeny threaten the stability of the white Christian hegemony.

Ferriss's narrator does not tell a straightforward linear narrative of the
abrogation of reproductive choice. We do learn that this case provided a
temporary rallying point for 'the dwindling voices wanting to return to
premillennial liberties', but the textual claim is that its actual effect was
eventually further to erode remaining choice:

all that resulted was a handful of legal abortions followed by the banning
of IVF procedures, and then the voices went silent. After the amnio law
was repealed, amnio itself came under attack; no use knowing what it's
too late to prevent, people said. Only the name, *misconceivers*, stuck –
both as a badge of pride, remembering the last battle, and as a stigma for
those of us who've supposedly got the whole miracle of conception ass-
backward.

(Ibid.)

The implied sequence of events is interesting, because it points to the eugenic
implications of some feminist pro-choice discourses, as well as to the controversial nature of all reproductive practices. Taken with later textual references
to the use of iconic representations of the unborn, there is also the implication
that IVF caused its own demise via the mythologisation of the foetus.

The role of the global foetus in undermining women's subjectivity

The 'global foetus' is Haraway's term. She claims that:

> Both the whole earth and the foetus owe their existence as public objects to visualizing technologies . . . The global foetus and the spherical whole earth both exist because of, and inside of technoscientific visual culture. Yet, I think, both signify touch. Both provoke yearning for the physical sensuousness of a wet and blue-green earth and a soft fleshy child. That is why these images are so ideologically powerful. They signify the immediately natural and embodied, over and against the constructed and disembodied.
>
> (Haraway 1997b: 174)

The use of iconic photographs of embryos in the service of the anti-abortion lobby is a key trope in *The Misconceiver*, as is the narrator's contestatory conceptualisation of unwanted foetuses/embryos as incubi; but it is clear that even the narrator has been largely convinced by this war of words and images, despite her continued practice of 'misconceptions'. Feminist theorists have mapped the history of this representational hegemony.

Rosalind Pollack Petchesky suggests that it was in the mid 1980s that defeats in the conventional political arena led the 'pro-life' movement to attack abortion rights in the terrain of mass culture and imagery, specifically around ideological struggle over the symbolic meanings of foetuses. This shift has also entailed the self-conscious use of medico-technical discourses rather than those of religion:

> in its efforts to win over the courts, the legislatures and popular 'hearts and minds'. But the vehicle for this shift is not organised medicine directly but mass culture and its diffusion into reproductive technology through the video display terminal.
>
> (Petchesky 1999: 172).

Petchesky constructs a genealogy of the construction of the foetus as a fetish, from the earliest appearance of photos of the foetus: 'in the June 1962 issue of *Look* (a major mass-circulation "picture magazine" of the period)' (ibid.: 174) through to the production and distribution of the anti-abortion film *The Silent Scream* in 1984, which, she claims: 'with formidable cunning . . . translated the still and by now stale images of foetus as "baby" into real-time video'. In 'The Virtual Speculum in the New World Order', Haraway (1997b) further fleshes out the constructed nature of this fetish with her account of 'the iconic form that has been made so familiar by the exquisite, internationally distributed images produced by the Swedish biomedical photographer, Lennart Nilsson'. Haraway suggests that:

The visible foetus became a public object with the April 1965 *Life* magazine cover featuring Nilsson's photograph of an intrauterine eighteen-week-old developing human being, encased in its bubble-like amniotic sac. The rest of the Nilsson photos in the *Life* story, 'The Drama of Life before Birth', were of extrauterine abortuses, beautifully lit and photographed in colour to become the visual embodiment of life at its origin.

(Haraway 1997b: 178)

As Haraway points out, these foetuses were neither represented nor seen as abortuses and instead 'signified life itself, in its transcendent essence and immanent embodiment' (ibid.: 225). In *The Misconceiver*, the narrator repeatedly refers to the power of this type of image, and instances the story of one abortionist who went insane and committed suicide when repeatedly subjected to images produced by anti-abortion lobbyists:

cute little not-born babies getting their skulls crushed. That these were skulls with bloated brains in them, or attached to spines that carried no messages from brain to body, or that the blood which ran in babykin's veins was going to kill both him and his mommy was not mentioned in the photo captions.

(Ferriss 1997: 97)

Deborah Steinberg makes explicit the link between the specular foetus, the new reproductive technologies and abortion:

Because IVF has made it possible to create embryos outside and (re)place them in women's bodies, it has significantly altered the terms of debate around pregnancy, abortion and childbirth and the role of medicine and the state in relation to all three . . . Moreover debates about abortion and women's right to choose have now become inextricably entangled with questions about IVF embryo research . . . Indeed, it can be argued that IVF has made material the ideological separation between woman and embryo that underpins anti-abortion ideology

(Steinberg 2000: 202–3)

and that had already been made part of the public imagination through visualisation technologies.

The Misconceiver is a an extremely credible extrapolation from the *fin de siècle* historical moment of its publication, as its narrator elaborates the imagined societal changes as being incremental consequences of the interrelated activism of a decentralised 'Coalition', rather than the work of one centralised agency. The use of a constellation of economic, legislative and popular discourses to effect the aims of the anti-abortionists and the harnessing of apparently pro-choice practices to their project is convincingly portrayed, as are the myriad of personal reasons for which individuals consent to or resist these changes. This could be seen as the dark reflection of the utopian coalition politics that are one version of the cyborg subjectivity envisioned by Donna Haraway (1991b).

The novel is profoundly disturbing for feminists because, even though it closes with its narrator assuming responsibility for her own choice to be a 'misconceiver' and her decision to contest these curtailments to women's reproductive rights, as part of a 'political clique' of 'feisty women', she seems to be too susceptible to the anti-abortionist lobby's characterisation of embryos as murdered children. She seems to theorise women's right to choose as a war against the incubus, her revisioning of the global foetus. This seems to be a retrograde step. As Poppema (1996: 122) points out:

> if society would just dare to frame the abortion conversation in terms of the *woman's* life, then it would have come a long way. The abortion controversy, after all, is much less about children than about control over what women may do with their own lives.

Medical and lay relations to reproductive technologies

Young women becoming sexually active since the legalisation of abortion in both the US and the UK have been relatively able to take a certain degree of sexual agency and reproductive autonomy for granted, within the context of the official health care system. So the opening passage of *The Misconceiver*, which contains a graphic description of an abortion, or misconception, carried out by a young woman of fifteen (on her sister; the woman who is training her in this practice) is deeply shocking for readers who have not shared Donna Haraway's experience of the 'eruption of the gynaecological speculum as a symbol in US feminist politics in the early 1970s' (Haraway 1997b: 193). Haraway elaborates:

> The repossessed speculum, sign of the Women's Liberation Movement's attention to material instruments in science and technology, was understood to be a self-defining technology. Those collective sessions with the speculum and mirror were not only symbols, however. They were self-help and self-experimentation practices in a period in which abortion was still illegal and unsafe. The self-help groups developed techniques of menstrual extraction, that is, early abortion, that could be practised by women alone or with each other outside professional medical control. A little flexible tubing joined the mirror and the speculum in more than a few of those sessions.
>
> (Ibid.: 193–4)

Haraway acknowledges the empowering experience of this practice, but also its insufficiency to contest the medicalised globalisation of the iconic foetus, and the absent presence of the maternal body as object of surveillance.

Poppema (1996: 68–73) also refers to the impact that similar experiences in women's groups and feminist medical communities had on her personal-political formation. As an abortion provider at the turn of the twenty-first century and a member of professional associations which educate and provide facilities to enable women to make decisions about their own reproductive bodies, she is part of the loose coalition that is contesting the valuation of the foetal super-subject over women conceived not as subjects but as foetal containers. Although she insists that abortion will never be made illegal again, her politicised response to the tactics of the right-wing anti-choice coalition has been to question what she would have done if she were practising medicine when abortions were illegal:

> I probably would have been part of a women's underground health collective, helping perform abortions for women rich and poor while maintaining a regular practice. And I'd also be one of the doctors who would be training lay practitioners to do the procedure. Properly trained lay practitioners, after all, did a great job during the years prior to legalization. They came up with innovative methods that probably helped improve the procedure after abortion rights were legalized.
>
> (Ibid.: 151–2)

It is terrifying to think that Poppema's attempt to insert herself, imaginatively, in a pre-legalisation history sounds so similar to the future history that Ferriss imagines, based on a remarkably similar social and political analysis of the US at the close of the twentieth century.

Human reproductive politics in the New World Order: feminist standpoints

In her discussion of 'human reproductive politics in the New World Order', Haraway (1997b: 204) contrasts the 'intensively cultivated foetuses, located at the center of national culture and portrayed as individuals from fertilization on, versus throwaway foetuses and dead babies, located "down there" and known only as "angels"'. The intensively cultivated foetuses to which she refers are the offspring of new and assisted reproductive technologies in the affluent West, while the throwaway foetuses are the 'missing and dead babies' of 'the poorest residents on earth'.

The Misconceiver focuses so closely on the situation in the future US that a global perspective on reproductive politics is precluded and is certainly absent from the narrator's consciousness. However, the tendency to represent/ produce the foetus as '*sacrum* ... an object in which the transcendent appears' which Haraway documents in 'The Virtual Speculum' has been taken to its logical conclusion in this future US with the criminalisation of abortion, and, indeed, it may be taken further if the Coalition succeeds in reinstating the 'old law about natal hierarchy' which would make it illegal to save a pregnant woman's life if such intervention caused the death of the baby (or abortion of the foetus).

In contrast, in explaining why she came to be an abortion doctor, Suzanne Poppema sets her decision precisely in terms of 'human reproductive politics in the New World Order'. She describes a period of politicisation beginning in the late 1970s when she travelled with her husband 'to some of the least developed regions on the globe', and 'witnessed firsthand the persistence with which little girls are undervalued compared with boys and how women are subjugated'. She adds:

> My odyssey of politicisation led me to Denver, where I worked in city clinics serving Mexican and Asian Americans. This experience showed me firsthand the forces that shape the limited options of the poor . . . In Denver and Seattle I witnessed the steady weakening of the social infra- structure by right-wing political administrations and their patriarchal admirers.
>
> (Poppema 1996: 23–4)

In the process of reflecting upon her experiences, and deciding in which way she could best use her professional skills to help alleviate some of the social inequality that she had witnessed in the heart of the US, as well as in devel- oping countries, Poppema explains:

> Gradually it occurred to me: In virtually every society where a wanted child is greeted by a healthy, accommodating family, that child can expect incredible life advantages – physically, emotionally, socially, and eco- nomically – compared with an unwanted child. My goal, then, became that of helping the women . . . who for whatever reason, would choose not to continue a pregnancy. If I could abort unwanted births, then I could help prevent unwanted children and help mitigate the human misery that attends them.
>
> (Ibid.: 24)

Although it would be very easy to critique the liberal, and even Malthusian, assumptions that underpin Poppema's narration, if we extracted phrases out of context, there are some very important messages to be taken from the way she describes her practice as a medical practitioner of abortion. Even though she writes as a wife and mother, as well as a doctor, and although a firm belief in the value of strong families to individuals and society permeates her text, she places her ideals in the context of a clear-eyed critique of local and global social inequality. And in the way she treats her patients, she is very different from Phoebe, the first-person narrator of *The Misconceiver*. She does not ask her patients if they want her to kill their baby. She refers to foetal matter at all times as 'tissue' and insists on the competency of her patients to make their own choices about treatment of their 'sovereign human bodies'. She has no discourse of moral censure towards women who choose abortion, and is indeed adamantly opposed to discourses – and social institutions – which suggest that women should suffer the consequences of sexual intercourse and that if they choose abortion it should be as painful a process as possible, morally and emotionally, if not physically.

Although the narrator of *The Misconceiver* acknowledges that the fictional trajectory of reproductive rights curtailment is 'tragic', she adds:

> Marie and the others had lived it while I hadn't. No matter how much information they handed me, no matter how many dates and movements and newsbites, I would never understand how tragic it all was . . . I was out in the world, trying to be a teenager, learning that straight hair and an engagement ring were coveted symbols and abortion a vile stain, a subhuman act . . . I understood the order Marie put things in, but it was all *steady-state* [italics added] for me, it was in the past. I helped Marie because she asked me to and because each woman that came in seemed to need us so desperately, that was all.
>
> (Ferriss 1997: 117–18)

This narrated reflection suggests that emotional investment in political resistance requires a very strong connection to lived experience, and that it is difficult to fight for something if you don't feel that you have been overtly deprived of it. If you are otherwise relatively advantaged by the status quo, and if you can't or won't critique your own experience in its social, historical and geographical context, it may seem unreasonable to demand what is represented as extreme in the commonsenses of the individuals, publics and institutions with which you do identify.

This is one of the preconceptions (or misconceptions?) that underline the importance of what Sandra Harding would call standpoint epistemologies and what Donna Haraway also refers to as situated knowledges:

> conducting an analysis of reproductive freedom from the point of view of *marked* groups – groups that do not fit the white, or middle-class or other 'unmarked' standard – is the only way to produce anything like a general statement that can bind us together as a people. Working uncritically from the view-point of the 'standard' groups is the best way to come up with a particularly parochial and limited analysis of techno-scientific knowledge or policy, which then masquerades as a general account that stands a good chance of reinforcing unequal privilege . . . .
>
> (Haraway, 1997b: 197)

In *The Misconceiver*, Phoebe is marked to some extent. Simply because she is a woman, certain behaviours are necessary or forbidden for her to avoid censure or punishment. However, as a white, middle-class professional – her official profession is computer programming – she is unmarked in comparison to the black women she treats who are bitter about their easy access to Norplant and tubal ligation, and who resist by risking pregnancy and managing their own bodies by enlisting the aid of misconceivers. As she has also ceased to menstruate, she imagines that she is immune from pregnancy, despite the assurance of medical professionals that there is no underlying pathology to account for her difference. So she does not have the personal investment in managing fertility that her clients do, and this may limit her political empathy. But Haraway argues that:

> *learning* to think about and yearn toward reproductive freedom from the *analytical and imaginative standpoint* of 'African American women in poverty' – a ferociously lived discursive category to which I do not have 'personal' access – illuminates the general conditions of such freedom. A standpoint is not an empiricist appeal to or by 'the oppressed' but a cognitive, psychological, and political tool for more adequate knowledge judged by the nonessentialist, historically contingent, situated standards of strong objectivity. Such a standpoint is the always fraught but necessary fruit of the *practice* of oppositional and differential consciousness. A feminist standpoint is a practical technology rooted in yearning, not an abstract philosophical foundation.
>
> (Ibid.: 198)

By the end of the novel, Phoebe, its narrator, does seem to have achieved some degree of political consciousness, and even early in the narrative she does remark on the difference that 'race' and other differences make to women's reproductive choices. However, she believes that the love and desire she feels for her male partner, and the centrality of that relationship to her subjectivity, weakens her will for activism. This tendency to focus on the individual and the closest of relationships and to decontextualise them from the larger societal webs in which they are enmeshed is represented as a temptation to disavow political analysis and avoid political activism, which is more likely to operate in positions of relative privilege. And it is this tendency that many feminist commentators on reproductive technology cite as a key barrier to developing any collective position on the benefits and pitfalls of the NRTs. Some feminists claim that we should not criticise the NRTs when they offer some benefits to some women, but rather that we should seek to extend the access to those benefits. Indeed, this may be part of the work that feminists need to do in the social arena of reproduction. But if Haraway is right, and: 'feminist knowledge is rooted in imaginative connection and hard-won political coalition – which is not the same thing as identity but does demand self-critical situatedness and historical seriousness' (ibid.), then it is not all that needs to be done. Simply making imaginative connection with those infertile women who want to avail themselves of high-tech interventions is not good enough. Their predicament needs to be set in the context of the scope of reproductive choices available to all women, in all places. The suggestion is not that women should or can step back from their deeply felt personal responses to their own reproductive bodies, rather that the work of feminist coalition demands that we take account of the full range of responses to and possibilities of reproductive bodies when we endeavour to produce knowledge about the social arena of reproduction. And speculative fiction can provide us with a template for the process of embodied imagination that will enable us to engage in this 'practical technology rooted in yearning'.

Conclusion

The ongoing challenge for feminist theory and feminist research is to hold in constant tension the need to conceptualise the theoretical research field in a maximally inclusive fashion while conducting research at suitable localised sites. As Haraway points out: 'looking for a feminist doctrine on reproductive technology in particular, or on technoscience in general, would be ludicrous' (Haraway 1997b: 191). The fields are in constant flux, always contested and contestable, and to attempt to construct a doctrine would be a hopeless attempt to freeze history, even if it were not politically dubious.

The strategic epistemological tools offered by the feminist science theorists like Harding and Haraway who suggest that we should make every effort to design research projects and set political agendas from the 'analytical and imaginative standpoint' of those marked as Other in our society, while resisting the attempt to fix or totalise categories, are key in this struggle. As Haraway points out, these are 'ferociously lived discursive categor[ies]' that require us to practise 'oppositional and differential consciousness'. In other words, just as we cannot presume to speak on behalf of others, neither should we take the easier option of minimising controversy by particularising research so much that it cannot contribute to a meta-project of developing an anti-oppressive feminist politics of women's reproductive rights. Steinberg (2000) proposes: 'an "anti-oppressive" feminist analysis of science, medicine and technology' which draws on Harding's formulations of postmodern feminist standpoint theory as well as the analyses of black feminists, including (but not limited to) Amos and Parmar, and Patricia Hill Collins. And if we can transpose the lessons of imaginative identification that we learn from speculative fiction into other research domains, perhaps we can achieve anti-oppressive feminist standpoints.

As Harding (1991b: 51) elaborates in her discussion of the requirements of strong objectivity:

> To enact or operationalise the directive of strong objectivity is to value the Other's perspective and to pass over in thought into the social condition that creates it – not in order to stay there, to 'go native' or merge the self with the Other, but in order to look back at the self in all its cultural particularity from a more distant, critical, objectifying location.

Applying this principle to the field of reproduction, Donna Haraway draws on Charlotte Rutherford's 1992 article, 'Reproductive Freedoms and African American Women' and Rutherford's articulation of what reproductive freedom would mean for contemporary African American women, to suggest that:

> all citizens would be better served by such a policy than from an approach to reproductive choice or rights that begins and ends in the well-insured sonographically monitored, Bell Telephone system-nurtured uterus with its public foetus.
>
> (Haraway 1997b: 198)

This might lead to the framing of research interests rather differently than they were in some of the earlier feminist empiricist approaches to reproductive technologies. As Steinberg (1999: 195) points out – with specific reference to Stanworth 1987a:

> To take infertile women as the starting-point in such studies has many ramifications . . . it seems to posit that the women who have the primary (or only) stake in (or will be affected by) IVF, are those who might or do undergo it.

Suggesting that women other than those undergoing IVF treatment might be affected by it does not deny the importance of taking the experiences of 'infertile' women seriously. Just as all women are implicated in the development of medical scientific practices that are directed towards women, so too are all women implicated in the specific innovations relating to IVF and their potential consequences, intended and unintended.

Both Harding and Haraway continually stress the importance of deconstructing hegemonic discourses as part of the project of standpoint epistemologies/situated knowledges/strong objectivity. If we are to avoid the dystopian excesses envisioned by Lucy Ferriss, one of the most important tasks facing feminists is to insist on feminists' competency to shape the discursive field of reproduction and not simply to respond to its shaping by medical professionals, legislators and other social and political groupings with investments in particular meanings of foetuses, mothers and reproduction.

Acknowledgements

Thanks to Caroline Vautier for the conversations that provided the environment for developing this chapter. Thanks also to the following for constructive feedback during the drafting process: Gillian Bendelow, Hannah Bradby, Amanda Hallsworth, Matthew and Monica Haran, Anne-Marie Kramer, Lisa Smyth, Lesley Spiers Meg Stacey, Deborah Lynn Steinberg. Special thanks to Gary T. Fleming.

Notes

1 *Why I Am an Abortion Doctor* is authored by Suzanne T. Poppema MD with Mike Henderson. The narrative voice is a direct address to the reader by Dr Poppema, and there is no textual explanation as to the part that Mike Henderson played in the production of the narrative.
2 According to Aurora Medical Services' website's biography of Suzanne T. Poppema MD:

> Dr Poppema is the medical director of Aurora Medical Services and a University of Washington School of Medicine Associate Clinical Professor. She is the president of the National Abortion Federation and has been on their board since 1991. Dr Poppema is recognized internationally as a leader in providing medical abortion in the United States. A graduate of Harvard Medical School, she has been practising family medicine and women's reproductive health care since 1975.

3 Sarah Lefanu took the title for her groundbreaking critical survey of the relationship between feminism and science fiction from a remark made in a short story by James Tiptree Junior (Alice Sheldon's pseudonym), which she quotes: 'What women do is survive. We live by ones and twos in the chinks of your world-machine' (Lefanu 1988: 126).
4 Peter Redman has drawn on narratology, psychoanalysis and the 'narrative turn' in contemporary social theory to account for the ways in which subjectivity is formed dialogically with narratives either in textual form or circulating culturally as commonsenses (Redman 1999: esp. chs 2 and 3).
5 In *Bodies That Matter*, Judith Butler (1993) analyses how subjectivity is constructed/enabled through a series of regulatory practices that produce bodies that matter at the cost of those who are othered or abjected. Racial discourses and the heterosexual matrix are some of those interarticulating regulatory practices.

References

Bordo, Susan (1993) *Unbearable Weight*, Berkeley, Los Angeles and London: University of California Press.
Butler, Judith (1993) *Bodies That Matter*, New York and London: Routledge.
Callahan, Joan C. (ed.) (1995) *Reproduction, Ethics, and the Law: Feminist Perspectives*, Bloomington: Indiana University Press.
Clarke, Adele E. (1998) *Disciplining Reproduction*, Berkeley, Los Angeles and London: University of California Press.
Daniels, C. (1993) *At Women's Expense: State Power and the Politics of Fetal Rights*, Cambridge, MA: Harvard University Press.
Farquhar, Dion (1996) *The Other Machine*, New York and London: Routledge.
Ferriss, Lucy (1997) *The Misconceiver*, Sceptre; New York: Simon and Schuster; UK edition, London: Hodder and Stoughton, 1998.
Gerber Fried, Marlene (1990) *From Abortion to Reproductive Freedom: Transforming a Movement*, Boston, MA: South End Press.
Goggin, Malcolm L. (ed.) (1993) *Understanding the New Politics of Abortion*, Newbury Park, CA, London and New Delhi: Sage.
Haran, Joan (2000) '(Re)productive fictions: reproduction and embodiment in Marge Piercy's science fiction', in John Moore and Karen Sayer (eds), *Science Fiction: Critical Frontiers*, London: Macmillan.

Haraway, Donna J. (1991a) *Simians, Cyborgs and Women*, London: Free Association Books.

—— (1991b) 'A cyborg manifesto', in Haraway, *Simians, Cyborgs and Women*, London: Free Association Books.

—— (1991c) 'Situated knowledges: the science question in feminism and the privilege of partial perspective', in Haraway, *Simians, Cyborgs and Women*, London: Free Association Books.

Haraway, Donna J. (1992, 1989) *Primate Visions* London & New York: Verso (first published by Routledge, Chapman & Hall).

—— (1997a) *Modest_ Witness@Second_ Millennium. FemaleMan© _ Meets _ Onco-Mouse^{TM}*, New York and London: Routledge.

—— (1997b) 'Fetus: the virtual speculum in the New World Order', in Haraway, *Modest_Witness@Second_Millennium. FemaleMan©_Meets_OncoMouse^{TM}*, New York and London: Routledge.

Harding, Sandra (1991a) *Whose Science, Whose Knowledge?*, Buckingham: Open University Press.

—— (1991b) ' "Strong objectivity" and socially situated knowledge', in Harding, *Whose Science, Whose Knowledge?*, Buckingham: Open University Press.

Hartouni, Valerie (1997) *Cultural Conceptions*, Minneapolis and London: University of Minnesota Press.

King, Katie (1994) *Theory in its Feminist Travels*, Bloomington and Indianapolis: Indiana University Press.

Kirkup, Gill, Janes, Linda, Woodward, Kathryn and Hovenden, Fiona (eds) (1999) *The Gendered Cyborg*, London: Routledge.

Lefanu, Sarah (1988) *In the Chinks of the World Machine: Feminism and Science Fiction*, London: Women's Press.

Petchesky, Rosalind Pollack (1999) 'Foetal images: the power of visual culture in the politics of reproduction', in G. Kirkup, L. Janes, K. Woodward and F. Havenden (eds), *The Gendered Cyborg*, London: Routledge.

Poppema, Suzanne T., with Mike Henderson (1996) *Why I Am an Abortion Doctor*, Amherst, NY: Prometheus Books.

Redman, Peter (1999) 'Boys in love: narrative, identity and the production of heterosexual masculinities', unpublished PhD thesis, University of Birmingham.

Rutherford, Charlotte (1992) 'Reproductive freedoms and African American woman', *Yale Journal of Law and Feminism* 4 (2): 255–90.

Sawicki, Jana (1991a) *Disciplining Foucault*, New York and London: Routledge.

—— (1991b) 'Disciplining mothers: feminism and the new reproductive technologies', in Sawicki, *Disciplining Foucault*, New York and London: Routledge.

Smith, Patricia (1995) 'The metamorphosis of motherhood', in J.C. Callahan (ed.), *Reproduction, Ethics and the Law: Feminist Perspectives*, Bloomington: Indiana University Press.

Smyth, Lisa (1998) 'Narratives of Irishness and the problem of abortion: the X case 1992', *Feminist Review* no. 60: 61–83.

Stanworth, Michelle (1987a) *Reproductive Technologies*, Cambridge: Polity Press.

—— (1987b) 'Reproductive technologies and the deconstruction of motherhood', in Stanworth, *Reproductive Technologies*, Cambridge: Polity Press.

Steinberg, Deborah Lynn, (1999) 'Feminist approaches to science, medicine and technology', in G. Kirkup, L. Janes, K. Woodward and F. Hovenden (eds), *The Gendered Cyborg*, London: Routledge.

Part II

Gender (in)equality and (emotional) division of labour

The 'two Adams' revisited?

5 What about the girl next door?

Gender and the politics of professional self-regulation

Celia Davies

Introduction

A profession, Eliot Freidson argued some 30 years ago, is an occupation of a very distinctive kind. It has gained a position in the division of labour that gives it autonomy and control over its own affairs. It has made a successful avowal to the public that there is an 'extra-ordinary trustworthiness' among its members. They can be relied upon to put their knowledge and skills at the service of the public. They will extend and develop their knowledge base in the interests of society as a whole. The profession will collectively vouchsafe that each of its members maintains the ideals of practice and will take the responsibility to ensure that newcomers are inducted in an appropriate way (Freidson 1970: xvii).

This kind of autonomy, and the self-regulation that accompanies it, Freidson warned, creates isolation. The flaw lies in the self-sufficiency of self-regulation, which:

> develops and maintains in the profession a self-deceiving view of the objectivity and reliability of its knowledge and of the virtues if its members. Furthermore it encourages the profession to see itself as the sole possessor of knowledge and virtue, to be somewhat suspicious of the technical and moral capacity of other occupations, and to be at best patronizing and at worst contemptuous of its clientele.
>
> (Freidson 1970: 70)

All this, the passage continues, leads a profession to insularity and to 'a mistaken arrogance about its mission in the world' (ibid.: 370).

These remarks have a painfully contemporary ring as case after case of the failings and failures of the medical profession hits the headlines in the British press. By the summer of 2000, with reports from the high-profile formal inquiries into the Bristol doctors and the Shipman case still to come,[1] media questioning was reaching a crescendo. Calls for reform were emanating from the health service consumer lobby too (NCC 1999a, 1999b). The Labour government, having come to power in 1997, at first saw self-regulation as a matter of 'streamlining' and making small adjustments. Three years on, in a changing political climate, it was becoming apparent that this might not be enough[2] and that an altogether more radical approach to professional self-regulation itself might be indicated.

What, however, of others who regard themselves as professionals in the health sphere? Freidson was clear that medicine's dominance in the health care division of labour left them in a markedly different and subordinate position. He acknowledged that they would seek professional status by creating many of the same institutions. What they achieved would be 'partial', 'secondhand' and 'limited by a dominant profession'. This was because 'the discriminatory power of full autonomy belies the value of using instead such institutional arrangements as training and licensing' (ibid.: 76). While analysis of these others in the health care division of labour was central to the working through of Freidson's understanding of the dominance of medicine, the nature and form of their subordination was not of interest in its own right. Furthermore, it would have been surprising, in 1970, if gender had been singled out as a critical and analytical tool.

These two themes, the significance of subordinated professions for an understanding of the institutions of regulation and the gendered division of labour, provide the twin bases for this contribution. This chapter draws on Margaret Stacey's insights into the closed culture and autonomy of medicine (Stacey 1992c). It considers the way in which it has been possible to build on these to provide a thought-provoking comparison of how the powers of regulation have been handled by the regulatory bodies in medicine and in nursing in Britain. Like Freidson, Stacey observes that regulation does not and cannot work in the same way as other professions in the health care division of labour. Stacey's pioneering unmasking of the 'gentleman's club', however, and the theoretical work which has followed leave us with more to do if we are to understand some of the dilemmas faced by the girl who sought to built a similar house next door.[3]

What is PSR?

Professional self-regulation (PSR) is a set of institutionalised practices whereby an occupational group gains the privilege of legislative recognition. It secures a statutory right to maintain a register of those it deems qualified to practise in a particular field and it is then able to decide criteria for admission to and exclusion from that register. Those excluded from the register are unable to call themselves registered and in most cases are effectively prevented from practising as members of the profession. If they falsely represent themselves as registered, they can be taken through a legal process and fined. It is a legally protected monopoly or market shelter.[4] In return for its privileged position, the profession makes an undertaking to act in the public interest. It will use its complex knowledge to set standards that work for the common good. It will also police its own members, removing from the register and hence preventing from practice those who fail to maintain those standards. PSR, in the words of the one major inquiry into its functioning in medicine, is best seen as a contract 'by which the public go to the profession for medical treatment because the profession has made sure that it will provide satisfactory treatment' (Merrison Report 1975: para. 4).

Regulatory bodies comprise a mix of elected and appointed members, the majority of whom traditionally have been drawn from the profession in question.[5] They are funded by practitioners who pay registration and, increasingly today, periodic re-registration fees. There is a number of separate bodies engaged in the practice of professional self-regulation in the health field in the UK. Regulatory bodies have long been established for doctors, dentists, opticians and pharmacists and have more recently been created for osteopaths and chiropractors. Nurses and midwives, having started separately, now share a unified regulatory structure and a single body; the Council for Professions Supplementary to Medicine offers a regulatory umbrella for a number of others (including, for example, occupational therapists, physiotherapists and radiographers).

All regulatory bodies set overall standards that the would-be practitioner must reach and in various ways oversee programmes of pre-registration education. All also have ways of reviewing individual cases of misconduct and, where it is deemed appropriate, removing practitioners from the register. There is considerable variation in the ways these bodies fulfil their functions. The publication of codes of conduct and practice has become common in recent years and the imposition of requirements for evidence of practitioners' actions to update knowledge and skills has become more widespread. The rather stronger notion that practitioners should be required to demonstrate continuing competence to such a body not only presents challenges of implementation but is, not surprisingly, deeply controversial among practitioners themselves.[6] So too is the question of the locus of a regulatory body in relation not to single episodes of serious misconduct but to poor performance.[7]

In terms of legislation, PSR is a patchwork, hard to grasp by those not intimately involved with it. Precise powers, organisation of functions and membership arrangements vary between bodies and are not well understood by practitioners, press and public (NCC 1999a, 1999b). The relevant statutes say little about the rationale of registration as such. A purpose or rationale for PSR tends to be given only in so far as legislation indicates an intention to set up and maintain a register. The crucial assumption of PSR, however, and the one firmly adhered to by regulatory bodies, is that self-regulation simultaneously provides guardianship of the standards of the profession and protection for the public. This claim to independence, to being 'trustworthy' in Freidson's terms, puts the profession in a position beyond that of the mere 'sectional' interest. It sees itself as 'above the fray' (Davies 2000), and this is what, in theory at any rate, distinguishes a regulatory body from the professional associations and trade unions with which it is often confused.

In her account of her time as a member of the General Medical Council (GMC), Margaret Stacey vividly conveys the sense of solemnity and tradition she encountered as she first entered the GMC building in 1976. She refers to the surroundings, with their nineteenth-century furnishings and busts of former presidents, as conveying a sense of continuity of tradition. She wrote of the careful preparation of new members, the shepherding into place on meeting days. She emphasised the formality and discipline – the hint indeed of pomposity which surrounds activities (Stacey 1992c: 70). Stacey also emphasised that gender, together with class and ethnicity, were key factors in creating this social reality and crucial to providing a sociological understanding of it. Early in the book, in a characteristic personal observation, she commented: 'I always felt somewhat marginal to the proceedings, a marginality stemming from my womanhood . . . and from my lay status' (ibid.: 6).[8]

Gender threads through this account in a number of ways. Stacey points out that the forerunner of today's GMC was composed entirely of men and underlines the battles that women faced in order to qualify and be recognised as doctors. She charts the first election of a woman to Council in 1933, the presence of a woman – but only one woman – on the GMC in the years from 1950 to 1970 and the slow increase of women members thereafter. Despite the changes that occurred in the 1970s and the substantial increase in overall numbers that she herself experienced, the Council, she observed, 'continues to be composed principally of an elite of white medical men' (ibid.: 84). Charting the debates that were held on the matter of tenure of the office of President, she recalls noticing that future presidents were always referred to as 'he'. She records that the entire Council collapsed in spontaneous laughter when she rose to ask whether a woman could be president, but that the President assured her that this was indeed possible (ibid.: 94).

It is in the final section of the book that the gender theme comes out most strongly. In a particularly memorable passage she writes:

> In 1858 the GMC was effectively a gentleman's club. Its promise that the public could trust those it registered amounted to ensuring that there were no 'bounders' in the medical fraternity [*sic*] who would do dastardly things such as no gentleman would do – or permit himself to be found doing. In the mid-nineteenth century committing adultery was a prime example of such inappropriate behaviour, as was making sexual advances to a patient or getting divorced. Committing murder was also not on. . . .
>
> When I joined the Council in the mid-1970s it still had some of that air of a gentleman's club about it. One felt that change was accepted reluctantly and that tradition dominated. It was a place for white men for whom good food and drink was provided as a proper accompaniment to the serious work that was undertaken.
>
> (Ibid.: 204)

She goes on at this point to say that the few women who were present in her time were treated with civility. There was 'no overt sexism or racism but a quiet acceptance of the superiority of white men and of the rightness of the established social order'. Stacey goes a long way in her final chapters towards describing the elements going to make up that sense of rightness and superiority that was part of the ethos of the GMC. It involved a strong sense of solidarity, a wish to bring the errant member back into the fold and a reluctance to admit those who were not 'one of us' and might let the side down. It involved a strong sense of difference which excludes and subordinates other health professions, displayed a remoteness even from its own rank and file, and did not recognise the interdependence of practitioners or the challenges from user and carer movements. She refers to false gods and collective illusions, to myths – of solo practice, clinical autonomy and expertise, and to a belief in cognitive exclusiveness – none of which serve the present age. It is an elite system, she remarks, that has not, and she strongly implies cannot, lived up to the trust it has been accorded and still seems to want from others. And she outlines features of a new professionalism to replace it.

A little later, and invited specifically to provide a feminist reflection on the GMC, Stacey (1994b) again emphasised the poor record of medicine in affording entry to women both to the profession as a whole and to its elite institutions. She pointed to the difficulty, in male-dominated professional conduct hearings, of conveying a woman's experience and perspective on sexual abuse and noted how, for example, being invited, as the only woman, to sit beside the president at dinner was both courteous yet patronising. She observed that the sense of superiority that pervaded the GMC was even at that point no longer going completely unchallenged, but she also noted how hard it was to begin to shift its masculinist ethos.

Intertwined as it is with a wide-ranging critique of forms and mechanisms of accountability and with a call for a public inquiry which is no less relevant today than it was when it was written, the gender dimension of Stacey's thinking is quite apparent. Yet it is not strongly foregrounded. Can this be taken further? More specifically, can the analysis be developed in such a way as to provide something to say about the dilemmas of creating institutions that are ostensibly equivalent in a world already structured by gender?

Taking a gender analysis further

Writing for a volume on feminist perspectives in health care law, Jonathan Montgomery (1998) has made a comparison between the GMC and the regulatory body for nurses, midwives and health visitors, the United Kingdom Central Council for Nurses, Midwives and Health Visitors (UKCC). His debt to Stacey is acknowledged at several points. His work represents a step beyond Stacey – though whether it is a step in quite the right direction needs to be examined.

Montgomery argues that concepts of professionalism and professionalisation cannot be understood without reference to gender: 'Both the male dominance of medicine from the second half of the nineteenth century, and the need for nurses and midwives to establish a registration system', he writes, 'can be linked with the move of health care from a predominantly domestic sphere to an occupation in the marketplace' (ibid.: 35). The footnote at this point refers to Stacey's 1988 text, *The Sociology of Health and Healing*. The major theoretical debts of his analysis are, on the one hand, to Witz (1992) and, on the other, to Gilligan (1982). Using these, he proposes two avenues of exploration.

First, there is the possibility that there may be a distinctively feminine conception of 'professionalism', emphasising corporate responsibility over individual autonomy. This would mirror the differences in approaches to moral reasoning identified by Carol Gilligan. Second, it may be that the form of professional registration is shaped by the economic and social position in which occupations find themselves. Witz argues convincingly that it is erroneous to conceive of professionalisation as a uniform strategy, and shows how it is more illuminating to think of individual professional projects in which particular professional groups adopt strategies that will succeed, given the limits and possibilities of their position (Montgomery 1998: 36).

From these starting points he draws out a contrast. The GMC, he argues, can be said to have used its powers to respect and protect the autonomy of doctors, whereas the UKCC has held more aspirational values and sought to impose these on the professions it regulates. Four distinct points of comparison relate to this. First, he underlines the power of the medical schools – institutions predating the formation of the GMC in the mid nineteenth century. The GMC, as Stacey had pointed out, regulates medical education with a very light touch. It has not by and large seen fit to inspect medical schools and has preferred to draw key people into its deliberations rather than impose requirements on them. The result is respect for academic freedom and a strong sense of what Montgomery calls entitlement. Schools are entitled to set their curricula; doctors, having successfully studied this, are entitled to register. This, he points out, not only resists any centralising power in the GMC but also prevents the NHS from requiring that doctors be educated in ways that meet immediate service needs. Nursing, by contrast, won its very recent place in higher education on the back of a regulatory body initiative. In this instance, there is some specification of the curriculum, a requirement to obtain approval of the statutory bodies – along with a dependency on the NHS to sponsor students and support clinical placements. Montgomery also makes much of the point that doctors automatically register whereas nurses have to satisfy a UKCC requirement for 'good character'.

In a second and closely related point, Montgomery links this difference to the form of drafting of the legislation. Medical Acts are framed in terms of entitlements and rights. They have taken the practising doctor as their point of reference and set limits around the powers of the regulatory body to interfere in the autonomy of the doctor. The Nursing Acts, as he puts it, 'assume sympathy with the regulator' and embrace regulation more. Making the Gilligan link he explains:

> The language of rights and entitlement, with its acontextual atomisation of individuals' positions, can be seen as a masculinist feature of the legal framework. It assumes that disputes will arise in a confrontational manner and delineates the positions of the parties. The drafting of the Nurses, Midwives and Health Visitors' Act 1997 assumes that the UKCC, the educational institutions and individual practitioners will usually co-operate with each other so that it is more important to set out what is expected of them than to describe the entitlements of parties should there be a dispute.
>
> (Ibid.: 40–1)

Distinctive approaches to ethics are then examined. While both bodies have the right to issue advice on conduct, this has been carried out differently. The UKCC sought to establish standards, setting out principles that a nurse should uphold and giving guidance not just on minimal standards but on good practice and practice improvement. The GMC's guidance, by contrast, has until recently emphasised hazards and how to keep out of trouble. The intention, Montgomery ruefully observes, 'seems to be less to protect the public from doctors than to protect doctors from the public' (ibid.: 43). Again the link to Gilligan is drawn:

> The guidance from the predominantly female professions displays a commitment to responsibility, stressing what is expected without regard to the sacrifices that it may require to deliver them. The individuality of each member of the profession is not highlighted. Rather the importance of working within relationships is stressed. Collaboration and co-operation, and appropriate reporting to those in authority are emphasised. Doctors are assumed to follow their consciences unless something untoward occurs.
>
> (Ibid.)

Fourth, turning to professional discipline and powers to sanction practitioners and remove them from the register, Montgomery puts forward a number of arguments to suggest that the UKCC operates a more punitive approach and attends to more of what he calls 'mundane details' than does the GMC.[9] He also contrasts the UKCC's insistence on a duty of whistleblowing with the more ambivalent approach of the GMC. In all, he concludes, the disciplinary procedure in nursing is seen as another opportunity to define professional norms and encourage good practice, whereas in medicine it is 'merely a mechanism for punishing those who breach the code of medical honour' (ibid.: 49). The distinct impression in all this, he points out, is that doctors are presumed to be trustworthy by their statutory body whereas nurses are not.

Both in relation to ethics and to discipline, it should be noted, Montgomery draws attention to change. Recent good practice guidance from the GMC moved in the UKCC's direction. It has adopted the language of leadership and instruction – what he calls the priest rather than the policeman. Recent moves to create opportunities to question medical performance represent a shift for medicine away from the presumption that practice will always be good practice towards the notion that practitioners are and will be in need of support and guidance.

In his conclusion, Montgomery offers strong support for the Gilligan thesis, suggesting indeed that the UKCC 'embodies a victory for a feminine ethic of responsibility over a masculinist hunger for power' (ibid.: 50). But he gives important support for the Witz thesis too. Medicine, he stresses, gained PSR from a position of pre-existing privilege. It did not need to justify itself or argue the logic of its status. In contrast, '[T]he women who sought similar privileges for their occupations had to justify them. Thus the expertise and high moral character of practitioners had to be demonstrated, not merely asserted.' Deriving directly from this, he proposes, the UKCC's 'strong grip' on practice is best seen as ' primarily a defence against those who argued that they were not truly professions and threatened to reduce their status (or frustrate the professional establishment's project to enhance it)' (ibid.: 51). In other words, without the granting of unquestioned status, the strategy has to be different – a lesson medicine today perhaps is in the process of learning.

Developing the gender agenda

Montgomery's analysis exemplifies some of the challenges of taking further the insights about gender and self-regulation bequeathed from Margaret Stacey's pioneering work on the GMC. He has done a very important service by teasing out these differences of approach between the UKCC and GMC. By holding to a contradictory position, however, by affirming the significance at once of Gilligan and of Witz, he has not provided the theoretical glue that will enable the whole to stick together effectively.[10] What then needs to be done? How can these gender analyses of Stacey and now Montgomery be taken further?

I should like to outline four theoretical points and provide a brief exemplification of their importance. First, Stacey and now Montgomery have offered key insights into the notions of masculinity that underpinned the creation of PSR and the specific form that it took. I would argue that Stacey's stress on the pre-eminent importance for doctors of clinical autonomy, their seeming reliance on an out-of-date notion of solo practice, their reluctance to admit diversity in membership, their sense of solidarity, and Montgomery's observations about rights and entitlement are of a piece. What binds them together and gives them meaning is a project of nineteenth-century middle-class masculinity: the forging of a place in the social order for a class who owed their position not to land or to trade, but to the provision of a service. I have argued elsewhere (Davies 1996) that the heroic journey of mastery of knowledge, the complex etiquette of fee-paying and referral, are all part of the same historical project. It is a project of forming a masculine identity as strongly separate and seemingly autonomous – creating a bounded, detached and deeply self-reliant notion of self as apart from other. What was emerging here was an identity as 'professional man'. Professional man could not provide for an array of dependants and employ a large retinue of servants and retainers in the manner of the land-owning country gentleman. He could maintain a middle-class household and provide for a leisured lady as its nominal head. He could, by dint of his hard work and learning, take up a position for himself as undertaking important, respected and valued work where the majority of members of the community would look up to him and the landed gentry too would be pleased to call upon his services. PSR underlines and endorses professional identity.[11] The notion that such a respected, self-respecting and exceptional group of men could and indeed must collectively regulate its own affairs, and the invention of a statutory recognised and professionally controlled register for this purpose, is a direct continuation of this thinking.

The connections are clearly visible in the review of medical regulation in the 1970s (Merrison Report 1975). Stacey locates this report in relation to the GMC of the time. In tracing its reception and the passage of subsequent legislation, she makes clear the political connections of the profession and just how much deference to doctors remained. In looking at the text of the report and its discursive content and strategy, however, two points stand out: one is the strong argument that undertaking its own regulation is crucial to the self-respect of the profession; the other is the conviction that a lay contribution notion can only be marginal and minimal given the knowledge base of the profession. There is in that report a sense of separation and self-reliance, confidence and superiority and of being apart from the ordinary mass of persons that, as a late twentieth-century woman, I have to struggle to understand. I can only understand it by seeing strong continuities with a moment of profession formation in the middle of the previous century (Davies 1996, 1999).

My second point, seeing an historicised and gendered identity project in this way, is that the way in which it becomes written into specific institutional forms needs to be brought into sharper focus. Stacey's observation, taken up by Montgomery, that the GMC never sought to control medical schools is important here. The aims of the GMC, said the Merrison Report, 'need to be disseminated not only on paper and in talk but in the minds of those who have taken part in the formative discussions' (Merrison Report 1975: para. 381). The strategy between self-respecting equals, in other words, is 'a word in your ear, old chap' and nothing more. The assumptions behind modes of disciplining doctors through the machinery of what is still called 'serious professional misconduct' deserve a paper of their own, where again Stacey's formulations have much to offer. Montgomery's comment that they are based on trust, on a presumption that few will go astray, is of a piece with the gendered and classed identity I have been endeavouring to tease out. The Merrison Report is again instructive. It was quite explicit that any form of 'large-scale continuous scrutiny' was distasteful. It is a sign of the times how much has changed and is in the throes of further change today (Irvine 2000).

The third point relates to what Stacey has for long years referred to as the gender order and the gender division of labour. A central tenet of my work on nursing in recent years has been to insist that we cannot understand masculinities apart from femininities, or the gendered health work of nurses apart from the gendered health work of doctors. Medicine and nursing are locked together in a binary relation, a relation that affirms the one and denies the other and that requires, but denies that it requires, a particular positioning of the denied group. That positioning is essential if medicine is to understand itself in the way that it does. Nursing, I have thus argued, is not a profession in the way that medicine is. To put it most simply and briefly, the preparation, cleaning and clearing, the mopping up of tears and fears is essential to preserve the fleeting encounter of medical diagnosis and advice (Davies 1995).

The third point, then, is this: if health work is characterised by binary 'othering', the institutions set up by those differently positioned by the binary divide can have the appearance but never the reality of equivalence. To treat the GMC and UKCC as similar organisations differing only in their strategies is to lock the analysis into one of two routes. The first leads to a position where the second organisation never quite lives up to the first, never quite succeeds, and by striving in that direction always teeters on the brink of an unmasking of its own self-interest. The second is a route that ends in essentialism: men and women really are such different creatures that, whatever it is, they do it differently. Montgomery, following Gilligan, advances along the second of these paths, though his reliance on Witz causes him constantly to pull back. Stacey, focused centrally on the GMC, does not need to take a decision as to which of these pathways to take.

If these points are accepted, point four is that comparisons between institutions of PSR in the health field become strategically important but tactically tricky. The UKCC is structurally in a position of subordination to medicine and struggles with the fact that the work it seeks to regulate has been constructed by gender. This does not mean today – as it has done so clearly in the past – that medical men are in a powerful position in membership of the Council and dominate proceedings. It means rather that the Council of a subordinated profession is positioned in a disadvantaged way and somehow or another it must grapple with this. Its strategies are gendered strategies not in the sense that they derive straightforwardly from the essential gender characteristics of their members; rather they are gendered in the sense that gender has been crucial to their social formation. I shall try briefly to illustrate the kind of interpretation and insight that this theoretical position might open up, taking the UKCC as my example.

Two forms of gender subordination[12]

Legislation in the 1979 Act created the UKCC and National Boards in each of the four countries of the UK. This brought together as many as nine previous bodies carrying out regulatory functions. It was a moment of flowering of PSR. A code of professional conduct was devised and issued and at once started to have a key place. There was considerable elaboration and development of the disciplinary machinery of professional conduct, particularly after new legislation in 1992 concentrated this function at Council level. There was a period of intense work on pre-registration education, followed by the development of the idea of the live register and demonstrable updating. These things meant that PSR was at its peak in the early 1980s. Interestingly, this was the very moment when the withdrawal of trust from professions in the public sector and the introduction of new forms of workplace control (at first through managerialism, later through markets) was at its most intense (Davies 2000). At the same time, there were distinct weaknesses in the initial legislation, there was a cumbersome and near unworkable structure and a tense relationship between Council and Boards, and between the professions and professional groups being regulated. The focus here, however, is on the tension between nurses and midwives within the UKCC and on the significance of them in terms of the politics of regulation and gender subordination.

How were these tensions manifested? The midwifery profession had remained unsure whether it wanted to throw in its lot with nursing in the long period following the Briggs Report in 1972 and the passing of the new legislation in 1979. Some vigorous and effective lobbying gained it a naming in the title of the Act and a statutory committee to which all 'midwifery matters' were to be referred. But midwives clashed with nurses on almost all the major policy challenges that the UKCC faced. On pre-registration education, the 2-year common foundation and 1-year specialist branches did not sit easily with midwifery's 18-month post-registration programme; nor indeed did the terminology of branches endear itself to a group whose retort was that they were not a branch but a tree! Presenting the new pre-registration education as creating more of an analytical and thinking practitioner was another flashpoint – midwives, with functions laid down in legislation, and a delimited sphere of autonomous practice, already thought of themselves as practitioners. Devising a framework for post-registration practice was another headache. Both the idea of regular updating and re-registration and the notion of specialist roles sat uneasily with the ways midwifery had developed. From a midwifery perspective, the proposals could too easily be read as bringing a danger not just of failing to recognise, but of diluting or even losing hard-won gains. When in the mid 1990s the issue of clinical supervision came on to the agenda, and the UKCC went as far as it could in face of employer prerogative in recommending it as good practice, the guidance document did not cover midwifery. Midwives had a form of statutory supervision already and this move seemed to cut across or even undermine it. The debate generated acrimony and no little confusion between the two groups.

I want to suggest that these differences need to be understood in terms of different histories of regulation, which are at the same time different modes of subordination. Midwifery gained a form of PSR nearly 20 years earlier than nursing. The doctors were divided about it. It was work that a doctor could do and work that if undertaken by a GP might well win the lifelong loyalty of a family and the augmentation of the patient list and the practitioner's income.[13] PSR in this context took a form that was closely rule-bound. The title, indeed the function, of midwife was set out in statute and protected (we might say circumscribed). Individual practitioners were closely monitored. They had to declare their intention to practise in a particular area and they had to submit to control by a local supervisor of midwives, appointed by the local authority, who was usually a health visitor, herself under the direction of the local Medical Officer of Health. Nursing, by contrast, had a very different form of PSR. Here the title 'registered nurse' was protected in statute but the function was not. A registered nurse was someone who had undertaken the prescribed training as a nurse. What the job was, how nursing was to be defined, was left to a long-running and still-running debate. There are two different forms of subordination here: the first means close rule-setting, putting boundaries around what the other is allowed to do; the second means bringing the subordinate into close and loyal relationship, influencing hearts and minds, creating the willing, deployable, all-purpose helper.

Two different histories opened up from this. The midwives came to know their rules and to see how they could make the rules work for them. Over the years, the insult of a supervisor of midwives from another professional group and of the policing function she carried out shifted towards a midwifery supervisor who could support practice and encourage professional development. When the issue of updating and demonstrating continuing competence to practise started to come on to the agenda, the midwives could say 'we do that already'. Nurses have taken a very different route. Without a framework of practice rules, on the face of it, they had more freedom. In reality, however, they did not. What PSR gave them was a lever to develop nurse education. Their battle through the years has been to improve educational entry programmes, to remove education from the clutches of the employer, to create a thinking nurse, able and eager to define and demonstrate the uniquely important contribution of nursing.[14] Their dilemma has been that they have never had the control in the workplace to carry this into effect. Their efforts have opened them to the accusation of being seen as hopeless status seekers, showing the worst sides of professionalism: its attention to itself, its inflexibility in face of change and its inattention to user needs. Each group, however, understands something of its own subordination but little of the subordination of the other. Each tries to work with its tried and familiar ways of bettering its position. The nurses' subordination is the classic gender subordination. It is the more deeply gendered – the more difficult one to name and struggle against. But putting nurses and midwives together only enhances the tensions. They have different histories, different positions in the health division of labour; they will inevitably see and respond differently. The UKCC, with both midwives and nurses under a single regulatory umbrella, has been subject to two quinquennial reviews, each carried out by a firm of management consultants (Peat, Marwick and McLintock 1989; JM Consulting undated). Both were deeply critical of the 'tribalism' they found in the UKCC, and insiders to some extent accepted this criticism. Neither report began to understand the dynamics of gender and gender subordination at the heart of PSR.

Concluding remarks

This chapter has sought to understand and theorise the dynamics of gender in ostensibly similar sets of institutions in the health care field. Drawing from the work of Stacey and Montgomery, and from an argument that profession represents an historicised and gendered ideal, it has explored some of the ways in which this has influenced the regulatory practice of nurses and doctors. A subordinated profession cannot secure the same level of institutional self-sufficiency and closure as a dominated one and it will not suffer from Freidson's 'flaw of autonomy' in the same way. At the same time, however, its experience of regulation is deeply problematic. There will be dilemmas of how to carry out key aspects of the regulatory task for which the established model offers no precedent. The experience generates internal divisions among the regulated and strong pressures among them to conform. Indeed, since nurses are frequently hierarchically subordinated in the workplace, and without the clinical autonomy and the access to resources of their medical colleagues, it may create, not the under-accountability of which the classic professions are accused, but an over-accountability in its demands that each individual is responsible for her or his professional practice.

This analysis does not regard nursing as a 'failed' or somehow 'lesser' professional project. It turns any notion of lesser importance on its head. Attending to the ambiguities of regulation for a subordinated group provides an important opportunity to reflect on both the dominant and the subordinated, and to illuminate the behaviour of each of them. If current regulatory practice is to be reformed and perhaps – as many are beginning to argue – unified across the health professions, then it needs to confront and transcend the gender legacies at the heart of its present institutional structures. This is task that Margaret Stacey pioneered when she sought to provide a feminist sociological analysis of her experience as a member of the GMC.

Notes

1 Lengthy GMC proceedings concerning the conduct of paediatric heart surgery at Bristol Royal Infirmary were conducted in a glare of adverse publicity. The final ruling in May 1998 was followed by a government decision to set up a public inquiry. Chaired by Ian Kennedy, this continued to attract attention and was due to report in autumn 2000. The trial of Dr Shipman in 1999, a GP accused of murdering fifteen women patients and convicted in February 2000, also raised questions about GMC actions and powers. Ministers again instituted an inquiry – designed to report at around the same time as the Kennedy inquiry. These along with the publication of a report on gynaecologist Rodney Ledward in June 2000 were the best-known of what seemed to be an unending series of cases reported by the press.

2 Labour policy can be traced through its White Paper on the NHS in December 1997, a consultative document on quality the following year and through the debates surrounding the Health Act, 1999. See Davies (2000), Davies and Beach (2000: ch. 9).

3 Stacey's work on the GMC arose from her experience of being a lay member and was not a topic she had chosen to focus on as strategically relevant to her theoretical thinking. She has provided, none the less, a substantial corpus of writing on this theme, which is not well known in the sociological community. Details are provided in the list of references for this chapter.

4 There are variations here in that the relevant legislation may protect the function, as in the case of midwifery, the common title, as in the case of medical practitioner (but not doctor), or the title registered (as in registered nurse, state registered chiropodist, and so on).

5 When Margaret Stacey joined the GMC, what she called truly lay membership was minimal. Lay membership of the UKCC has also been very small; equally if not more important, however, have been changes in patterns of involvement in and participation in the work of the Council by those seen as 'consumers'. See Davies and Beach (2000, ch. 8).

6 Nursing implemented a new standard for maintaining registration in 1995 which included five days of mandatory study over three years (see Davies and Beach 2000: ch. 6). The GMC took a decision in 1998 to implement a regular demonstration of up-to-dateness and ability to maintain a good standard of practice. Consultation on the detail of this is still ongoing (see Irvine 2000).

7 Stacey has critically explored this topic for medicine. See, for example, Stacey (1992a, 1992b). A brief discussion of the problem that poor performance presents for PSR in nursing can be found in Davies and Beach (2000: ch. 5). A new stage in the debate was marked by the publication in November 1999 of a consultative document prepared by the government's Chief Medical Officer. *Supporting Doctors, Protecting Patients* proposed new procedures within the NHS to deal with poor performance of doctors in the NHS. These included use of the disciplinary machinery for matters of personal misconduct (theft, violence, harassment, as well as failures to fulfil an NHS contract) and new Assessment and Support Centres to deal with clinical performance. What the document called 'serious clinical problems/mistakes' would still go direct to the GMC.

8 Equally characteristic is her deliberate setting out of the values she sought to promote in her membership. She was the lay member who felt a responsibility to speak on behalf of the public and interpret popular views. She was the social scientist with an interest in how social science was placed in the medical curriculum. She was someone committed to opposing racial discrimination and hence interested in the problems of overseas doctors and the recognition of overseas medical schools. Yet, with all these, she was also the woman interested in how

women doctors and women patients fared, and, as the book was to reveal, the woman sociologist able to interrogate her unease and reveal the masculinity of the setting in which she had found herself.

9 This is one of the points where the problems with a form of theorising that attempts to hold the Gilligan and Witz positions simultaneously is particularly marked. I would want to argue that the key point about the Hefferon case which Montgomery uses is that there is and can be *no comparator* for medicine. It thus exemplifies the problems of treating gendered institutions as equivalent – a point that I amplify in the next section.

10 Some of its problems are contained in an early passage where he says: 'It is not that professionalism is a male-dominated concept, nor that professionalisation is necessarily a battle between gender groups, but that the working of these concepts cannot be understood without reference to issues of gender' (ibid.: 35). If the last part of that sentence is true, then why the caution in the first parts? My position, exemplified in the remarks which follow, is that we must accept that profession is a male-dominated concept – it stands for a particular masculinist identity. And it affirms that identity through self-regulation.

11 An attempt to explore dimensions of gender, class and race in relation to this argument can be found in Davies (1998).

12 This section builds on Davies and Beach (2000: ch. 7). I should like to acknowledge my debt to Abigail Beach for a major part in bringing this material together and helping to develop an interpretation of it.

13 Witz (1992) is particularly helpful on these historical points.

14 Rafferty's work (1996) on the General Nursing Council in the interwar years is illuminating on this matter.

References

Davies, C. (1995) *Gender and the Professional Predicament in Nursing*, Buckingham: Open University Press.

—— (1996) 'The sociology of professions and the profession of gender', *Sociology* 30 (4): 661–78.

—— (1998) 'Gender and race, class and age: the decomposition of the professional ideal', paper presented to the session 'Gender and Professions' (WG02), International Sociological Association Congress, Montreal, July.

—— (1999) 'Rethinking regulation in the health professions in the UK: institutions, ideals and identities', in I. Hellberg, M. Saks and C. Benoit (eds), *Professional Identities in Transition*, Gothenburg: University of Gothenburg/Swedish Humanities and Social Sciences Research Council.

—— (2000) 'The demise of professional self-regulation: a time to mourn?', in G. Lewis, S. Gewirtz and J. Clarke (eds), *Rethinking Social Policy*, London: Sage.

—— and Beach, A. (2000) *Professional Self-regulation: A History of the UKCC, 1969–1998*, London: Routledge.

Freidson, E. (1970) *Profession of Medicine: A Study of the Sociology of Applied Knowledge*, New York: Dodd, Mead.

Gilligan, C. (1982) *In a Different Voice: Psychological Theory and Women's Development*, London: Harvard University Press.

Irvine, D. (2000) 'Medical regulation: modernisation continues', *Consumer Policy Review* March/April.

JM Consulting Ltd (undated) *Report on a Review of the Nurses, Midwives and Health Visitors Act 1997*, Bristol: JM Consulting Ltd.

Merrison Report (1975) *Report of the Committee of Inquiry into the Regulation of the Medical Profession*, Cmnd 6018, London: HMSO (Chairman: Dr A.W. Merrison FRS).

Montgomery, J. (1998) 'Professional regulation: a gendered phenomenon?', in S. Sheldon and M. Thomson (eds), *Feminist Perspectives on Health Care Law*, London: Cavendish.

National Consumer Council (NCC) (1999a) *Models of Self-regulation: An Overview of Models in Business and the Professions*, London: NCC.

—— (1999b) *Self-regulation of Professionals in Health Care: Consumer Issues*, London: NCC.

Peat, Marwick and McLintock (1989) *Review of the United Kingdom Central Council and the Four National Boards for Nursing, Midwifery and Health Visiting*, commissioned by Department of Health, Scottish Home and Health Department, Welsh Office, Department of Health and Social Services, Northern Ireland. Crown copyright.

Rafferty, A.M. (1996) *The Politics of Nursing Knowledge*, London: Routledge.

Stacey, M. (1988) *The Sociology of Health and Healing: A Textbook*, London: Unwin Hyman.

—— (1989a) 'The GMC and professional accountability', *Public Policy and Administration* 4: 12–21.

—— (1989b) 'A sociologist looks at the GMC', *Lancet* 1 April: 317–21.

—— (1990) 'The British GMC and medical ethics', in G. Weisz (ed.), *Social Science Perspectives on Medical Ethics*, Dordrecht: Kluwer.

—— (1992a) 'For profession or public? The new GMC performance procedures', *British Medical Journal* 305: 1085–7.

—— (1992b) 'Medical accountability: a background paper', in A. Grubb (ed), *Challenges in Medical Care*, Chichester, Sussex: John Wiley.

—— (1992c) *Regulating British Medicine: The GMC*, Chichester, Sussex: John Wiley.

—— (1993) 'Self regulation or public regulation?' (guest editorial), *AVMA Medical and Legal Journal* 4 (3): 1–2.

—— (1994a) 'Collective therapeutic responsibility: lessons from the GMC', in S. Budd and U. Sharma (eds), *The Healing Bond*, London: Routledge.

—— (1994b) 'Feminist reflections on the GMC: recreation and retention of male power', in S. Wilkinson and C. Kitzinger (eds), *Women and Health: Feminist Perspectives*, Brighton, Sussex: Falmer Press.

—— (1994c) 'From being a native to becoming a researcher: Meg Stacey and the GMC', in R. Burgess (ed.), *Qualitative Methodology*, London: JAI Press.

—— (1994d) 'Medical accountability', in G. Hunt (ed.), *Whistleblowing in the Health Service: Accountability, Law and Professional Practice*, London: Edward Arnold.

—— (1994e) 'The power of lay knowledge: a personal view', in J. Popay and G. Williams (eds), *Researching the People's Health*, London: Routledge.

—— (1995) 'The British General Medical Council: from Empire to Europe', in T. Johnson, G. Larkin and M. Saks (eds), *Health Professions and the State in Europe*, London: Routledge.

Witz, A. (1992) *Professions and Patriarchy*, London: Routledge.

6 Reflections on women's unpaid health work

Selective use of packages of care

Gillian Lewando Hundt

Introduction

This chapter takes as its starting point the work which Stacey developed on the concept of unpaid health work in discussing the role of both patients and carers (Stacey 1984, 1988). She argued that patients are actors and negotiate care, and that they, along with carers, are in effect unpaid health workers. She also drew attention to the interface between paid and unpaid health work in the hospital, clinic and home (Stacey 1988: chs 14 and 15). Others have developed this view further (Graham 1984), particularly in relation to carers of children and older people (Read 2000). The unpaid health work of pregnant women and mothers is the focus of this chapter and primary research data from the Middle East illustrates the general argument.

The central notion of women as unpaid health workers is explored in the context of reproductive health care, in particular childbirth and prenatal foetal screening. A second conceptual theme within the chapter is how professional concepts of risk are embedded in the packages of care that are developed and how lay concepts of risk underpin the way in which women choose to use them. The main argument is that women, when presented with packages of care such as hospital childbirth or prenatal screening, often choose components of these packages of care rather than the whole package. They utilise them selectively and the rationale and careful choices they make are part of their unpaid health work. The focus of this chapter is on the complexities of acceptance and refusal of components within packages of care and is in line with the view that 'the relationship between women and medical expertise is fluid and complex' (Abel and Browner 1998: 322). It focuses on the way women exercise agency and power by refusing components within packages of care.

So, in the main, women do not reject a total package of care but only certain elements of it. Rather like a discriminating shopper in a supermarket, each woman's basket or trolley of goods is different and based on a complex web of decision making, particular to her situation and life experience, her household, her socio-cultural background and her economic resources. Researchers looking at the field of complementary medicine have established that patients rarely reject biomedicine in its totality but often use multiple healers and systems of care (Sharma 1992). The choices have a clear rationale but may differ from the professional biomedical view of what is desirable.

The women figuring in this chapter are Negev[1] Bedouin who are part of the Palestinian minority living in Israel. They in a sense are part of the group of forgotten Palestinians in that their families chose to remain in Palestine in 1948 whilst many of their relatives became refugees in the Gaza Strip, Lebanon or Jordan. They are Israeli citizens and live in the Negev, a semi-arid area in southern Israel within the pre-1967 borders. I have lived, worked and conducted research with the Negev Bedouin over a period of 30 years between 1971 and 1999, and the chapter is illustrated by primary data from two different periods of research. The first example concerns women's select-ive use of hospital childbirth and is from fieldwork carried out in the early 1980s as part of my doctoral research[2] (Lewando Hundt 1988) together with some data from the infant feeding study which my fieldwork supplemented. The second example involves women's selective uptake of diagnostic tests in prenatal screening. This is from a larger research project concerned with the evaluation and improvement of maternal and child preventative health care services carried out in the 1990s, which was recently published[3] (Lewando Hundt *et al.* 2001).

Palestinian Israelis: the Negev Bedouin

The Negev, two-thirds of the land area of Israel, contains 7 per cent of the population, and the Bedouin comprise 23 per cent of the population of the Negev. In 1980, the population was 49,200 (*Statistical Abstract of Israel* 1981) (see Table 6.1). By 1995, the population of the Negev Bedouin Arabs was officially reported to be 88,300 (*Statistical Abstract of Israel* 1996) (although this is considered by many to be an underestimate and that the true figure in 1995 was between 90,000 and 95,000). Prior to the establishment of the State of Israel in 1948, it was estimated that there were between 50,000 and 70,000 Bedouin Arabs in the Negev. During the war of 1948, many Bedouin left the area for Egypt and Jordan and became Palestinian refugees. Approximately 11,000 remained (Marx 1967) and became Israeli citizens. They form part of the minority Palestinian Arab population of Israel today. They are Sunni Muslims.

Bedouin have been in the Negev since the sixth century, having migrated from the Arabian peninsula. Negev Bedouin were semi-nomadic and lived from herding sheep, goats and camels and the growing of winter barley and wheat. It has become increasingly difficult to live a semi-nomadic life, as much of the Negev is given over to agriculture, industry, towns and areas for military manoeuvres, including three airports. As a consequence, Negev Bedouin have increasingly entered the labour market, mostly as unskilled or skilled labourers.

Many Bedouin in Jordan, Syria and Egypt are under a process of

Table 6.1 Demographic trends of Bedouin and Jews in the Beersheva[1] sub-district

	1980		1995	
	Bedouin	*Jews*	*Bedouin*	*Jews*
Size of population	49,200	226,600	90,200	325,900
Population 14 years and under (%)	53.8	35.7	55.3	29.3
Birth rate per 1000	52	22	55	19.8
Infant mortality per 1000	28.3	14.1	13.5	5.5

Sources: *Statistical Abstract of Israel* 1981 and 1998.

sedentarisation in agricultural villages, whereas in Israel, in the late 1960s, the Israeli government began implementing Bedouin settlement in planned towns. The transition from tent to house has been underway for over 30 years but it is gradual. In 1982, there were two planned towns with two more under construction. The Bedouin Infant Feeding Study, which took place in 1981–2, had a sample of 1552 mothers who had given birth to babies in those years. Only 29 per cent of them were living in houses, 50 per cent were living in huts and 22 per cent were living in tents (Naggan *et al.* 1991). In 1991 a sub-sample of this group was followed up and it was found that 74 per cent were living in houses, 20 per cent in huts and 6 per cent in tents (Forman *et al.* 1995). By 1995 there were seven planned towns housing about 50 per cent of the population. The other 50 per cent still lived in shanty towns in huts and houses (with no planned infrastructure of water, electricity, sewage disposal, paved roads), or in small encampments in huts and tents. Government policy does not allow the building of permanent structures outside of the planned towns. An estimated 5 per cent are migratory within the national boundaries of Israel, but return seasonally to a permanent home base in the Negev.

The Negev Bedouin have a high birth rate and large families, so the majority of the population is young. The infant mortality rate has dropped between 1980 and 1995 but still remains twice as high as the Jewish infant mortality rate in the Negev. This reflects the living conditions and socio-economic disparities between the two groups. The women marry young and bear children throughout their reproductive years. Family planning is generally used on completion of family size but there is an increasing use of modern contraception for child spacing. The general fertility rate is 282 per 1000 women of childbearing age per year. This compares with a fertility rate of 154 per 1000 for the total Muslim population of women in Israel (calculated from data in the *Statistical Abstract of Israel* 1996). The general fertility rate for Jordan in 1990 was 168 per 1000 women (*Jordan Population and Family Health Survey* 1992) but there was variation between the urban and rural populations. The total fertility rate of married women in towns between 1988 and 1990 was 4.75 whilst amongst rural villages and Bedouin it was 6.85 (Gilbar 1997).

The Bedouin is a socially disadvantaged population, many of whom live on low incomes and in poor housing and there is a relatively high rate of unemployment compared to other groups in Israel. Many of the women have no formal education or only primary education. An increasing number attend high school and some go on to teacher training college or university. Girls started attending school in 1972 so most of the mothers in the 1980s data had not been to school. More of the mothers in the 1990s data had some formal education.

Although an articulate group within their own socially isolated community, Bedouin mothers' viewpoints are yet to be addressed by health professionals and administrators. Indeed, Bedouin women are in double jeopardy, in terms of their gender and ethnicity, and as a minority group within Israel their voices are muted (Ardener 1997; Bowes and Domokos 1996) as they are subject to both Palestinian Bedouin and Israeli patriarchy.

Selective use of hospital for the management of childbirth

The management of childbirth and obstetric care has been the subject of considerable sociological and anthropological research since the 1970s (Macintyre 1977; Oakley 1979). There has been research which looks at the history of professions in this field (Oakley 1976), anthropological research which emphasises beliefs and cultural practices (Jordan 1988), sociological research which analyses lay patient and professional service provider inter-action (Comaroff 1977; Graham and Oakley 1981), and research which analyses the impact of technology on the management of labour (Arney 1982). More recently, the body as a social construction (Martin 1989) and the role of medical technology has become more of a dominant theme in research, in particular in relation to the new technological means of reproduction, such as IVF, and diagnostic tests.

Pregnancy is an ambiguous state in the sense that it can be considered normal and natural or an illness (Mackinlay 1972; Hern 1975). Israel has a pro-natalist policy as have other countries in this region and this is shared as a value by the Palestinian minority as part of a woman's role and a way of ensuring the survival of their families and people (Anthias and Yuval Davis 1983). There is statutory maternity leave and substantial child benefit allow-ances. Women continue paid work up to the time of delivery unless given sick leave owing to complications. Within Bedouin society women also continue herding, tending livestock and carrying out domestic work until delivery and rest in the 40 days *post partum* period. Fertility and children are highly valued and a married woman is called a 'girl' (*bint*) until she has given birth to her first child when she is called a 'woman' (*hurma*).

During the Turkish and British mandates of Palestine, Palestinians gave birth at home and were attended by lay midwives. In Israel, during the 1950s and 1960s a vigorous policy of hospital childbirth was pursued as part of the development of health care and the pro-natalist policy. Women were encour-aged to give birth in hospital by this being free of cost for all citizens. These were not reclaimed costs. Delivery and hospital care subsequent to delivery were free to all. In addition, a small amount of money called the birth allowance was given to every mother. It would purchase a small fire or some baby clothes. Prior to the option of delivery in hospital, the Negev Bedouin women gave birth at home, in the squatting position, often holding on to a tent pole and being supported by other women. This was similar to the birthing practices of other Palestinian women most comprehensively recorded by Gramquist (1947). Hospital childbirth only became an option for women in the Negev area of Israel from the mid 1950s when a hospital was established in the main town, Beersheva. Thus, as hospital delivery attended by doctors and professional midwives became a national policy in Israel implemented by the Ministry of Health, so Negev Bedouin women began from the 1960s onwards to deliver in increasing numbers in hospital rather than at home.[4]

Table 6.2 shows that the percentage of home births increased rapidly over a decade. In the tribe where I carried out my fieldwork in the 1970s and 1980s, the first woman to deliver in hospital did so during the 1967 war and the baby was called *Harba*, which means war. The majority of Negev Bedouin lived within a 50 kilometre radius of the city of Beersheva and were served by the Soroka Medical Centre, the teaching hospital of Ben-Gurion University of the Negev. Over 96 per cent of Bedouin births took place in this hospital in the 1980s (Guptill *et al.* 1990; Forman *et al.* 1991).

Table 6.2 Place of delivery of Negev Bedouin women over a decade

Year	Soroka Hospital		Home		Total	
	No.	*%*	*No.*	*%*	*No.*	*%*
1972	1183	62.6	706	37.4	1889	100
1973	1225	66.0	631	34.0	1856	100
1977	1732	83.3	347	16.7	2079	100
1981	2215	96.5	80	3.5	2295	100

Sources: For 1972, 1973 and 1977: Harlap *et al.* (1977); for 1981: NIH feeding study database – hospital records of women giving birth in Soroka and tribal registrars.

Few Bedouin women today prefer home births. The younger women who have not delivered at home frequently say that they could die in childbirth (*ana bamoot fil beit*) and that they know that they and the baby would be safer in hospital if something goes wrong.[5] Older women have experienced both home and hospital confinements.

Obstetric history of a mother who had home and hospital deliveries

'My first four children were born at home. I was married when I was thirteen and I was fourteen when I had my first child (1958). My eldest was born at home and my mother-in-law helped me. When my second child was born I was alone for it was night-time. I gave birth to her and swaddled her without washing her and lay down and went to sleep after trying to cut the cord in the way my mother-in-law had done with the first. I find that giving birth lying down is more comfortable for me, although I know that many women squat when delivering babies at home. I delivered the third baby alone too and with the fourth I sent my husband to get a car to take me to hospital. When he arrived with the car, he came with my mother. The baby was almost out, so my mother cut the cord and dealt with everything. I then had two miscarriages. I went to the hospital for one and stayed at home for the other. During my fifth pregnancy, I didn't feel well. I felt tired in a way I hadn't before. I worried that maybe something was wrong. So I went to the clinic in the village for the first time and went to the hospital to have the baby' (1976) (conversation held in August 1984 when the mother was 40 years old).

Bedouin live in a 50 kilometre range of the hospital in towns, villages and shanty towns and encampments. Although almost all women gave birth in the hospital in 1982, some delivered on the way to hospital (see Tables 6.3 and 6.4).

The women most likely to give birth on the way to hospital were multipara

Table 6.3 Place of birth according to parity in 1982 of 403 mothers

Place of birth	1st–2nd		3rd–6th		6+		Total	
	No.	%	No.	%	No.	%	No.	%
Home	0	0	5	2.5	2	1.6	7	1.8
Hospital	79	97.5	182	91.5	112	91.1	373	92.5
On the way	2	2.5	12	6	9	7.3	23	5.7
Totals	81	100	199	100	123	100	403	100

Notes

1 The sub-sample of the 1982 cohort of normal birthweight babies in the Bedouin infant feeding study 1981–3 who were followed up at 2 and 9 months was 412, but parity was unknown for five home births, three hospital births and one delivered on the way to hospital so there are data on 403 of the mothers.

2 The z test of proportions demonstrates that at the 0.05 per cent level there is a significant difference between first and second births as compared to higher parities.

Table 6.4 Place of birth by planned town or shanty town/encampment of 412 mothers in 1982

Place of birth	Planned town		Shanty town/ encampment		Total	
	No.	%	No.	%	No.	%
Home	2	1.2	10	4.1	12	2.9
Hospital	164	95.9	212	88.0	376	91.3
On the way	5	2.9	19	7.9	24	5.8
Totals	171	100	241	100	412	100

with shorter labours or women living in shanty towns and encampments. It is clear that living in a town enables a woman to get to the hospital in time (there may be a confounding of parity and age, for the population of the planned towns was younger and therefore more likely to be having their first or second child). Superficially, it follows that the further away from a road, the longer the journey to a hospital; however, I would argue that the timing of arrival at the hospital was not just a matter of distance, but part of a strategy to avoid medical intervention in labour. In other words, women were deciding to manage their own labour, but to go to the hospital for delivery.

First, getting transport to hospital was not easy whether you lived in a town or an encampment. The vehicles are owned by the men in the family; they also need to be at home if they are to transport a woman in labour to hospital. Women described telling their sisters-in-law, husbands or brothers-in-law that they needed to get to the hospital and had to wait until a vehicle was found. For example, one woman living in a small encampment, who was having her second child, told her husband she wanted to get to the hospital. He walked 2 kilometres to the road in order to hail a passing Bedouin-owned vehicle and returned two hours later with a car to find that his child had been born. Although this may appear to be a clear case of delay owing to distance and difficulties of access, there may also be more complex explanations. Women related repeatedly that they waited at home until labour was well advanced before they made public the fact that they were in labour and needed transport to the hospital. A false alarm would cause so much bother and expense and would be shameful (*ayb*), and also arriving late discouraged medical intervention, as one woman explained: 'I wait at home and keep walking up and down and go to the hospital at the last minute. That way they can't do things to you.' Another claimed: 'A few years ago you would have been sent home if it wasn't time to give birth. Now you're put into that ward A2.'

There is a widespread fear and dislike of Caesareans because they involve an operation and limit a woman's fertility. In one instance, there were over twenty women present on a congratulatory visit to woman in her home after childbirth. Five of these women had had one or two Caesareans, including the mother of the newborn baby, but two others, when told they needed a Caesarean section, had refused to sign for one, and both of them had delivered normally. One young mother of three had had a Caesarean with her first and third child, another had had one with her first child and then subsequently delivered vaginally. There was a general consensus that although Caesareans were sometimes necessary, they were to be avoided. Some women felt that it was preferable to lose the baby and retain unlimited fertility.

It could be asked whether the hospital had an interventionist approach to labour in the 1980s. As we know, Caesarean rates vary within and between hospitals and countries. In 1983 the rates in the US were 20.3 per cent and in Britain were 10.1 per cent (Savage 1986: 83–4, 86). The Soroka Medical Centre had become a teaching hospital with the opening of a medical school in the mid 1970s and foetal monitors were installed for use in the delivery room from the late 1970s. Published data from 1977 show that, whereas Jewish women had a rate of 4.3 per cent of Caesarean sections, Bedouin women had a rate of only 1.8 per cent. In general there was a lower level of interventions in Bedouin births than in Jewish births and these differences are not explained on the basis of lower risk because the recorded complication rates show that Bedouin differed little from Jews in this respect (Harlap *et al.* 1977: 525–6).

By 1982, the rate of Caesarean section had increased to 4 per cent of Bedouin deliveries, bringing it close to the rate for Jewish deliveries in 1977. Other interventions had increased such as induction of labour, forceps delivery and vacuum extraction. Out of 1780 births during 1981 and 1982, 47 per cent were being monitored during labour and only 41 per cent had no intervention whatsoever (Forman *et al.* 1991). This would seem to indicate that the hospital management of labour had become more active and more typical of a high-technology approach of a teaching hospital rather than a low-technology approach of a district hospital.

The ability to bear children is supremely important to Bedouin women, as it defines a woman's status to a large extent. She does not control her own fertility and her children belong to her husband's family. If she cannot conceive she may be divorced, and if she has too few children or not enough sons her husband may take a second wife. A Bedouin woman needs therefore to protect her fertility and a Caesarean threatens this by putting a limit on the number of future births she can have. There is no conflict of interest between Bedouin men, Bedouin women and medical staff on the common goal of delivering healthy babies. The conflict arises when intervention involves limiting fertility and when hospital childbirth means controlling and managing labour. Therefore Bedouin women attempt to retain control of their labour and their fertility by trying to arrive when labour is well advanced. Midwives commented that Bedouin women often arrive in the second or third stage of labour nearly fully dilated, in contrast to Jewish women, who arrive in the early stage of labour. By arriving late in labour, the women certainly avoided shaving, enemas, monitoring, lying horizontally and immobile during labour strapped to a monitor (routine practice in the early 1980s) and, in their view, possible surgical intervention. I would argue that Bedouin women perceive the hospital as a place to give birth but believe that labour should be managed at home, provided it is not problematic. Therefore they developed a pattern of selective use of the hospital obstetric and labour wards in line with their own priorities and values.

Selective use of prenatal foetal diagnostic screening

Health professionals are increasingly screening healthy women, a procedure that, within sociology, is conceived of as a form of surveillance (Howson 1998; Armstrong 1995). Screening is carried out on a routine basis to detect both treatable and non-treatable conditions. Prenatal screening is an area of health care in which advances in medical technology have enabled an increasingly precise knowledge of foetal development. Hence prenatal care now includes not only monitoring a mother's health during pregnancy through checking her blood glucose, haemoglobin and blood pressure levels, but also an increasing number of procedures aimed at screening the development of her foetus.

The issues of screening and the detection of abnormalities are connected to the debate on contrasting medical and social assessments of risk and danger. Multiple understandings of risk are an important area of debate within public health today. The statistical, medical and lay assessments of risk are arrived at in very different ways and are often contradictory. As Lupton (1993) points out, the notion of statistical risk was derived from mathematical probabilities and was neutral. The meaning of 'risk' has changed as it has become part of social and political discourse. In her essay 'Risk and Danger', Mary Douglas writes: 'the idea of risk is transcribed as unacceptable danger' (1994: 39), and suggests a concept of risk that takes into account the cultural as well as the political context of risk perception. This should include assessing whether the risk is 'integral or peripheral' to the individual and the community, and how it is thought to affect the individual and the collective community (ibid.: 46).

Recent work in the sociology of the body views the body as a social construction (Shilling 1993) or a phenomenological entity understood through lived experience (Turner 1992; Nettleton and Watson 1998). Other current sociological and anthropological work in the area of childbirth and prenatal care contrasts 'authoritative knowledge', usually of health personnel (Sargent and Bascope 1996), to the 'embodied knowledge' of women. Recent research has begun to explore women's views of prenatal screening and their rationales for being screened and taking the subsequent decisions on whether or not to proceed with their pregnancies (Rapp 1993, 1998; Browner and Press 1995). The recent development and delivery of new reproductive technologies in prenatal screening to detect foetal abnormalities has highlighted this area of health care research.

Browner and Press found that 90 per cent of the women they studied in California accepted diagnostic tests such as alpha-fetoprotein (AFP) blood tests which screen for neural-tube defects and the possible presence of Down's syndrome as a routine part of prenatal medical care partly due to the way in which it is routinised in clinic routine and in the language used: namely, a 'simple blood test' (Browner and Press 1995: 309). Rapp has explored patterns of amniocentesis use and rejection by women, and highlighted how their decisions are influenced by aspects of their own social context: religion, social networks, significant others or past reproductive history. She has maintained that 'pregnant women are thus positioned as ethical gatekeepers *vis-à-vis* this technology. They are at once moral pioneers and cultural conscripts in a social drama played out upon an uneven and shifting terracing on which reproductive technologies are routinized in a multi-cultural, class and gender stratified world' (Rapp 1998: 165).

Prenatal care

Routine preventative maternal and child health care services in Israel are provided by a national network of community maternal and child health (MCH) clinics, the majority of which are run by the Ministry of Health. Public health nurses are the primary care givers in the MCH clinics, with physician support provided through periodic visits to the clinics by paediatricians and obstetricians. These clinics operate according to national guidelines established by the Public Health Service of the Ministry of Health for providing prenatal and well-baby preventative care. A service charge of US$50 per family gives coverage for six months of prenatal and well-baby care. Families who receive income support from the government can obtain an exemption from the payment of fees. Fee-for-service care is available to citizens and non-citizens.

In 1995–6, there were ten MCH clinics in planned Bedouin settlements, one in Beersheva and four in Jewish development towns serving Bedouin women and children. The majority of the twenty-seven nurses working in the MCH clinics serving the Bedouin were Jewish. Among the twenty-seven nurses, four were Arabs from central or northern Israel and five from the local Bedouin community.

In 1996, the following specific screening services were available in Israel:

- Ultrasound screening at 18–22 weeks was free of charge for all women who were covered by curative health insurance and usually included full foetal screening.
- The maternal serum alpha-fetoprotein (AFP) test was available through routine referral to all women at a cost of US$12 at 16–19 weeks. This screened for neural-tube defects and the risk of Down's syndrome. The AFP test was recommended to all women, while those over 35 years of age might be referred for an amniocentesis without it.
- Amniocentesis was recommended to all women 35 years of age or older and paid for by the Ministry of Health. Younger women were referred for an amniocentesis or third-level sonography when earlier screening test results indicated the possibility of a problem. The costs of these referrals were covered by health insurance, otherwise an amniocentesis cost $300. This test primarily detects Down's syndrome and other chromosomal anomalies. It can also be used to detect specific genetic mutations.

The clinic could be attended for a variety of purposes including confirmation of pregnancy, foetal screening and the monitoring of maternal health. The data indicate that women pick and choose services from the package of prenatal care. Women who register early may not do so in order to undertake foetal screening: they may come to have a urine test to find out if they are pregnant and may not return to the clinic for prenatal care until much later in pregnancy.

Preventative maternal and child health clinics in Israel provide care on payment of a six-monthly fee of about US$50. As a socially disadvantaged population, this payment for immunisation of their children and prenatal care is, for many Bedouin families, a significant expenditure and is often paid for out of the state child benefit allowance (Beckerleg *et al.* 1997). One way of minimising the payments and maximising the care is to register in the third trimester of pregnancy so that the first three months of the child's immunisations are covered. Alternatively women could register for prenatal care and confirmation of pregnancy whilst covered for the immunisation of their previous child. In addition, apart from financial constraints, local 'embodied knowledge' may encourage women to register in the second trimester. There are two words used to denote pregnancy in the colloquial Palestinian Arabic of the Bedouin. *Mehlife* is used to describe the state of the mother during the first few months before the foetus moves and before the pregnancy shows. Once this stage is over, between 12–16 weeks, the mother is said to be *Hamile* and the pregnancy becomes public knowledge. This terminological distinction may indicate complex local conceptions about the nature of pregnancy and foetal development and this may affect prenatal care utilisation.

This discussion of the selective use of foetal screening draws on two sources of data: clinic record extraction and semi-structured interviews (Lewando Hundt *et al.* 2001). The logbooks of all Ministry of Health MCH clinics serving the Bedouin population in the Negev were examined to identify all infants born in January 1994 and in January 1995: 701 infants were identified. However, only 537 (77 per cent) of their mothers attended MCH clinics for prenatal care and they comprise the sub-sample upon which the data extraction part of the study was based. The following information was abstracted: date of clinic registration; uptake of screening tests; characteristics of the family (consanguinity, maternal and paternal education, parity, death of a previous child). There were no data on the prenatal care of 23 per cent of the mothers who did not attend the clinics.

The data show that in this group of 537 women who attended the clinics for prenatal care, 91.6 per cent had at least one ultrasound at some point during pregnancy. However, uptake of screening tests for congenital malformations and hereditary disease was considerably lower. Our data indicate that few of the women referred for maternal serum alpha-fetoprotein (AFP) tests, amniocentesis or specifically for ultrasound at 18–22 weeks, when foetal screening may take place, actually undertook the tests.

The most popular test for detection of congenital anomalies is ultrasound, but the rates of uptake of referrals for ultrasound performed at 18–22 weeks when foetal screening tests, if indicated, are carried out, are relatively low. Data show that women who come early (before week 13) and those who come later (after week 23) are less likely to have any of the tests; 17 per cent of women who had registered by week 17 took up the referral to carry out an MSAFP (mothers must register for prenatal care in the first trimester if they are to be referred by the MCH nurses for the MSAFP test) (Lewando Hundt *et al.* 2001: table 1).

Analysis showed that none of consanguinity, maternal age or maternal or paternal education was associated with the uptake of tests. Parity had a curvilinear association with test uptake; primipara, on the one hand, and women with nine or more previous births, on the other, had the highest test uptake. The only strong and significant predictor of test uptake was the death of a previous child: mothers who had lost a child were more likely to undergo foetal screening (ibid.: table 2).

In-depth interviews were held in the homes of sixteen mothers who had been participants in an earlier phase of the larger research project. These mothers were selected as key informants because they appeared to be articulate and open to discussion. The in-depth interviews picked up four broad themes relating to women's exercise of choice and control over their own bodies and lives. One of these themes concerned ideas about the nature of risk in relation to screening tests during pregnancy. The following quotes from interviews reveal the rationales which explain why women use prenatal care but do not take up diagnostic foetal screening tests; in other words, they use the prenatal care on offer selectively. The women showed a keen awareness about the nature of prenatal foetal screening and that marriage within the family may possibly but not always cause problems, as the following quotes show:

> The tests at the clinic are more important if the couple is from the same family and tribe because their children are more likely to have problems or be disabled.

> Everybody these days knows the dangers of marrying within the family but nobody takes action. This kind of marriage is still preferable according to custom. If any outsider comes asking for the hand of any girl in the tribe, her parents won't agree. Thus the tests at the clinic are very important because there is a big chance of having a deformed foetus in this situation.

> They asked me to go to the hospital for a blood test. They wanted to know whether the child was deformed or not. I refused to go there because women told me that this is a difficult test and the foetus's life is endangered because they pass the needle inside the womb to reach the foetus and pull out some of its water. So I didn't go – I delivered and everything is fine, thank God.

> The last time the nurse asked me to do the blood test and to check the foetus's headwater, I didn't want to do these tests. Firstly my children are fine with no problems. Secondly my husband and I are not from the same family and thirdly I am still young [35 years old].

We have men who didn't marry their cousins. Our neighbour's wife, for example, is not from his tribe but, despite that, their daughter has some health problems, while others have married their cousins and have healthy children. Everything is from Allah and it is his will and everything is luck (*naseeb*). I have heard many times that if a couple is from the same family, their chances of having a deformed infant are higher.

In our tribe there is no difference between children whose parents are related and those children whose parents are from different families. Both are healthy and fine. However, I can see the difference in other families when there are couples from the same families who have children who are disabled. We cannot guess, or foresee this happening, everyone has their own fate. Some couples have healthy children despite being from the same family, and some couples who are not from the same family have children with disabilities.

Parallel cousin marriage is the socially preferred marriage pattern in the Middle East amongst Muslim communities. The Negev Bedouin is no exception to this general pattern, men preferring to marry their father's brother's daughter (*bint amm*). This used to enable property in the form of herds and land to be kept within the family. In addition, women are protected by marrying relatives as they continue to live near their natal family and are thus able to visit their parents, siblings and cousins. Indeed, the term used to designate an unrelated possible husband is 'foreigner' or outsider (*ajnabee*).

Marrying within the family is a regional pattern perpetuated for reasons of economy, security and property. The Negev Bedouin is a displaced population of whom only a small fraction remained in Israel after the war in 1948 to face an uncertain political future with few resources. Those who remained sought mutual support and protection, achieved by continuing to marry relatives even if the pool of potential spouses was now small. After the 1967 war, the borders between Israel and the Occupied Territories of the West Bank and Gaza Strip were opened and marriages were contracted with kin who had left the Negev and become refugees in the Occupied Territories. Thus, kin links were revived. Today, families reckon that they can protect and support their daughters better if they are married to relatives. They live near their own parents and siblings and their families and so the extended family is strengthened and honour is upheld, even if herds and land are no longer shared. The risks of marrying out and living amongst foreigners are significant: mothers-in-law can be oppressive and husbands have more freedom to be abusive to unrelated wives, for there is less social pressure to maintain a harmonious relationship (Lewando Hundt 1984).

An indication of the rate of consanguineous marriage amongst the Negev Bedouin at the time of the study in the mid 1990s can be derived from the analysis of 148 home interviews undertaken six months after childbirth. These showed that 58 per cent of the mothers were married to relatives, while

42 per cent were married to unrelated men. Of the 58 per cent who were married to relatives, 26 per cent were married to first cousins. Marriages are arranged between families and the girls are increasingly consulted.

Perception of 'false alarms'

> This is a sensitive issue and everything is God's will. Once my neighbour became pregnant and the doctors told her that the foetus was deformed and advised her to have an abortion. The foetus was a boy and she had four girls. So she and her husband refused to have an abortion. They were very worried during the pregnancy. She was sick, ate little and kept on crying. When she gave birth, we all had a big surprise for the boy was normal and healthy and is now two years old today. . . . My sister also had an ultrasound of her foetus and they told her that he had no spinal column at all. My sister kept the foetus, and after she gave birth we found that the baby girl was completely healthy. She is four years old now.

Bedouin women understand that consanguinity can lead to the birth of impaired children. But they also argue that both the consequences of consanguinity and the tests are uncertain in their outcome. Bedouin women frequently cite false alarms as a way of illustrating how wrong the results of screening can be. Women's expectations regarding the accuracy of the tests are gleaned largely from information given to them by health providers. For example, according to the policy of the Ministry of Health, the result of an AFP test that puts a woman at the risk of having a Down's syndrome baby at 1 in 380 entails a recommendation for diagnostic amniocentesis. The semi-structured interviews clearly indicate that the statistically increased chance of having an abnormal foetus is interpreted by women as a definite diagnosis. Consequently, the tests are perceived as imprecise and the results often wrong.

Women recognise that not all offspring of consanguineous unions are adversely affected, and that the probability of bearing an impaired child is actually quite low. Analysis of the record review data found no relationship between consanguineous marriage and the uptake of screening tests during pregnancy. Nevertheless, women appeared to be well aware of the problems that may sometimes occur as a result of consanguineous marriage and of the role of screening in detection. This knowledge may be derived from personal experience or from observation, as the excerpts from the interviews indicated.

An additional reason for not taking up a referral for a foetal screening test is the fact that these tests could lead to a request by the medical staff for the pregnant woman to have a termination when the pregnancy is well advanced, which is not considered permissible.

Religion and abortion

> The religious view is still a problematic matter. If I was pregnant and doctors told me I had a deformed foetus, I would not agree to an abortion because this is against our religious principles. I personally could not do it for religious reasons, because I consider it to be killing a soul.

> In our society it would be too late to do anything about that because the woman is not allowed, according to our religion, to have an abortion. Hence there is no point in doing tests during pregnancy. It's only a waste of time, money and effort. Only if the woman herself has a severe health problem during pregnancy would it be worth doing the tests. According to the religion, if her life is at risk because of the pregnancy, she is allowed to have an abortion.

> I believe abortion is not prohibited if it is done in the first four months of pregnancy because during this period the foetus has no soul.

Within Islam, there is a plurality of views concerning the permissibility of abortion. Some scholars and their followers argue it is not permitted at all. Others say that it is permitted up to seven weeks, while some argue that abortion is permitted up to 120 days after conception, or according to some other scholars, until the foetus quickens in the womb (Hathout 1997). A recent *fatwa* (interpretative ruling of Islamic texts and legislation by a religious authority) from the Mufti of Jerusalem (the highest Islamic judge in the area) allows abortion up to 120 days after conception if the mother's health is at risk or if the baby is deformed. Earlier testing would enable women to have the pregnancy terminated before the end of four months so that Islamic rulings would be obeyed and before the pregnancy was public knowledge.

The data indicate that those who use the clinics do so selectively with regard to foetal screening. MSAFP and amniocentesis are seen as possibly leading to the recommendation to have an abortion, which many women do not consider a viable option. A similar lack of uptake of referrals for these diagnostic tests occurs amongst religious Jews. The in-depth interview findings reported here indicate that Bedouin women may be more likely to agree to a termination of pregnancy if this is performed within 120 days of conception. A study of parental choice amongst the Negev Bedouin suggests that couples are more likely to opt for termination if the anomaly is detected early in pregnancy (Sheiner *et al.* 1998). Earlier terminations would possibly be more acceptable if women who had registered for prenatal care very early in their pregnancy (weeks 10–11 of gestation) could be offered chorionic villus sampling (CVS), which is not currently available.

In the main, assessment of levels of risk is a conceptual issue, viewed differently by health providers and Bedouin women. Bedouin women have a local understanding of the related concepts of danger or risk, chance and luck. The women interviewed made frequent references to God's will (*kull ishee min Allah*) and to the role of luck or chance (*naseeb*), and thus articulated the view that the birth of a healthy or disabled child is beyond their control. What is within their control is the decision not to take up diagnostic foetal screening tests.

The selective use of prenatal diagnostic tests is understood by Israeli health personnel as a reluctance among women to have abortions if a potential problem is detected. Nevertheless, they continue to encourage the uptake of tests, as Browner and Press (1995: 320) point out: 'Once a test exists, whether a woman accepts it is not a neutral act: refusal carries the explicit rejection of technical expertise and implies a reluctance on the part of the expectant mother to do everything in her power to assure the health and well-being of her developing foetus.'

Conclusion

The selective use of screening tests reported here demonstrates that the medicalisation of prenatal care with the use of advanced technology does not simply result in the mechanistic domination of the service user. Decisions concerning the take-up of screening are not solely guided by individual concerns. Lock (1998: 231), in her research on the use of genetic testing by women in Japan, has pointed out that 'communities and families often expect to influence reproductive decisions made by young couples' and that this is typical of 'community-based family types'. Further research in this area could explore the involvement of others in the family and the community in decision making regarding reproductive technologies.

The women reported in this study make rational choices regarding the appropriate level of surveillance of their bodies and acceptable levels of medical intervention, as do women in Japan and the US (Lock 1998; Rapp 1998). However, their 'embodied knowledge' may conflict with the 'authoritative knowledge' of medical staff (Browner and Press 1996). Health professionals, along with much of 'Western' society, appear to be trying to minimise risk in all its manifest forms. However, the tests cannot fully achieve this, and perhaps women service users realise more fully than health professionals that risk is an integral part of life.

These are two examples of unpaid health work resulting in the selective use of health care. The first is the avoidance of medical interventions in labour whilst simultaneously choosing to go to the hospital for childbirth. The second is the avoidance of prenatal foetal diagnostic tests whilst simultaneously accepting other aspects of routine prenatal care. These women wanted to safeguard both their chances of having a healthy baby and their future unlimited fertility. Their selective use of health care and specific aspects of medical technology is an indirect use of power. They rarely directly refuse the care. They take the referrals for the foetal screening tests but do not use them. They arrive late at the hospital rather than refuse procedures, although do so when it is unavoidable. This indirect pattern of selective use is related to the fact that these women are from a socially and economically disadvantaged group who are a minority within Israel. They are disadvantaged by ethnicity, gender and class within the wider Israeli society and are muted within their own Bedouin society. They exercise power indirectly (Lewando Hundt 1984). They are not part of a primarily middle-class, educated, organised group such as the National Childbirth Trust. They are selectively using the care on offer, despite often speaking little of the dominant language of the health care providers (Hebrew) and are thereby safeguarding their fertility, the health of their children and themselves through their unpaid health work.

This unpaid health work of challenging medical hegemony and particular aspects of medical technology or elements of health care is not unique to Palestinian Bedouin. The current 'low' uptake of the triple measles, mumps and rubella (MMR) vaccine in England owing to anxieties about possible ill effects is another example of selective use of health care. There are many examples of selective use. The choices made are not only due to problems of access or information: they are the result of careful rationales and examples of unpaid health work.

Acknowledgements

I should like to thank the women who gave their time and thoughts so generously. The infant feeding study was funded by the National Institute of Child Health and Disease 1981–3 and carried out collaboratively with the Faculty of Health Sciences, Ben Gurion University of the Negev. The fieldwork was carried out by me. The research on foetal screening presented here was part of a larger study financed by the European Commission Avicenne Initiative Grant CT93A12–031 administered from DG XII 1995–9 on the maternal and child health care to Bedouin in the Negev and Palestinians in Gaza.

Notes

1　There are some differences in Hebrew and Arabic names for both the Negev/ Negeb and Beesheva/Beersheba. In Hebrew a v replaces the b. In Arabic there is no v. The Hebrew letter used (Bet) can be pronounced either as a b or v. In biblical and Victorian literature the town is referred to as Beersheba. In this paper the contemporary pronunciation as used in Hebrew is used.

2　This chapter contains data from my PhD thesis which was undertaken at the University of Warwick. When I was looking for somewhere to consolidate and complete a PhD, I wrote to Meg Stacey about whether it would be possible to spend this time as a mid-career break in the Sociology Department. She replied that, although she could not supervise me, there would be plenty of people to talk to at Warwick who were interested in issues of gender, ethnicity and class in relation to health. The inclusive atmosphere of engaged intellectual debate and commitment which she fostered remains. So it seemed fitting to write this around a key concept within her work with primary data from that period when so many people were debating aspects of ethnicity, gender and health.

3 The data on prenatal screening has been published as 'Knowledge, action and resistance: the selective use of prenatal screening among Bedouin women of the Negev, Israel', *Social Science and Medicine* (2001) 52 (4): 561–776. The authors are myself as first author, Shoham Vardi, who undertook all the statistical analysis and some of the preliminary qualitative data analysis with me, Kassem, who carried out the interviews, and Beckerleg, who also worked on the writing of the paper with me. The drafts were reviewed by all the authors whom I acknowledge – Shoham-Vardi, Beckerleg, Kassem, Abu Jafar and Belmaker and Abu Saad. Excerpts from this paper are reprinted with permission from *Social Science and Medicine*.

4 There are hardly any home deliveries in Israel. Midwives work in hospitals. This is in great contrast to a plural system of delivery in Gaza, where around 40 per cent of births are in hospital and the rest either in clinic settings (United Nations Relief and Works Agency – UNRWA – or private) or at home with a lay or professional midwife.

5 Medical staff and other Jewish Israelis have often told me that Bedouin women give birth in hospital in order to receive the small birth grant. No Bedouin woman has ever told me this. The idea that the hospital is used for childbirth for primarily financial gain is, in my view, mistaken.

References

Abel, E.K. and Browner, C.H. (1998) 'Selective compliance with bio-medical authority and the uses of experiential knowledge', in M. Lock and P.A. Kaufert (eds), *Pragmatic Women and Body Politics*, Cambridge: Cambridge University Press.

Anthias, F. and Yuval-Davis, N. (1983) 'Contextualizing feminism: gender and class divisions', *Feminist Review* 15: 62–75.

Ardener, E. (1977) 'Belief and the problem of women and the "problem" revisited', in S. Ardener (ed.), *Perceiving Women*, London: Dent.

Armstrong, D. (1995) 'The rise of surveillance medicine', *Sociology of Health and Illness* 17 (3): 393–404.

Arney, W.R. (1982) *Power and the Profession of Obstetrics*, Chicago: University of Chicago Press.

Beckerleg, S., Lewando Hundt, G., Belmaker, I., Abu Saad, K. and Borkan, J. (1997) 'Eliciting local voices: the use of natural group interviews', *Anthropology and Medicine* 4 (3): 273–88.

Bowes, A.M. and Domokos, T.M. (1996) 'Pakistani women and maternity care: raising muted voices', *Sociology of Health and Illness* 18 (1): 45–65.

Browner, C.H. and Press, N.A. (1995) 'The normalization of prenatal diagnostic screening', in F.D. Ginsburg and R. Rapp (eds), *Conceiving the New World Order: The Global Politics of Reproduction*, London: University of California Press.

—— and —— (1996) 'The production of authoritative knowledge in American prenatal care', *Medical Anthropology Quarterly* 10 (2): 141–56.

Bullock, C. and Khalid, F.N. (1995) 'Health issues related to customary consanguineous marriages among Pakistanis', *Health Promotion International* 10 (3): 209–18.

Comaroff, J. (1977) 'Conflicting paradigms of pregnancy: managing ambiguities in antenatal encounters', in A. Davies and G. Horobin (eds), *Medical Encounters: Experiences of Illness and Treatment*, London: Croom Helm.

Davis-Floyd, R.E. (1990) 'The role of obstetrical rituals in the resolution of cultural anomaly', *Social Science and Medicine* 31 (2): 175–89.

Douglas, M. (1994) 'Risk and danger', in M. Douglas, *Risk and Blame: Essays in Cultural Theory*, London: Routledge.

Forman, M.R., Berendes, H.W., Lewando Hundt, G. *et al.* (1991) 'Perinatal factors influencing infant feeding practices at birth: the Bedouin infant feeding study', *Paediatric and Perinatal Epidemiology* 5: 168–80.

——, Lewando Hundt, G., Berendes, H.W., Abu-Saad, K., Zangwill, L., Chang, D., Belmaker, Abu-Saad, I. and Graubard, B.I. (1995) 'Undernutrition among Bedouin Arab children: a follow-up of the Bedouin infant feeding study', *American Journal of Clinical Nutrition* 61: 495–500.

Gilbar, G.G. (1997) *Population Dilemmas in the Middle East*, London: Frank Cass.

Graham, H. (1988) *Women, Health and the Family*, Brighton, Sussex: Harvester Press.

—— and Oakley, A. (1981) 'Competing ideologies of reproduction: medical and maternal perspectives on pregnancy', in H. Roberts (ed.), *Women, Health and Reproduction*, London: Routledge and Kegan Paul.

Gramquist, H. (1947) *Birth and Childhood Among the Arabs: Studies in a Mohammedan Village in Palestine*, Helsinki: Sodestrom.

Guptill, K., Berendes, H.W., Chang, D., Sarov, B., Naggan, L. and Lewando Hundt, G. (1990) 'Seasonality of birth among Negev Bedouin women in Israel', *Journal of Biosocial Sciences* 22: 213–23.

Harlap, S., Prywes, R., Grover, N.B. and Davies, A.M. (1977) 'Bedouin and Jews in southern Israel: maternal, perinatal and infant health in Israel', *Journal of Medical Sciences* 13 (5): 514–28.

Hathout, H. (1997) 'Islamic views on some reproductive issues in cultural and religious attitudes towards genetic issues', in A.S. Teebi and T.I. Farraj (eds), *Genetic Disorders Among Arab Populations*, Oxford: Oxford University Press.

Hern, W.M. (1975) 'The illness parameters of pregnancy', *Social Science and Medicine* 9: 365–72.

Howson, A. (1998) 'Surveillance, knowledge and risk: the embodied experience of cervical screening', *Health* 2 (2): 195–216.

Jordan, B. (1988) *Birth in Four Cultures: A Cross-cultural Investigation of Childbirth in Yucatan, Holland, Sweden and the United States*, 4th edn, Montreal: Eden Press.

Jordan Population and Family Health Survey 1990 (1992) Amman and Columbia, MD: DS & IRD/Macro International.

Lewando Hundt, G. (1984) 'The exercise of power by Bedouin women', in E. Marx and A. Shmuelli (eds), *The Changing Bedouin*, Brunswick, NJ: Transaction Inc.

—— (1988) 'Health inequalities and the articulation of gender, ethnicity and class amongst Negev Bedouin Arab mothers and their children', unpublished PhD thesis, University of Warwick.

—— (1999) *Evaluation and Improvement of Maternal and Child Health Services for Palestinians in Gaza and Bedouin in the Negev*, Final report on CT93AV12–031, Brussels: European Commission, DG XII.

—— and Forman, M.R. (1997) 'Autonomy, access and care: a study of Palestinian Bedouin of the Negev in Israel', *Social Sciences in Health* 3 (2): 96–112.

——, Shoham-Vardi, I., Beckerleg, S., Belmaker, I., Kassem, F. and Abu Jafar, A. (2001) 'Knowledge, action and resistance: the selective use of prenatal screening by Bedouin women in the Negev, Israel', *Social Science and Medicine* 52 (4): 561–76.

Lock, M. (1998) 'Perfecting society: reproductive technologies, genetic testing, and the planned family in Japan', in M. Lock and P.A. Kaufert (eds), *Pragmatic Women and Body Politics*, Cambridge: Cambridge University Press.

Lupton, D. (1993) 'Risk as moral danger: the social and political functions of risk discourse in public health', *International Journal of Health Services* 23 (3): 425–35.

Macintyre, S. (1977) 'The management of childbirth: a review of sociological research issues', *Social Science and Medicine* 3: 477–84.

Mackinlay, J.B. (1972) 'The sick role: illness and pregnancy', *Social Science and Medicine* 6: 561–72.

Martin, E. (1989) *The Woman in the Body: A Cultural Analysis of Reproduction*, Milton Keynes: Open University Press.

Marx, E. (1967) *Bedouin of the Negev*, Manchester: Manchester University Press.

Naggan, L., Forman, M.R., Sarov, B., Lewando Hundt, G., Zangwill L., Chang, D. and Berendes, H.W. (1991) 'Factors influencing the duration of exclusive and partial breastfeeding over the first 18 months: the Bedouin infant feeding study', *Paediatric and Perinatal Epidemiology* 5: 428–44.

Nettleton, S. (1995) *The Sociology of Health and Illness*, Cambridge: Polity Press.

Nettleton, S. and Watson, J. (1998) *The Body in Everyday Life*, London: Routledge.

Oakley, A. (1976) 'Wisewoman and medicine man: changes in the management of childbirth', in J. Mitchell and A. Oakley (eds), *The Rights and Wrongs of Women*, Harmondsworth, Middx: Penguin.

—— (1979) 'A case of maternity paradigms of women as maternity cases', *Signs: Journal of Women in Culture and Society* 4: 607–31.

Rapp, R. (1993) 'Accounting for amniocentesis', in S. Lindenbaum and M. Lock (eds), *Knowledge, Power and Practice*, London: University of California Press.

—— (1998) 'Refusing prenatal diagnosis: the uneven meanings of bioscience in a multicultural world', in R. Davis-Floyd and J. Dumit (eds), *Cyborg Babies: From Techno-sex to Techno-tots*, New York and London: Routledge.

Read, J. (2000) *Society, Family and Disability: Listening to Mothers*, Buckingham: Open University Press.

Sargent, C. and Bascope, G. (1996) 'Ways of knowing about birth in three cultures', *Medical Anthropology Quarterly* 10 (2): 213–36 (special issue).

Sharma, U. (1992) *Complementary Medicine Today: Practitioners and Patients*, London: Routledge.

Sheiner, E., Shoham Vardi, I., Weitzman, D., Gohar, J. and Carmi, R. (1998) 'Decisions regarding pregnancy termination among Bedouin couples referred to third level ultrasound clinic', *European Journal of Obstetrics and Gynaecology and Reproductive Biology* 76: 141–6.

Shilling, C. (1993) *The Body and Social Theory*, London: Sage.

Stacey, M. (1984) 'Who are the health workers? Patients and other unpaid workers', *Health Care, Economic and Industrial Democracy* 5: 157–84.

—— (1988) *The Sociology of Health and Healing*, London: Unwin Hyman.

—— (ed.) (1992) *Changing Human Reproduction: Social Science Perspectives*, London: Sage.

Statistical Abstract of Israel (No. 33) (1981) Jerusalem: Central Bureau of Statistics.

Statistical Abstract of Israel (No. 47) (1996) Jerusalem: Central Bureau of Statistics.

Statistical Abstract of Israel (No. 49) (1998) Jerusalem: Central Bureau of Statistics.

Turner, B. (1992) *Regulating Bodies: Essays in Medical Sociology*, London: Routledge.

Zola, I.K. (1972) 'Medicine as an institution of social control', *Sociological Review* 20: 487–504.

7 Shouldering the burden

Health work in the locality: the case of funeral directing

Anne Murcott

Introduction

Most British locality studies are silent on that essential of neighbourhood health services, the burial of the dead. To say this, however, not only begs several questions, it is also insufficiently precise. For the concern here is not so much with the burial of the dead; rather it is better expressed as *the work* of burying the dead.[1] Laying out and removing the body, digging the grave, shouldering the coffin, conducting[2] the funeral – tasks that are, and have been, part of the work of burying the dead in one form or another for centuries – it is these which are largely missing from British locality studies. It is also these which are mostly missing from other specialist fields of British sociological enquiry: they barely register in the sociology of health and illness, even in its now venerable sub-speciality of the sociology of health professions and trades, and are virtually absent from the sociology of work and occupations. Only very recently – seen as part of what for many is a belated interest in death, dying and mortality[3] – has there been a growth in the empirical sociological study of the work of dealing with the dead.

This chapter draws on an inspection of that newly emerging British literature, paying attention to the cognate contribution of social historians, in order to enlarge on one or two themes in the sociological study of this form of health work. In the present context, it should be noted, 'work' refers to the expenditure of human effort in order to accomplish some identifiable activity, without prejudging whether the activity in question is represented in a nameable occupation, is even distinctively named, and certainly without prejudging whether it is rewarded in any material sense whether the reward be describable as gift exchange, as barter, or paid for as a wage that is part of a contract of employment. What is presented here is part of a larger project, enthusiasm for which was originally fired some 30 years ago, but which is relatively newly initiated and is intermittently under way. This is one of those regrettable pieces that isn't: it has yet to end, is highly selective, and so can make no pretence at a comprehensive account or developed analysis. It also postpones several things, including discussion of the type of health work funeral directing is. The point of departure is a brief discussion of British community – or locality – studies, not just in some contrived deference to this special occasion[4] but by way of deriving a fresh insight into the topic. The chapter then pauses to dwell on this slightly different angle to suggest that there are very particular implications of the word 'locality' for the burial of the dead, before moving on to reflect on the two main themes. The first is the relation between unpaid and paid work and the, largely one-way, historical development of the former towards the latter; related to this is the second theme: unsurprisingly perhaps, the question of the gendered division of labour. One small point to emerge along the way is an awareness that in some fashion the line between paid and unpaid work cannot always be drawn that sharply.

Funerals and the dead in locality (community) studies

One a way of detecting the period when a sociologist was reading for her or his first degree is to discover how s/he construes the notion of 'community'. Directing the first ever British re-study between 1966 and 1969 of a smallish town – Banbury in north Oxfordshire – faced Margaret Stacey and her team[5] with several thorny methodological problems. Chief among them was determining what, if anything sociologically special, the word community was to mean. Tackling it led Stacey (1969) to prefer using the term 'locality' studies to 'community' studies. As noted in the next section, her preferred nomenclature is instructive, though perhaps not in a way she expected. First, however, the claim with which this chapter opened – that this group of British studies is largely silent on the burial of the dead – needs a little substantiation.

In passing, it might be added that although this chapter is unashamedly parochial in electing to confine its attention solely to the British literature, a nice little point noticed in checking back on the literature on community is too good to miss. In his confident proclamation of the defining characteristics of 'The little community', Robert Redfield itemises four of them. The last of these is self-sufficiency – the 'little community' as a form of what he calls the 'organised life of man' providing for all or most of the needs or activities of its members. Offering a neat irony for the present discussion, he summarises his point with the ringing declaration: '[T]he little community is a cradle-to-grave arrangement' (Redfield 1960: 4). Few of us – at least in Britain[6] – seem to have noticed.[7]

Examining the British community studies for evidence of attention to death is not original. Tony Walter (1993) has blazed this particular trail in his review of the limited contribution British sociology has made to the literature on death. His concern, however, is with all kinds of manifestations and representations of death, asking 'how British society manages the dying, the corpse and the bereaved' (Walter 1993: 268). He divides the discipline into familiar sub-specialties, including 'community studies' to which he finds he can devote little more than half a page. Of a sociological generation seemingly untroubled by what community is to mean, he observes that unlike anthropological studies of what he calls 'pre-modern communities', which do pay substantial attention to 'members' mortality', as he puts it, this is not true of British community studies – apart, he casually and inaccurately remarks, from 'a couple of pages on coffin-handling and burial' in W.M. Williams's study of Gosforth (ibid.: 275).

While the re-inspection of this literature made for present purposes is bound to concur with Walter's overall conclusion that there is singularly little attention to death, the present focus on the *work* of dealing with the dead – what, following Charmaz (1980) (who uses it as two words) or Smale's (1985) PhD title, Walter dubs 'deathwork' (1993: 276) – can find a little more of interest in this group of studies than he allows. Firmly giving Walter his due, this interest is more in the nature of small analytic straws in the wind than major contradictions of his position. In part, though, Walter overlooks the implications of his own, and undoubtedly apt, comparison with the work of (social) anthropologists. In the process, he bypasses two important considerations he could have picked up from re-reading Williams's study of Gosforth. The first is to realise that what he dismissively calls those 'couple of pages' are part of a chapter on aspects of the 'life-cycle of the countryman'. It is a life, remarks Williams (1956: 66), which 'ends very much as it began, with a large gathering of friends and relatives, a church ritual and a feast', which he then goes on to describe. There it is: evidence of the way 'the dying, the corpse and the bereaved' are managed – the very focus, translated back into his own words, of Walter's interest. There it is: reference to the social arrangements in which emotional and practical support is offered to the bereaved and which provide for the spiritual/religious/magical obeisance due to the dead. Elsewhere Williams returns to the point that a death in the village evokes good neighbourliness both symbolic (e.g. sending a wreath) and practical (e.g. helping prepare food the for the mourners), earlier having noted that, in several manifestations, social class in Gosforth carries through to death and the funeral.[8]

Features – literal and metaphoric – of social life run through and across social death – sacred and profane – not just in Williams's study, but in the study of his teacher, Alwyn Rees: the second consideration that re-reading Gosforth permits. Death is certainly evident in Rees's (1950) study of Llanfihangel, in his chapter on religion, and on politics – in the guise of disputes about the cemetery that followed a shortage of land for burial at the turn of the last century.[9] And death is notably evident under the headings of kindred and neighbours. Much like Williams, Rees describes the reciprocity between neighbours:

Death brings further manifestations of kindliness. In the interval between death and burial the bereaved family leaves much of the housework to other people. In particular it is experienced neighbours who prepare the corpse for burial, and prepare food for those who have come a long way to the funeral.

(Ibid.: 92–3)

The key difference between Rees's report of the matter and Williams's – and an important point taken up again in the next section – is that Rees records that there are those living locally who are experienced in preparing both the corpse and – so his text seems to read – the food. The work of Rees, a geographer, as well as that of Williams, is clearly well settled in a recognisable anthropological tradition of the period. It is, incidentally, mildly surprising that Walter missed out on taking lessons of social anthropology rather further and, as a result perhaps, devoted no section in his review to family and kinship – *prima facie* a social arena in which coping with dying and the bereaved might just be found. He would have picked up a good deal about death if he had looked, for instance, at Firth *et al.*'s (1969) strangely neglected study of middle-class kinship in 1960s' London.

That said, there is a couple of other small and admittedly oblique points of interest to be found in the community studies. Both have to do with occupations. Neither Margaret Stacey (1960) in her first study of Banbury nor James Littlejohn (1963) in his study of the Cheviot parish to which he gave the name Westrigg was concerned with the study of occupations *per se*. Both, however, looked carefully at the range of occupations they found represented in each location. Littlejohn reports that in one of his earlier periods of fieldwork in 1946 he made his own census of the Westrigg population, 326 people in all, and produced a list of occupations represented. Note for the moment that 'joiner' and 'handyman' are listed, and so too are 'Minister' and 'nursing attendant' – but there is neither doctor nor undertaker.

Like Williams and Rees, Littlejohn also covers the question of mutual aid. But setting his work apart from other British studies of rural areas, Littlejohn sought to develop a more thoroughly grounded historical analysis of the parish.[10] He reports the now extremely familiar trends towards the reduction in mutual aid and in the exchange of neighbourly services, and records the alterations in the nature of social relationships such that no longer did everyone know of the existence of everyone else. Yet once, the important events in an individual's life – birth, christening, marriage and death – were announced in church, and as everyone went to church, everyone knew of them (Littlejohn 1963: 49).

Littlejohn also reports concomitant changes in the occupations of the parish: the disappearance of the bootmaker and the miller, the tailor saved from going out of business by clothes rationing during the war – when his services were in demand for mending – and the joiner and his assistant still plying a steady trade, but in all sorts of casual jobs instead of joinery. The implications are echoed in Stacey (1960) as a central feature of her book. Tradition and change – its very title – are reflected, she proposed, in shifts in the occupational and industrial structure. Thus tradition and allegiance to the local, along with long-established trades and skills – plush weaving, coach building – were giving way to something more modern that derived from factories and cities beyond the town (ibid.: 30), observable in the emergence of trades and job titles new to the locality now taking their place alongside the recognisably traditional occupations of doctors or priests (ibid.: 14). She does not happen to mention undertaker.

Locality and the body

Present purposes allow us to sidestep those thorny questions about what community is to mean that plagued so many sociologists three decades ago. But present purposes prompt us to pick up on the implications of locality and the local. Along with much else that is biologically material – the physiological need to eat, excrete and sleep, the imperatives of disease and infirmity – death is bound to be local. Unlike the famished, exhausted or sick, the dead cannot move – however painfully – in an attempt to deal with their own predicament. Indeed, they are no longer capable of dealing with what remains of their self on earth, abandoned at the site of their death. The predicament of the dead belongs not to them but to the living. For the dead, telling the living about whatever predicament they now face is beyond them – though the living are inclined to believe there are duties to be performed that will intercede on the dead's behalf.[11] In several respects, the dead get in the way of the living. The king is dead (so too is grandma, dad or Aunt Bessie): long live the king (grandson, daughter and nephew Joe). In this sense, the dead interrupt a continuity that is life. Death is not only bound to be local – bound in space – it is also bound in time. Like those other material facts of biological life, eating, sleeping, disease and so on, death has a temporality. Dying may well be more and less successfully described in terms of trajectories, temporally speaking (Glaser and Strauss 1968). So too must death, in the temporality of decomposition; decay entails a process, a further trajectory, or maybe a continuation of the one begun before death, during dying, at birth even.

The dead have to be dealt with there and then. When they are not, the consequences intrusively, unbearably, become apparent to the living. The consequences signal something devastating, something profoundly improper, times appallingly out of joint, no matter what the culture.[12] The sacred and the profane, in exquisite conjunction, are both at stake. But what is also at stake is the mundane. This is what is local about death. The dead cannot be left; the dead have to be attended to, on the spot. There is a practical task to be – it may as well be said – undertaken.

Dealing with the dead: work, paid and unpaid

It is perhaps appropriate that James Littlejohn has already been mentioned, for his name is included in the acknowledgements to Erving Goffman's *The Presentation of Self in Everyday Life* (1971). Goffman's is a book which might well be responsible for the first introduction to Britain – or more likely initially only to Scotland[13] – of a study in which dealing with the dead is analysed as work, and paid work at that. The study is by Robert Habenstein, a fellow graduate student of Goffman's at the University of Chicago, who was awarded his PhD in 1954, a year after Goffman; a study which appears to have influenced greatly Goffman's analysis of performances[14] (see appendix to this chapter). What makes that study of prime interest in the present context lies in Habenstein's concern to investigate dealing with death as work – deathwork, if one must. It is also, incidentally, the source of the present interest in death initiated more than 30 years ago, generated, it so happens, by a course on 'Occupations and institutions' (in the Department of Social Anthropology at Edinburgh University) which Littlejohn himself ran in the academic year 1965–6 (see Murcott 1996).[15] In this respect, the reason for embarking on the present line of enquiry is rather different from those suggested by Walter, who speculates (and adduces a little evidence) that an interest in death among British sociologists is commonly sparked by their own personal experience, for example, of bereavement or of funerals (Walter 1993: 287).

It may have taken three decades and more since Habenstein's thesis, but there is now some – not a lot – British empirically based sociological study of the modern work of dealing with the dead. Several of the themes of Habenstein's study are enduring and are treated in the more recent British studies. Notable among these is the question of the nature and status of the undertaker's trade: whether indeed it is to be called undertaking or funeral directing; whether indeed it is 'merely' a trade or whether this has been overhauled with obvious signs of professionalisation (Howarth 1996). There is too an inbuilt inevitability: one that requires the management of 'dirty work' – Hughes's (1971) expression – the impression of management needed to engage in dirty work but avoid being occupationally and personally besmirched by it. Dirty work here, of course, refers to dirt both literally and metaphorically – dirt, defined, as Mary Douglas (1966) so decisively put it, as 'matter out of place'.

Dirty work also refers to Everett Hughes's sociological shorthand to denote a class of morally repudiated, physically repugnant, polluting and/or culturally dangerous activities of various kinds. Although the following quotation comes from his essay on those outrages committed by the National Socialist Government of Germany which he describes as 'the most colossal and dramatic piece of social dirty work the world has ever known' (Hughes 1964: 23), his point applies more widely: 'Almost every group which has a specialized social function to perform is in some measure a secret society, with a body of rules developed and enforced by the members and with some power to save its members from outside punishment' (ibid.: 35). Arising out of his prewar teaching on what he says came to be known as 'Hughes on the Nazis' (Hughes [1951] 1971: v) he gave that essay the poignant title 'Good people and dirty work'; and he used the same shorthand in several other essays on work and occupations noting, in 'Work and self', that '[D]irty work of some kind is found in all occupations' (ibid.: 343).

No doubt it can safely be said that dealing with the dead represents some of the dirtiest work imaginable in all human societies. In the parochial British case under discussion here, no more than the first, simple questions of enquiry into this dirtiest of dirty work are at issue for now: questions such as what is the work? who is to do it? and when does, and did it, become paid work? For, as already indicated, the present discussion draws on only a selection of the literature, examining the record of a one-way historical trend for some three centuries, that is, a trend from the unpaid to the paid, but ending by entering a tiny question mark as to whether and how far that trend is completed or even shows signs of being reversed. It is a familiar history of a shift from the domestic and unpaid, combined with the local and incidentally paid for, to the commercial, the socially organised in terms of a named occupation. But it is also one that historians propose has taken place unevenly around the country at different rates in different places, such that one or two tasks involved in dealing with the dead are recorded as continuing unpaid well into the last century. The rest of this discussion is devoted to illustrating just some of these features. It begins with the consideration of undertaker as occupation.

Eighteenth-century trade cards provide visual evidence of the shrewd observation Everett Hughes makes about named occupations: 'The names are tags, a combination of price tag and calling card' (Hughes [1951] 1971: 338). One such (illustrated in Habenstein 1955: 173) named, advertised and illustrated trades in the plural: carpenter, joiner, dealer in second-hand goods, upholsterer, as well as undertaker. Most probably serving those of the 'middling sort', the newly emerging middle classes, he was successor to William Boyce who opened a shop *c.*1675 under his sign of the White Hart and Coffin (Litten 1991: 19) also in the City of London at what was apparently known then as the Great Old Bailey. There is possibly some disagreement as to whether Boyce was the first known undertaker: according to Julian Litten he is the 'first recorded person trading as an undertaker *per se*' (ibid.: 19), whereas Clare Gittings has William Russell, also a painter and coffin maker, as 'the first known undertaker', who appears in the historical record as making an agreement with the College of Arms in 1689 (details of which are omitted here for want of space).

Social historians give a strong impression that the inauguration of undertaking as an occupation is quite readily datable. They claim that at first it was only found in London (Gittings 1984: 94) – although just possibly this might be due to London's documentary record being particularly rich – and that initially and in many other areas of the country (are they in effect talking only of England?) it was a part-time occupation; or, put another way, it was a part-occupation, a sideline to others. They do not need to mention that the names of those engaging in that named occupation were men. It is with this, the question of undertaking as a sideline, in mind that attention was paid above to Stacey's and Littlejohn's itemising of occupations in Banbury in the 1950s and Westrigg in the late 1940s. Now, it may already be too late, even for the oral history that would throw light on this little detail, to discover whether the roadman or joiner in Westrigg or the Banbury born-and-bred cabinet maker, carpenter or wood machinist (Stacey 1960: 31) was also involved in some aspect of the funeral trade. But, either running against Gittings's apparent claim that undertaking was a sideline to other occupations especially in rural areas, or underlining the way that Dagenham at the turn of the century could not be counted as London, there is an oblique view of the growth of a twentieth-century undertaking firm found in the autobiography of the proprietor.

Jack West built up the Dagenham firm as a dedicated funeral business. He published his autobiography, a set of reminiscences as late as 1988, when he himself was seventy-eight. He appears to assume that his readers will not need to be told that his father undertook funerals too, a father introduced as a 'builder, surrounded by yard and workshop' in which as small children he and his siblings were privileged to play:

> with its floor covered with crisp wood shavings to romp about in . . . be tempted to try out the carpenter's planes, only to be reprimanded for damaging the edges. I could only have been about three years old, when I wandered out into the workshop and pulled a pail of boiling pitch over, that had been prepared to line a coffin. I have no memory of it, except what my parents told me . . .
>
> (West 1988)

This is West's first mention of the sideline to his father's trade, and he does not dwell on it at that point in his book, discussing instead the small but lifelong scar on his face.

So we have the emergence of a named occupation, which over centuries can be documented to co-exist with other named occupations. There is a *prima facie* plausibility for such co-existence. In many rural areas (as Gittings, 1986: 94, implies) there may simply not have been the volume of undertaking work to support a full-time undertaker – part of the import of death's character as local, this is the obverse of the dead's having to be dealt with there and then. Undertaking emerges as an occupation in which the suppliers' control of the rate of demand – both the volume and evenness of flow – is comparatively low. That dealing with the dead has its own imperatives does, though, imply that, within reason, it makes sense to have some of the accoutrements ready to hand: the time between death and disposal can be short for several reasons, including the practicalities of the preservation techniques available as well as the spiritualities governing the decencies. With this in mind, let us turn to consider a small selection of the tasks involved.

Part of the early, seventeenth-century impetus to the development of the named occupation of undertaker is the sheer number of tasks deemed appropriate to a funeral, at least for the well-to-do or minor gentry. Litten (1991) implies, incidentally, that in this century, it is the length of the list of tasks that is responsible for use of the name funeral director: a collection of tasks to be directed, orchestrated and stage-managed. And Gittings (1986: 95) makes the following observation:

> The rationale for relying on a single purveyor of all things necessary for a funeral was, in itself, sound and apparently beneficial to hard-pressed executors. For instance, to organise the funeral of Sir Hannibal Baskerville of Sunningwell, Berkshire, in 1670, 17 different suppliers had to be contacted for goods ranging from mourning hats and rings to cakes and beer; and this figure did not include ordering the coffin and shroud or making arrangements with the minister, gravediggers, ringers and so forth.

For now, consider only a few of these tasks – just those associated with laying out the body. These few are selected for several reasons: in part because they present a particularly acute form of making mundane, routine and matter-of-fact that which is potentially simultaneously both sacred and profane; and in part because they lie at the core of the immediacy, the imperatives, of dealing with them that the dead present to the living.

These tasks are, of course, also those where the management of dirty-work is involved in an equally acute fashion. And they take place very close to the time and place where the transition from life to death occurs. Indeed, the very first task is to establish that the body really is a corpse. Gittings (ibid.: 108) has it that from the seventeenth century, in cases where foul play or accident was suspected, those paid to watch the dead until the coroner could attend were also 'on hand in case the "deceased" revived'. Fear of being buried alive recurs in the historical record – quite apart from Edgar Allan Poe's fearsome stories – in the most wonderful nineteenth-century contraptions devised as coffins with breathing tubes or other means of surviving premature entombment. In her lovely study of the interwar neighbourhood layer-out in a working-class area of north Coventry, Sheila Adams (1993: 157) notes a case reported to her in which the body 'sat up in bed and asked for a glass of water'. She also suggests that the layer-out, a woman living locally, also certified death for many working-class families, thereafter informing the medical practitioner who issued the certificate. For, as the 1964 *Manual of Funeral Directing* reminded the reader early in its chapter on 'Care of the body', the legal position is that unless cremation is intended: 'a doctor who has attended a patient need not see the body after death . . . every funeral director, therefore, should be able to satisfy himself . . . that death has actually taken place' (National Association of Funeral Directors 1964: 48). Several signs of death are listed, along with three tests for death including the classic mirror test, applying one of which is advised as 'wise and convincing'.

One way we know that it was women who for several centuries were engaged in shrouding the body is as a by-product of attempts to support the English (and Welsh?) economy. The Act of 1678 required that the dead were buried not in linen, silk or cotton, which had to be imported, but in wool and wool only. An affidavit was required to attest to the fact (although there is evidence of systematic and perhaps widespread evasion: see Litten 1991 and Gittings 1984). As Gittings (ibid.: 113) notes, many of these documents survive 'signed by the women who shrouded the corpse'.[16]

The set of tasks involved next (see, for instance, but also compare, the descriptions provided in Wright 1981, Hockey 1990 and Howarth 1996) offer a neat sidelight, less immediately on the relation of unpaid and paid work, as on the relation between the same set of tasks that comprises paid work in two named occupations, tasks which overlap between them. Nowadays, the work of laying out a corpse is, in principle, the same for the hospital nurse as for the undertaker. Wonderfully echoing the way the two occupations have come to abut one another, when the tasks of laying out the deceased are performed in hospital they are known as 'last offices' but when carried out at the funeral director's premises they are described as 'first offices' (Harris 1995: 77). Possibly no historical record survives that would help date when this terminological distinction arose: apart from territorial disputes between occupations leading to a court of law, it is not easy to imagine the circumstances that would give rise to its being documented. Glennys Howarth (1996: 156), however, does imply that nowadays there is some disagreement between each occupation's judgement of the adequacy of the other's performance of these tasks.

There is a long sequence of tasks that nowadays comprise laying out the body (see, for example, Wright 1981; Howarth 1996; also National Association of Funeral Directors 1964). These tasks together represent the literal and metaphoric conversion of the corpse – bearing whatever marks remain of the kind of life and the manner of death – to the body, presented and presentable in whatever state deemed at the period to be viewed – assuming viewing is itself deemed appropriate – and suitable for the manner of disposal. Then, a doctor sewed Charles I's head back on to his torso in preparation for his burial (Litten 1991). Now, heart pace-makers need to be removed if there is to be a cremation; they explode in the heat and blow up the cremator.

These then are among the tasks in dealing with the dead that have been noticeably gendered. It is not simply a matter of distinctions, as Howarth implies exist between occupations that are predominantly male or female, or jobs at the modern funeral director's mirroring the dual labour market at large (women office cleaners, receptionists or typists; men embalmers, morticians and hearse drivers). It is not simply a matter, either, as explicitly asserted by Adams (1993), of the informal organisation of care of the dead by the female working-class neighbourhood layer-out being replaced with the formalised organisation for the treatment of the dead body by the male mortician. At some point, though again the historical record is liable to be hazy, the assumption is that these are among the tasks that eventually cohered into those of the neighbourhood wise woman, midwife and nurse that tend to be thought of as at some rather earlier era being carried out, unpaid, as a matter of family duty, of household responsibility, part of the social obligations of women as kin and/or members of a household.

These claims deserve continued efforts at substantiation, as do other suggestions of much more modern fine-grained divisions of labour. Tantalisingly, recalling Rees's note that neighbours helped prepare the body, we may not be able to discover whether this was a service rendered for money, whether it was part of enduring neighbourly reciprocity – repayment of, or repaid by, the provision of some other specialist service in the past or future – or whether it involved a conventionally understood exchange of gifts or goods. However, we do have Elizabeth Roberts's (1989) fine discussion of the reports of the ways of death in the earlier years of this century by elderly people in three Lancashire towns whom she interviewed in the decade from 1971. Her data are of an urban rather than a rural area, so care is needed not to leap to unwarrantable conclusions, though the household and neighbourly economies of rural and working-class urban areas at the period may have been associated with parallel reliance on mutual aid in all kinds of crises.[17] Roberts (ibid.: 196) reproduces verbatim part of an interview with Mrs Armstrong (Rose, denoted below by her initial), who was layer-out for the street where she lived. She talked of the way they never accepted any form of recompense, monetary or otherwise:

R: . . . We never used to take anything off them, never bothered, but now today everything is altered and the undertaker does all that.

E.R: Would people give you a present, were they grateful for what you did, or just take it for granted?

R: No, they would ask you and try to offer you summat or buy you summat. They hadn't the money and we used to say 'No'. I never took nothing off them and it used to be our good deed for them, we were good neighbours.

And additional, timely, oral history may well allow following up the note on laying out in the 1964 *Manual of Funeral Directing* (National Association of Funeral Directors 1964: 49): 'It is usual for the funeral director to have trained assistants, *usually lady assistants*, for these duties. Nevertheless, the funeral director should know what is required and be prepared to perform these Offices if need be' (emphasis added). The funeral director reading the *Manual* is assumed to be male and, in the ordinary way of things, a gendered division of labour is assumed such that he is not going to be responsible for laying out.

By way of artificial conclusion to this chapter – artificial for, as was advised at the outset, this is a chapter which has no end, not yet anyway and is a long way off returning to its original case, that of the funeral director him- or herself – a few points will be drawn, together with a couple of further illustrations. Dealing with the dead illustrates, right into this century, instances, however few, however fleeting, of variation in the manner in which the associated work is socially organised. It ranges from work that is a side-line, thus representing intermittent paid work of the part-time male undertaker/builder or part-time prewar female neighbourhood layer-out; it is evident in what is typically comparatively low-paid work of women who make up the vast majority of the nursing profession. Also into this century are two other facets of the social organisation of work.

Both concern the accoutrements deemed necessary to a funeral. Burial in a shroud is a long established English (British?) practice – longer probably than burial in a coffin. Even with twentieth-century techniques and technology, sewing a shroud that is anything other than a length of fabric simply wound round the body takes its own time. Being able to lay hands on a supply when needed would appear prudent if not efficient. Also deserving to be examined is the rise of the supply wholesale to the retail undertaker. One of the most successful wholesalers in the early part of the twentieth century was also a London firm. Dottridge Brothers (mentioned, though misspelled, by Jack West) was founded by Samuel Dottridge. Born in 1811 he also began in the building trade, added funerals to this business, and then moved from retail across to wholesale trade. Dottridge Brothers was of sufficient prominence to have an official history,[18] compiled by way of celebrating its centenary in 1935. Archived locally with that history is one of its price lists *c*.1922. Here then are the prices of what are described as 'complete inside sets', which include the shroud: the Gladstone, satin throughout, cost 5 guineas, with the silk version 5 shillings dearer; the Kitchener was down a notch, in flannel trimmed with satin, at 45 shillings.

Now, set this successful wholesale enterprise of the capital city against the record of two sisters living, by the 1920s, only about two hours away on the London underground (the Metropolitan line is overground much of the way but runs out to their part of Hertfordshire). Litten (1991: 75) reminds us that acquiring one's grave clothes did not need to wait till death: 'many a young bride-to-be, especially in the more remote country areas, included such items in their trousseaus, either buying them ready-made from one of the known outlets, or having them made by a local seamstress, or producing them her-self'.[19] In other words, commercial producers supplied the general public as well as the specialist retailer. More entrancing is Litten's (ibid.) adding, apparently of an instance personally known to or reported to him, that 'the tradition continued throughout the nineteenth century and well into the twentieth. Alice Shelley (d. 1960) and Minnie Shelley (d. 1966), two nona-genarian sisters of Cheshunt, Hertfordshire, were buried in shrouds which they had themselves made.'

Litten is one of many who, over the two or three centuries' history of the undertaker, has a none too complimentary view of the funeral trade; he is extremely sniffy about the quality of modern funeral accoutrements, declar-ing he has 'no intention of being dispatched in a multi-density fibre board veneered coffin with plastic handles and Terylene lining' (ibid.: 4). But then, as his own history testifies, for some three centuries it has been possible for anyone, for a price, to specify in advance the quality and the lavishness of one's funeral. And there is nothing to stop Julian Litten or anyone else organising a friend's or relation's funeral, or his having a friend or relation promise to organise his own, without recourse to any paid-for services of a funeral director. Anyone in doubt as to how to go about doing so need only turn to the Which? consumer guide, *What to Do When Someone Dies*. The book is written by Paul Harris, the business manager of a firm of funeral directors in Salisbury, who has some 30 years' experience of conducting funerals. Harris (1995: 101) does warn that 'there can be considerable snags and difficulties, but with knowledge and determination, these can be overcome'. Does this parallel the advice about house purchase and the law that a solicitor might offer to anyone thinking of doing their own conveyancing? Heed might be taken, however, of his hints about the collapse of home-made chairs or shelves, and of his very severe warning that '*no one* should contemplate beginning a d-i-y career by making a coffin' (ibid.: 104).

Other moves may be afoot. There is talk of ecologically friendly disposal. The familiar pair of trade declarations, 'Family Firm', 'Low Cost Funerals' was noted[20] on the shop front below the firm's name, 'Green Undertakings'. And, putting a temporary stop to this discussion, an entrepreneurial example was carried by the *Independent* on 14 June 1997 under the headline: 'All-woman funeral directors cash in on a dead original concept'. Widowers, these entrepreneurs claim, prefer a woman undertaker, assuring thereby that no man other than themselves ever touch the body of their newly deceased wives.

Appendix: The Goffman/ Habenstein introduction

As part of his opening chapter on 'Performances', Goffman discusses the manner in which work is to be dramatised. He exemplifies the contrast between surgical nursing staff, who have no problem in displaying their skills: 'changing bandages, swinging orthopedic frames into place' are visible and readily understood as valuable and important; unlike medical nursing where in the process of stopping to chat with a patient, the skilled observation of the 'shallowness of the breathing and color and tone of the skin' (Goffman 1958: 20) is simultaneously but invisibly being carried on. In a parallel, but not an identical, instance, Goffman points out that the undertaker faces a problem in displaying – and also being able to charge for – skills which are not displayable.

His point is developed in a later chapter on 'Regions and region behaviour'. Members of an occupation engage in control of the backstage as part of the process of what Goffman (ibid.: 70) calls 'work control'. The amount of work needed, the mistakes made in the process, and other activities about which the purchaser of the service might want to enquire, if not quibble, in deciding whether the fee charged is reasonable, all are more comfortably performed out of sight of everyone except fellow members of the occupation.

If the bereaved are to be given the illusion that the dead one is really in a deep and tranquil sleep, then the undertaker must be able to keep the bereaved from the workroom where the corpses are drained, stuffed and painted in preparation for their final performance (ibid.: 71). Goffman adds a footnote to a point made by 'Mr Habenstein . . . in seminar':

> about the way that in some states the undertaker has a legal right to prevent relatives of the deceased from entering the workroom where the corpse is in preparation. Presumably the sight of what has to be done to the dead to make them look attractive would be too great a shock for non-professionals and especially for kinsfolk of the deceased. Mr Habenstein also suggests that kinsfolk may want to be kept from the undertaker's workroom because of their own fear of their own morbid curiosity.
>
> (Ibid.: 71)

Here is a beautiful instance of the back region that is kept closed to members of the audience, a 'widely practised technique of impression management' (ibid.: 70). By the time Allen Lane published *The Presentation of Self* in Great Britain in 1969,[21] Habenstein's chapter in Rose's pathbreaking collection *Human Behavior and Social Processes* had appeared, first published in Great Britain in 1962.[22] Placed in the collection immediately after a paper by Eliot Freidson on 'Dilemmas in the doctor-patient relationship' and before Robert Dubin's 'Industrial workers' worlds: a study of the "central life interests" of industrial workers', Habenstein's is entitled 'Sociology of occupations: the case of the American funeral director'. It is squarely located in the study of work, paid work, work consisting of a set of tasks, responsibilities and activities that has cohered into a nameable occupation, one that has a job title, recognisable on both sides of the Atlantic. His chapter title is purposely echoed in the subtitle of this chapter: it is intended to underline its interest in death, and its dealing with death as work.

Notes

1 And more exactly, if less euphoniously, expressed as the legal disposal of the dead, thus including cremation and excluding the nefarious.
2 Note that the verbs 'remove', 'shoulder', 'conduct' remain part of the everyday technical vocabulary of the funeral director.
3 If the titles of edited collections (e.g. Clark 1993) or journals (*Mortality*, launched in 1996) is anything to go by.
4 I am grateful to the organisers for the invitation to present a paper at 'Gender, Health and Healing: Reflections on the Public/Private Divide: an International Conference in tribute to Emeritus Professor Meg Stacey', University of Warwick April 1999.
5 Consisting of a research fellow – Colin Bell – and two research assistants – the late Eric Batstone and me.

6 A venerable North American exception is, of course, Lloyd Warner. His 1959 study in the Yankee City series predates this particular pronouncement of Redfield's.

7 Or, if we did, made nothing of it. I have not spent the time to re-read the book, so cannot be sure whether it was included or not, but during the two years of field-work for the second study of Banbury, I distinctly remember Colin Bell describing (and feeling sore that I'd missed) seeing the funeral of a gypsy matriarch with a floral tribute made into a miniature version of her chair – see Okely (1983: 219) for an extensive discussion of the management of death, dying and bereavement among traveller-gypsies.

8 This and several other points made in the present section might suggest that in the work of some sociologists, the question as to whether we want a specialism called the sociology of death and dying or should seek to introduce human mortality into every facet of sociology, with which Walter ends his review, is already answered for him by those following the example of British social anthropologists.

9 It is not clear whether the exclamation mark below represents Rees's own opinion or his report of his informants' outrage. He records objections to some of the land offered for the creation of a new burial ground: 'some Nonconformists insisting that the ground acquired by the Church was quite unfit for burial, that is was so rocky that people were being buried with their heads down!' (Rees 1950: 157). That certainly tells us something about the management of death.

10 As well as an arguably far more thoroughly theorised analysis of class.

11 For example, the medieval burial guilds could be said to represent a social organ-isational response to the thirteenth-century belief within the Church 'that masses said on behalf of the dead would shorten the length of time a soul spent in purgatory' (Litten 1991: 6).

12 It is not just the whole literary canon, not just classical mythology, never mind the place of death or resurrection in the great religions, but the sum total of human knowledge about human cultures and cosmologies that testifies to the point being made here. There are those news reports of the police or ambulance staff who have to break the door down after neighbours report an intolerable smell and the maggot-ridden body of another social isolate is found. And there are also occa-sional hints – are they no more than urban myths? – that Bates in Hitchcock's *Psycho* is not quite fictitious in being or becoming unhinged upon, or by, the death of a close kinsperson, whose body is retained – it remains, so to speak, to keep them company.

13 Although it is likely to have had quite limited circulation since it was initially published privately by the University of Edinburgh in 1956; my own copy is a second impression dated 1958.

14 He acknowledges the 'forthcoming dissertation' and seminar report 'describing the undertaker's work as the staging of a performance' (Goffman 1958: 21) in the Edinburgh version, and acknowledges the completed PhD dissertation adding: 'I owe much to Mr Habenstein's analysis of a funeral as a performance' (Goffman 1971: 42).

15 Never mind providing a key reference on the social organisation of death used in 20 years' teaching sociology to medical and nursing students from 1971.

16 Were they literate? Gittings does not say whether the women actually signed the documents or made their mark – although it is recognised that even the otherwise illiterate do sign their name. Perhaps this altered over the century and more that the legislation was in force.

17 Perhaps the normal crises of the life course are those more likely than, certainly as likely as, other types of crisis to be associated with an element of the establish-ment, the institutionalisation, the social and practical codification, of social arrangements for dealing with them.

18 No author is given, and it cannot be detected from the text who compiled/wrote it.
It is quite probable that it was an in-house production.
19 Litten (1991: 75) goes on, a trifle hodiecentrically: 'It was a dismal yet necessary
task, and whilst one can imagine a young woman's producing such items for
herself and her future husband, it is more difficult for us to accept that she probably also fashioned one or two smaller versions at the same time, for infant mortality was high.' He perhaps ought to have remembered what no doubt the young
woman herself knew only too well that she too was at risk of an early death in
childbirth.
20 From a bus in Taunton, Somerset, Sunday 4 August 1996.
21 The Penguin paperback edition appeared in 1971.
22 Reprinted and first published in paperback in 1971.

References

Adams, Sheila (1993) 'A gendered history of the social management of death in
Foleshill, Coventry, during the interwar years', in D. Clark (ed.), *The Sociology of
Death*, Oxford: Basil Blackwell.
Charmaz, Kathy (1980) *The Social Reality of Death*, Reading, MA: Addison-Wesley.
Clark, D. (ed.) (1993) *The Sociology of Death*, Oxford: Basil Blackwell.
Douglas, Mary (1966) *Purity and Danger*, Harmondsworth, Middx: Penguin.
Firth, Raymond, Hubert, Jane and Forge, Anthony (1969) *Families and Their Rela-
tives: Kinship in a Middle-class Sector of London. An Anthropological Study*,
London: Routledge and Kegan Paul.
Gittings, Clare (1984) *Death, Burial and the Individual in Early Modern England*,
London: Routledge.
Glaser, B.G. and Strauss, A.L. (1968) *Time for Dying*, Chicago: Aldine Press.
Goffman, Erving (1958) *The Presentation of Self in Everyday Life*, Edinburgh: Social
Sciences Research Centre, University of Edinburgh.
Goffman, Erving (1971) *The Presentation of Self in Everyday Life*, Harmondsworth,
Middx: Penguin.
Habenstein, Robert W. (1971) 'Sociology of occupations: the case of the American
funeral director', in Arnold M. Rose (ed.), *Human Behavior and Social Processes:
An Interactionist Approach*, London: Routledge and Kegan Paul.
Harris, Paul (1995) *What to Do When Someone Dies*, London: Which? (rev. edn of the
1994 new edn).
Hockey, Jennifer L. (1990) *Experiences of Death: An Anthropological Account*,
Edinburgh: Edinburgh University Press.
Howarth, Glennys (1996) *Last Rites: The Work of the Modern Funeral Director*,
Amityville, NY: Baywood.
Hughes, Everett C. (1964) 'Good people and dirty work', in Howard S. Becker (ed.),
The Other Side: Perspectives on Deviance, New York: Free Press.
Hughes, Everett C. ([1951] 1971) 'Work and self', in *The Sociological Eye: Selected
Papers*, Chicago: Aldine Atherton.
Litten, Julian (1991) *The English Way of Death: The Common Funeral since 1450*,
London: Robert Hale.
Littlejohn, James (1963) *Westrigg: The Sociology of a Cheviot Parish*, London:
Routledge and Kegan Paul.
Murcott, Anne (1996) 'Old boundaries and hybrid identities: a footnote to "Social
anthropology type B"', unpublished paper presented at 'Boundaries and Identities:

a conference to celebrate fifty years of social anthropology at the University of Edinburgh', October, University of Edinburgh.

National Association of Funeral Directors (1964) *Manual of Funeral Directing*, London: National Association of Funeral Directors.

Okely, Judith (1983) *The Traveller-Gypsies*, Cambridge: Cambridge University Press.

Redfield, Robert (1960) *The Little Community*, Chicago: Chicago University Press.

Rees, Alwyn D. (1950) *Life in a Welsh Countryside: A Social Study of Llanfihangel yng Ngwunfa*, Cardiff: University of Wales Press.

Roberts, Elizabeth (1989) 'The Lancashire way of death', in Ralph Houlbrooke (ed.), *Death, Ritual and Bereavement*, London: Routledge.

Rose, Arnold M. (ed.) (1971) *Human Behavior and Social Processes: An Interactionist Approach*, London: Routledge and Kegan Paul.

Smale, B. (1985) 'Deathwork: a sociological analysis of funeral directing', unpublished PhD thesis, University of Surrey.

Stacey, Margaret (1960) *Tradition and Change: A Study of Banbury*, Oxford: Oxford University Press.

Stacey, M. (1969) 'The myth of community studies', *British Journal of Sociology* 20 (2): 134–147.

Stacey, Margaret, Bell, Colin, Batstone, Eric and Murcott, Anne (1975) *Power, Persistence and Change*, London: Routledge and Kegan Paul.

Walter, T. (1993) 'Sociologists never die: British sociology and death', in D. Clark (ed.), *The Sociology of Death*, Oxford: Basil Blackwell.

Warner, W. Lloyd (1959) *The Living and the Dead: A Study of the Symbolic Life of Americans*, New Haven, CT: Yale University Press.

West, Jack (1988) *Jack West Funeral Director*, Ilfracombe, Devon: Arthur H. Stockwell.

Williams, W.M. (1956) *The Sociology of an English Village: Gosforth*, London: Routledge and Kegan Paul.

Wright, Monroe (1981) 'Coming to terms with death: patient care in a hospice for the terminally ill', in Paul Atkinson and Christian Heath (eds), *Medical Work: Realities and Routines*, Farnborough, Hants: Gower.

8 The archaeology of psychiatric disorder

Gender and disorders of thought, emotion and behaviour

Joan Busfield

Introduction

This chapter is offered as a tribute to Meg Stacey, who has done so much to put the issue of gender on the sociological map in Britain, especially in relation to health, illness and medicine. In it I want to return to a set of issues that have preoccupied me over a number of years concerning the intersection of gender, psychiatric disorder and mental health practice.[1]

My focus here is on the gendered distribution of identified psychiatric disorder and on understanding this distribution. Though it is not the topic of this chapter, I am also interested (see Busfield 1999) in examining and understanding the gendered distribution of mental health practitioners – psychiatrists, clinical psychologists, psychiatric social workers and psychiatric nurses – who are part of the 'psy complex' (Castel *et al*. 1984). When looking at these two areas it is tempting to talk of a feminisation of mental health work over the twentieth century, since there has been a growing proportion of women amongst those with identified psychiatric disorder and a growing proportion of women in the mental health labour force. The psy complex appears increasingly to be a female complex. Yet such a conclusion is oversimple. In particular, as I shall show, there is a growing emphasis in mental health practice in recent years on male patients. I want to begin by outlining the broad features of the distribution of psychiatric disorder by gender. I distinguish three main types of psychiatric disorder – disorders of thought, emotion and behaviour – and explore changes in the mapping of these disorders over time, their differential relation to gender, and the reasons for this.

Understanding the gendered distribution of psychiatric disorder

Epidemiological data on the gender of those with identifiable psychiatric disorder represent a snapshot taken at a particular time and place. What we observe is the product of a complex range of ideas and practices, particularly those of mental health practitioners and policy makers, of the social institutions in which they are located, including the health services and the pharmaceutical industry. To make sense of any set of epidemiological data we have to look at the contemporary ideas about psychiatric disorder, including the ways in which its boundaries are set, the institutions and social relations in which mental health practice is embedded that structure its practice, as well as the social conditions that give rise to psychiatric disorder as it is constituted at that particular time and place. The diagnostic categories used by psychiatrists and other mental health practitioners, which define the boundaries of psychiatric disorder and are incorporated into epidemiological data, are the intellectual map psychiatrists have developed to make sense of the range of problems with which they deal. My concern in this chapter is not with the adequacy of this map or with the value of medical approaches to mental disorder, though they have been widely contested. Rather it is with the way in which the intellectual map defines and frames (Rosenberg 1992) the terrain of psychiatric disorder and, consequently, structures the observed gender differences. As Phil Brown (1990: 385) contends: 'Diagnosis is integral to the theory and practice of psychiatry, yet it is loosely studied by social scientists.' What is needed therefore is an archaeology of the way in which psychiatric disorder is framed and of the relation of different disorders to men and women and the reasons for them.[2]

The gendered landscape of psychiatric disorder in advanced Western societies which is visible from the epidemiological data is by now reasonably familiar, and is exemplified by the data given in Table 8.1 from a British study of psychiatric disorder in the community carried out by the Office for Population Censuses and Surveys (OPCS).

First, there is a group of disorders where the balance of male and female rates tends to be more or less equal, especially if cases are measured by means

Table 8.1 Prevalence of psychiatric disorders in Britain by gender, adults 16–64

Rates per 1000 in past week	*Female*	*Male*	*Radio F/M*
Mixed anxiety and depression	99	54	1.8
Generalised anxiety disorder	34	28	1.2
Depressive episode	25	17	1.5
All phobias	14	7	2.0
Obsessive-compulsive disorder	15	9	1.7
Panic disorder	9	8	1.1
All neutoric disorders	195	123	1.6
Rates per 1000 in past year			
Functional psychoses	4	4	0.0
Alcohol dependence	21	75	0.3
Drug dependence	15	29	0.5

Source: Meltzer *et al.* (1995: table 6.1).

Note: It is important to note that the two sets of rates cannot be added to give an overall figure since the figures for neuroses are rates per 1000 in the previous week whereas those for psychosis and substance use disorders relate to the past year.

of community surveys rather than the use of mental health services, so making the data less subject to the processes that influence selection into treatment. This group consists mainly, though not exclusively, of the more severe disorders such as schizophrenia and the various types of dementia, mostly the various senile dementias such as Alzheimer's. In Table 8.1 these severe disorders are represented only by category of functional psychoses, of which schizophrenia is the most important. Dementias are not included since the OPCS study surveyed people aged 15–64 and most dementias develop at later ages.[3]

Second, there is a group of disorders where there tends to be a marked female predominance. Notable here are various forms of depression, anxiety states and phobias, many studies showing more marked difference than those in Table 8.1, whether these are identified via community surveys or from in-patient populations (see Goldberg and Huxley 1980: 24–5).

Finally, there is a group of disorders where there tends to be a clear male predominance, a predominance that is usually found both in community surveys and in studies of treated cases. This group consists mainly of the behaviour and personality disorders. The only disorders in this group that are included in Table 8.1 are the two 'substance use disorders' of alcohol and drug dependence.

In order to illuminate the gendered landscape more starkly, we can say that in Western societies it is a landscape in which there tends to be a roughly even gender balance in disorders structured around thought, a female predominance in disorders structured around emotion, and a male predominance in disorders structured around behaviour. This typology of disorders of thought, emotion and behaviour, though it does not question official definitions of specific disorders, does not correspond exactly to the major groupings used within current psychiatric classifications. However, it has an important analytic value in understanding gender differences in psychiatric disorder. Of course, most psychiatric disorders involve diverse symptoms that refer to thought, emotion and behaviour, and the differentiation of these three domains is often easier in theory than in practice. None the less, the weight attached to the different symptoms varies for different disorders, and frequent reference to thought, emotion and behaviour in mental health literature suggests that such distinctions are routinely made.

The marked variation in the gender balance for different types of disorder means that the precise gender balance identified in any epidemiological study depends on the disorders under consideration. A survey of problems seen by general practitioners is likely to find more women than men with problems identified as psychiatric, since most of the psychiatric problems brought to medical attention will be less severe and there will be a high proportion of depression and anxiety, where women tend to predominate. Similarly a community survey designed to measure psychiatric disorder which largely lists symptoms of anxiety and depression is equally likely to find more psychiatric disorder in women (Busfield 1996: 82–90). In contrast, where the focus is on substance use and personality disorders the picture is likely to be very different, with men becoming more predominant. Of course, there is a considerable variation between women according to class and ethnicity in the level and type of disorder just as there is between different groups of men, and it is important to be aware of this variation. For example, Hollingshead and Redlich's classic (1958) study in the US, which examined all those undergoing some form of psychiatric treatment, showed higher levels of mental disorder, particularly of the more severe disorders, amongst those of the lowest social class. It also showed class variation in the gender differences, with the largest difference in the lowest social class where far more men than women were in treatment (see Busfield 1983: 117).[4]

Given this varied gender landscape, we need to consider the general mechanisms that generate gender differences in mental disorder before examining each group of disorders in more detail. I want to identify six main mechanisms. The first three mechanisms accept the boundaries of specific psychiatric disorders and of psychiatric disorder as a generic category as given at a particular time and place. First, either men or women may have higher levels of a particular disorder because they face more *exposure* to its causes as a result of their social situation. Amongst physical illnesses an example is the higher levels of AIDs in men, arising from gender differences in sexual behaviour which affect levels of exposure to the virus. Amongst psychiatric disorders an example would be higher levels of depression in women, arising from particular features of women's social situation. Second, either men or women may have higher levels of a particular disorder because they are more *vulnerable* to the causes of that disorder, either by virtue of biology or because of their social situation. Amongst physical illnesses an example would be coronary heart disease, where genetic differences between men and women which affect hormone levels in adulthood (along with differences in health-related behaviours which are linked to their social situation) lead to greater male vulnerability to coronary disease. In the case of psychiatric disorder an example might be a greater vulnerability to disorder as a result of biological changes associated with childbirth (although social factors may be equally important). Third, a gender difference in levels of a given mental disorder may arise because of the way in which mental processes and behaviour are shaped by social expectations, so that underlying psychological disturbance is *expressed* in different ways, as when, for instance, women react to difficulties by turning feelings inwards and becoming depressed.

The next three mechanisms relate to the processes involved in the identification of psychiatric disorder. Fourth, a gender difference in the levels of a given mental disorder may occur because of the biases in the assessment of the presence or absence of symptoms in the individual case. For instance, emotional states may be presumed on the basis of gendered assumptions despite the lack of clear evidence. Fifth, a gender difference can arise because of gendered biases in what is selected as *the* problem, as, for instance, when conduct is treated as criminal or wicked in a man but it is viewed as a product of psychiatric disorder in a woman.[5] And sixth and finally, gender differences in the levels of disorder may arise because of gender biases in what comes to be constituted as psychiatric disorder. This source of gender difference relates to the third point about the expression of psychological difficulties. However, instead of accepting the given boundaries of psychiatric disorder, here they are called into question not at the level of the individual case (as in the previous mechanism), but at the societal level. Gender can intersect with the way in which certain problems are framed as psychiatric problems and others as problems of deviance and morality, or with the way in which some phenomenon is seen as problematic or not, as when sexual violence, which is more common in men than women, is treated either as normal or a matter of bad behaviour rather than as indicative of psychological pathology.

I now want to use this framework to examine the three groups of psychiatric disorder in detail – disorders of thought, of emotion and of behaviour. I start with disorders of thought since historically these have been at the centre of mental health practice.

Disorders of thought

Psychiatry emerged as a new medical speciality from the second half of the eighteenth century in the context of the new asylums for lunatics. These asylums, first voluntary and then public, were established as a solution to the problem of lunacy – a lay rather than a medical concept which was applied to the disturbed, difficult and dangerous, whose problems were judged to result from some disturbance of reason (see Foucault 1967). Lunacy and madness – the two terms were used interchangeably – was a judgement of mind rather than of body or behaviour, though it had to be deduced from behaviour and action (including what people said). Or put another way, whilst body and behaviour were involved, mind was the key referent (Busfield 1996: 53–4).[6] And the mental processes in question were primarily thought and reasoning, not emotions and feelings.

The reasons for the establishment of asylums are complex but they satisfied a range of perceived needs and motivations: the need to keep secure those considered dangerous and disruptive who, because of their irrationality and unpredictability, were difficult to manage in workhouses and houses of correction (in the asylums all were detained on a compulsory basis); the desire to cure those who could be returned to health so that they could lead productive lives and no longer be a social and economic burden on others (including the local poor law); and the desire to provide a place of rest and asylum for those driven mad by the pressures of the world.

As the nineteenth century progressed the new asylum doctors, as part of their professionalising endeavours, put increasing effort into the task of mapping different disorders of mind in order to assist both the management and treatment of inmates. The spectrum of long-established medical labels for mental disorders included mania, dementia, hypochondriasis, hysteria (which from the seventeenth century had increasingly been seen as a problem of mind rather than body), epilepsy and melancholia. However, whilst new disease categories were being introduced – moral insanity and general paresis are two examples – throughout most of the century the longstanding polarity between two main types of insanity, mania and melancholia, predominated. Descriptions of the symptoms of the disorders combined reference to mind as well as to body and behaviour, with no very clear demarcation between the three. But while the descriptions did refer to the emotions, the contrast between the two disorders was made first and foremost in terms of thought and reason, and only secondarily in terms of emotion. In *Madness and Civilisation* Foucault (1967) discusses the binary opposition between mania and melancholia in detail, referring to the work of Thomas Willis, an English physician of the second half of the seventeenth century. Foucault (ibid.: 125–6) has this to say:

> Willis opposes mania to melancholia. The mind of the melancholic is entirely occupied by reflection, so that his imagination remains at leisure and in repose; the maniac's imagination, on the contrary, is occupied by a perpetual influx of impetuous thoughts. While the melancholic's mind is fixed on a single object, imposing unreasonable proportions upon it, but upon it alone, mania deforms all concepts and ideas; either they lose their congruence, or their representative value is falsified; in any case, the totality of thought is disturbed in its essential relation to truth. Melancholia, finally, is always accompanied by sadness and fear; on the contrary in the maniac we find audacity and fury. Whether it is a question of mania or melancholia, the cause of the disease is always in the movement of the animal spirits. But this movement is quite particular in mania: it is continuous, violent, always capable of piercing new pores in the cerebral matter, and it creates, as the material basis of incoherent thoughts, explosive gestures, continuous words which betray mania.

As this extract suggests, thought and reason were at the centre of the distinction between mania and melancholia. Whereas mania involved 'a perpetual influx of thoughts' and 'deforms all concepts and ideas', melancholia imposed 'unreasonable proportions' on a single object. Mania was, in effect, the medical term for the lay concept of madness, and in lay understandings it was evidenced by the frantic behaviour, excessive talk, odd laughter and the threat or carrying out of some unacceptable action, behaviours that suggested in combination disturbed thought and irrationality (MacDonald 1981). It was the label used most frequently for those admitted to an asylum or private madhouse. For instance, Parry-Jones, as part of his study of private madhouses, analysed the diagnostic labels applied to those admitted to two private madhouses in the 5-year period ending in 1843. He showed that well over half received a diagnosis of mania (Parry-Jones 1972: tables xii and xvi), a reflection no doubt of the fact that disruptive social behaviour was a key factor leading to admission to a madhouse.

The gender balance of inmates identified as having mania or melancholia seems to have varied. In Britain in the sixteenth and seventeenth centuries, when small private madhouses were almost the only specialist institutions for lunatics, there were somewhat more male than female lunatics in madhouses, houses of correction and workhouses (MacDonald 1986), and probably rather more with a diagnosis of mania than melancholia. This gender balance undoubtedly reflects in part the contingencies that determined whether an individual ended up in an asylum or not, with more men than women being disruptive and difficult and therefore liable to charges of lunacy. However, by the nineteenth century, when the public asylums were being set up and the numbers confined were increasing rapidly, there was a more even gender distribution of inmates. By this time the term melancholia was somewhat more likely to be applied to women than men, although in the sixteenth and seventeenth centuries it had had strong associations with men, being viewed as 'the affliction of gentlemen and scholars' (ibid.: 268).

By the end of the nineteenth century the mapping of psychiatric disorders began to change quite radically with the dismantling of the old opposition between mania and melancholia. Emil Kraepelin, a key figure in the new classificatory work, argued that mania and melancholia should be viewed as different forms of a single disease group, manic-depressive psychosis (Jackson 1986: 190), which he contrasted with dementia praecox (renamed schizophrenia by Eugen Bleuler in 1911).[7] For Kraepelin the key feature of the contrast between manic-depressive insanity and dementia praecox was that the former did not involve an inevitable deterioration of intellectual functioning whereas the latter did. But this related to another feature of the new opposition: that whereas the symptoms of dementia praecox focused on features of thought and reasoning, the key symptoms of the various types of manic-depressive insanity related to the emotions, though they could, when severe, involve hallucinations and delusions. The new grouping of manic-depressive disorders provided the foundation for the present-day group of 'mood disorders' in the two most influential current psychiatric classifications, the American Psychiatric Association's *Diagnostic and Statistical Manual of Mental Disorders*, now in its fourth edition (1994), and the World Health Organisation's *The ICD-10 Classification of Mental and Behavioural Disorders* (1992). The preference for the term 'mood' over 'emotion' is interesting and may reflect the desire to move away from the more familiar and evocative lay term, emotion, to an apparently rather more detached language of mood states.

Though the use of the term schizophrenia was slow to take hold (Loughlin 1996), by the 1930s it began to be more widely used and it came to represent the archetype of madness in the twentieth century just as mania had done in the previous centuries. Although the symptoms include some mention of mood, as in the reference to the 'flattening of affect', many relate to thought, including hallucinations, delusions, breaks or interpolations in the train of thought, thought insertion and thought withdrawal. And though there were often gender differences in levels of treated cases, most of the evidence from community surveys indicates that there is little in the way of a gender imbalance in identified cases (American Psychiatric Association 1994: 281–2; Goldstein 1992), though it also shows that the average age of onset and the content of disturbed thoughts and ideas differs between men and women (psychiatrists emphasise that it is the nature of the thought processes that is at issue in judgements of pathology, not their content). Community surveys also show little evidence of a gender difference in levels of dementia once allowance is made for differences in survival rates (Myers *et al.* 1984).[8]

The lack of an overall gender imbalance for most community survey populations in levels of schizophrenia is interesting. It suggests in the first place that there is no gender difference in genetic or environmental vulnerability to the condition as it is currently framed and no gender difference in exposure to the key environmental factors (there is evidence that both genetic and environmental factors play a part in its aetiology). It also suggests that fundamental processes of thought are being judged, which are not themselves subject to much in the way of differential social expectations and social shaping according to gender. In this respect the thought disorders differ markedly from the disorders of emotion and behaviour where social shaping plays a crucial role. Consequently, it suggests that the judgement of pathology of thought demarcated through concepts such as schizophrenia and the various dementias manages to get to the heart of thought processes that are shared between men and women.

Yet further examination of the data on levels of identified schizophrenia in different ethnic groups indicates that this picture needs to be qualified. For instance, data on ethnicity and schizophrenia show especially high levels of schizophrenia amongst Afro-Caribbean groups, especially men, which might appear to suggest the importance of the social shaping of behaviour. However, data from community surveys yield rather smaller differences (Nazroo 1997), indicating that much of the difference in identified levels in this instance is due to biases in the processes of identification and selection.[9] It is also important to note that the use of the concept of schizophrenia has varied over time and between countries. In the US, for instance, the category has had broader boundaries and gender differences in levels have been noted more frequently.[10]

The situation with Kraepelin's manic-depressive group of disorders is rather different. Significantly Kraepelin thought this group was more common in women than in men, and this is true of the mood disorders taken as a whole today. However, whereas a female predominance is typical of all types of depression, including major or psychotic depression, there is no gender difference for manic-depression itself (American Psychiatric Association 1994: 353), a condition characterised by alternating states of mania and depression now termed 'bipolar' disorder. This finding qualifies the claim of a particular linkage between women and disorders of emotion. As with schizo-phrenia, genetic factors make a significant contribution to its aetiology and it may be that this accounts for the absence of a significant gender difference in the levels of the disorder.

Kraepelin's grouping of a range of mood states under the broad umbrella of the manic-depressive insanity was an important step in the greater atten-tion to disorders of emotion that we find in the twentieth century. However, his focus was on asylum populations and he believed that, except for milder cases, treatment should be carried out in the asylum, where precautions could be taken against the dangers of suicide and the appropriate regimens of diet, exercise, baths and drugs could be provided (Jackson 1986: 193). It was doctors working outside the asylum in private practice whose activities gave increasing prominence to disorders of emotion and played an important part in widening the terrain of official psychiatric disorder.

Disorders of emotion

Outside the asylum the use of doctors for advice and treatment by those who were 'troubled in mind' was long-established. Michael MacDonald (1981), in his excellent study of the case records of the physician, Richard Napier, who practised at the beginning of the seventeenth century, shows that large number of his patients had less severe mental problems that did not justify labels of mania or insanity.[11] And unlike those with the more severe disorders, where thought and rationality were affected, who were usu-ally brought to the attention of doctors through the complaints of others, such individuals tended themselves to judge that they were disturbed: 'the sufferers *themselves* frequently judged that their emotions were abnormal' (ibid.: 149). As this comment indicates, emotions were often at the heart of these problems, individuals feeling that 'the sheer intensity of their moods was abnormal' (ibid.). Significantly Napier found that such problems occurred more frequently in women than men. Though men and women sometimes attributed their disorder to the work of the Devil or to being bewitched, they also mentioned a range of environmental causes with troubled courtships, marital problems, bereavements and economic difficul-ties being the most frequently mentioned (ibid.: 5). Since this list covers difficulties to which men and women were exposed it suggests a greater female vulnerability to these problems. This could be, as subsequent analysis has indicated (see Kessler and McLeod 1984), because of women's greater involvement in, and attachment to, their families. Equally it could be a consequence of women's subordinate position within the family which made it more difficult to ameliorate or escape from difficulties they faced. Mac-Donald (1986: 274) comments: 'Some sympathetic men and many miserable women recognised that subordination of wives to their husbands made them more vulnerable to misery and madness.' Another factor may have been gender differences in social expectations, which determined, from the earliest years, the way in which men and women handled their troubles and expressed their underlying feelings.

Apart from terms such as melancholia or hypochondriasis, the medical language used to differentiate such problems was limited. Napier used the lay language of the emotional life, referring to people being 'troubled in mind' or 'mopish' (a more plebeian and less medical concept than melancholia), as well as using terms such as sad and fearful. However, during the seventeenth and eighteenth centuries the link between the nerves and moods became a greater focus of medical attention and the language of 'nerves' increasingly framed lay discussions of the less severe mental disorders (Oppenheim 1991). This medical interest was reflected in the emergence of another medical speciality, neurology, focused on the nerves and nervous disorders, which was to some extent in competition with the developing specialism of psychiatry focused on the new group of asylum doctors.[12]

But it is not until the second half of the nineteenth century that we find much in the way of any greater medical differentiation of the territory of these less severe problems, which typically concentrated on the emotions. Again we can see the changes which occurred in the second half of the nineteenth century as part of the professionalising endeavour of the new medical specialists, sometimes doctors who worked in the new asylums as well as in their own consulting rooms, and sometimes the neurologists who worked outside the asylums.

An influential new category in the second half of the nineteenth century was that of neurasthenia or nervous exhaustion, introduced by G.M. Beard, an American neurologist working in private practice. The condition was characterised by a loose list of ill-defined symptoms:

Insomnia, flushing, drowsiness, bad dreams, cerebral irritation, dilated pupils, pain, pressure and heaviness in the head, changes in the expression of the eye, neurasthenic asthenopia, noises in the ears, atonic voice, mental irritability, tenderness of the teeth and gums, nervous dyspepsia, desire for stimulants and narcotics, abnormal dryness of the skin, joints and mucous membranes, sweating hands and feet with redness, fear of lightning, or fear of responsibility, of open places or of closed places, fear of society, fear of being alone, fear of fears, fear of contamination, fear of everything, deficient mental control, lack of mental control, lack of decision in trifling matters, hopelessness, deficient thirst and capacity for assimilating fluids, abnormalities of secretions, salivation, tenderness of the spine, and of the whole body.

(Beard [1881] 1972: 7)

This list shows the same mixture of elements concerning body, mind and behaviour that featured in earlier characterisations of mania, with no exclusive attention to emotional states. But the emotions are included, not only in the reference to 'hopelessness', which could also be a symptom of melancholia, but also in the list of fears, which features quite strongly. In addition, a number of the physical symptoms are ones associated with emotions including anxiety, a term that has tended to suggest physical as well as emotional experiences. Interestingly, in its early formulations, the category of neurasthenia was particularly associated with men, and, like melancholia in the sixteenth and seventeenth centuries and hypochondriasis in the same period, it was viewed by some as almost a mark of civilisation – a situation encouraged by the fact that it was mainly the affluent who could afford to bring such problems to medical attention.

Equally important to the delineation of emotional disorders was the concept of shell-shock, a term coined by C.S. Myers (1915) in the First World War for the disturbances of sensation, movement and vision, the loss of memory, loss of self-confidence and obsessional thoughts that he initially thought arose from the physical shock of shells exploding near soldiers. To some extent, the new disease was assimilated to older categories, with doctors differentiating two types of shell-shock: a hysterical form common amongst the lower ranks and a neurasthenic form more common amongst officers. But efforts to understand and treat shell-shock helped to secure a wider acceptance for Freudian claims about the psychogenic origins of disorders of the mind. For, though there was great debate about the causes of shell-shock, many began to concur that the disorder was essentially psychological, not in the character of its symptoms, which again included a mixed and ill-defined list of symptoms, but in its causation. Freud termed such diseases the psycho-neuroses to make clear the psychological origins of the disorders, distinguishing them from the 'actual neuroses' which involved some pathological functioning of the nervous system itself. They were also increasingly contrasted with the psychoses in psychiatric classifications, with the latter frequently being assumed to have physical causes and also to be more severe.

The concept of psycho-neurosis consequently incorporates, though it does not make explicit, a second conceptualisation of disorders of emotion. In the first sense, represented by the mood disorders, the disorder is viewed as a disorder of mood or emotion because the key symptoms refer to particular emotional states. To some extent neurasthenia belongs in this category because of the focus on fear, and in present-day psychiatry so do the various phobias. In the second sense, the disorder is viewed as a disorder of the emotions because it is the person's emotions and feelings that give rise to the symptoms. In that respect shell-shock is an emotional disorder because of the assumption that it is psychologically generated.[13] Of course, there is an elision here between 'psychological' and 'emotional' causes, but psychodynamic accounts of mental life have frequently tended to stress the role played by the emotions, particularly love and hate.

Within the framework of Freudian thought one of the most important neuroses (the prefix was gradually abandoned and the term neurosis took on the new psychodynamic meaning) is anxiety neurosis, an emotional disorder in both senses, since anxiety, the key symptom, is an emotional as well as a physical state, and anxiety neurosis was held to have psychogenic causes. Freud himself gave rather less attention to depression than to anxiety, but under the influence of his ideas for much of the second half of the twentieth century a contrast was made between endogenous depression – a psychosis – and neurotic or reactive depression, the latter, unlike the former, held to have clear psychological causes. In fact the balance between anxiety neurosis and neurotic depression, disorders which are in practice often hard to differentiate (Goldberg and Huxley 1992: 57), has changed according to the changing value attached to psychodynamic ideas and treatment. In the decades following the Second World War, the development of new drug treatments for depression by the pharmaceutical companies encouraged the use of this diagnosis at the expense of anxiety states (Blum 1978; Healy 1998).

Whilst the balance of the two conditions has fluctuated, since at least the middle of the twentieth century anxiety and depression (in its milder forms) have been the most important and most commonly diagnosed of the less severe mental disorders – the common colds and flu of psychiatry – though this parallel is not intended to diminish the unpleasantness of the experience for sufferers. The frequency with which they have been identified has resulted from a set of social processes in which psychiatric work on classification and treatment and the expansion of mental health services have reinforced each other. On the one hand, new professional work on these disorders has encouraged more individuals to bring such problems to doctors and mental health practitioners. This work includes new forms of treatment, such as the various forms of psychotherapy under the influence of psychodynamic ideas, and then new forms of drug treatment in the second half of the twentieth century, work increasingly encouraged by the activities of the drug companies. On the other hand, the improved access to medical care for wider sections of the population has enabled more people to bring these types of problem to medical attention in the search for help, support and treatment and this has helped to expand medical work in this field.

An important further development has been the attempt in the final decades of the twentieth century to exclude the language of (psycho-)neurosis from official psychiatric classifications on the grounds of its aetiological assumptions (and one suspects the hostility of many biologically-oriented psychiatrists to its Freudian connotations). This move has been largely successful but the distinction is still quite widely used in practice, not least because the psychotic-neurotic contrast provides a shorthand way of differentiating 'more severe' and 'less severe' disorders. One consequence has been to separate milder (neurotic) depression from anxiety states in classifications, notwithstanding the affinity between the two conditions. Depression, whether severe or mild, is located in the group of mood disorders. In contrast, the different types of anxiety have their own separate grouping which includes various phobias.

The exclusion of aetiological assumptions from psychiatric classifications is, however, by no means consistent. Not only does the DSM-IV retain the

category of organic mental disorders for conditions that have clearly established physical causes, it also includes the category of post-traumatic stress
disorder (a condition with affinities with the earlier shell-shock), the one
disorder where a psychogenic origin is explicit in the label. The inclusion of
this term, which is listed as an anxiety disorder in the DSM-IV, followed a
campaign by American veterans of the Vietnam War and their supporters
(Young 1995). Notwithstanding this exception, the overall effect of the exclusion of the category of neurosis from official classifications has been that
psychogenic aetiology and psychological processes are downplayed.[14]

Almost all the disorders of emotion except manic-depression show a
female predominance, and I have already suggested that the normative social
shaping of emotional expression in relation to gender is one important factor
generating the marked gender imbalances in emotional disorders. Notions of
femininity have made it more acceptable, even desirable, for women in many
Western societies to display fear, anxiety and sadness and to talk about such
inner feelings. In contrast, notions of masculinity have encouraged the control of such emotions and their discussion, although other emotions such as
hate and anger are more acceptable in men than women. In addition, alongside the importance of this social shaping of emotional expression is the
framing of the categories of psychiatric disorder themselves. What is striking
about the terrain of emotional disorders defined in terms of symptoms is that
it is relatively narrow. Only certain emotions – sadness, fear and anxiety –
have been incorporated into the psychiatric lexicon through the disorders of
depression, phobia and anxiety states. Other candidates for inclusion, most
obviously jealousy, anger and hate, though they may be mentioned as symptoms and now receive some attention in treatment programmes, are not
framed into distinct disorders.[15] Instead it is the behaviours with which
they are associated, particularly violence, which have been identified as
problematic.

This selectivity undoubtedly contributes to the gender imbalance of the
emotional disorders since historically it is the emotions particularly associated with women that have been pathologised. When people talk of women
being more emotional than men they are in fact focusing on particular emotions that have come to define what it means to be 'emotional', which is
usually read as showing more sadness, anxiety and fear. Men's emotional
nature has frequently been manifest in different ways which are far less likely
to be read as emotional, and are seen in terms of behaviours rather than
underlying emotions. Historically these behaviours when considered
unacceptable have been interpreted through the language of badness,
immorality and delinquency rather than of psychiatric disturbance. However,
during the twentieth century there has been an increasing tendency to treat
these behaviours as types of psychiatric disorder rather than as simply
socially unacceptable, though this is subject to the vagaries of legal, political
and lay attitudes and contingencies.[16]

Disorders of behaviour

The behaviour and personality disorders, which have extended the terrain of official psychiatric classifications in the twentieth century, have their antecedents in nineteenth-century categories. Of particular importance was the notion of moral insanity introduced by the English physician J.C. Prichard in 1833. Distinguishing between disorders 'of feeling or sentiment, the understanding, and the will' (see Hunter and MacAlpine 1963: 837), he regarded moral insanity as combining a disorder of feeling with a disorder of 'active powers and propensities'. The 'active powers' were conceived by Prichard in terms of mind – the will – but the concept at the same time introduces a focus on behaviour, as we see in the following description of moral insanity:

> The moral and active principles of the mind are strongly perverted or depraved; the power of self government is lost or greatly impaired and the individual is found to be incapable not of talking or reasoning upon any subject proposed to him, but conducting himself with decency and propriety in the business of life.
>
> (Quoted in Ramon 1987: 215)

In the twentieth century, the concept of moral insanity has been replaced by a wide range of behavioural and personality disorders, disorders in which the judgement of pathology is based first and foremost on behaviour. An influential concept has been that of psychopathy, a term with a wider meaning in other European countries than in Britain or the US (Manning 2000: 622). The term is still in use in current British mental health legislation, although in official classifications it has been replaced by categories such as conduct disorder or anti-social personality disorder. The DSM-IV uses both, differentiating them primarily according to the age of the individual concerned (whether the person is under 18 or not). It begins the description of conduct disorder, a category only applicable in the schema to young people, in the following way: 'The essential feature of Conduct Disorder is a repetitive and persistent pattern of behavior in which the basic rights of others or major age-appropriate societal norms or rules are violated' (American Psychiatric Association 1994: 85). It then refers to the frequency of aggression, violence and theft and gives a similar picture of anti-social personality disorder, the equivalent category for adults. Alcohol and drug dependence, as well as sexual disorders, are further examples of behaviour disorders. Whether they should be regarded as psychiatric disorders, given psychiatry's initial focus on disorders of the mind, has long been contested (see Wootton 1959).

Historically, the behaviour and personality disorders have not made a major contribution to in-patient psychiatric populations.[17] Though perceived dangerousness was an important criterion in admission to an asylum and continuing detention there in the nineteenth century, most of those considered dangerous were individuals in whom the danger was associated with a loss of reason (in the psychotic sense), and this situation continued with the expansion of asylum numbers in the first half of the twentieth century. However, with the introduction of policies of community care and the marked decline in the number of psychiatric residents, along with the growing attention to behavioural problems that are not deemed the product of a loss of reason, they have become of increasing importance in psychiatric in-patient populations. For instance, services for those with drug and alcohol problems have expanded while other services have been cut back.

A key factor in recent decades has been the growing emphasis on risk and public safety. As I have already indicated, issues of public safety have always been a factor in the detention of those with disturbed behaviour who are considered potentially dangerous and disruptive of the social order. However, there is now greater attention to various forms of risk across society, and a belief that dangers must and can be controlled and prevented (Beck 1992). Given the widespread association in the public mind between psychiatric disorder and violence, increasing efforts have been put into controlling the risk of violence from such people.[18] This is despite the fact that the developments in psychotropic medication have themselves provided a means of controlling dangerousness and so have arguably reduced the overall threat of violence posed by those with some psychiatric disturbance. Unfortunately, however, it is the perceived, not actual, risks of violence that have a crucial impact on mental health policy.

The majority of the behaviour disorders has been more frequently identified in men than women. There are two major reasons for this. First, as I have already argued, men's and women's responses to difficulties in their lives tend to be rather different, with men tending to turn their problems outwards in disruptive and difficult behaviour and women turning them inwards, so that they find expression in depression and anxiety. Second, there has been a reluctance to treat these behaviours as psychiatric problems rather than as forms of delinquency precisely because of their link with difficult, disruptive behaviour. This is both at the level of identifying the character of the problem in the individual case (mechanism 5) and at the level of determining whether a particular problem is more psychiatric than one of socially unacceptable conduct (mechanism 6). As a result they tend to be kept out of the psychiatric frame.

Changing patterns

As will be clear from the analysis so far, the gendered landscape of psychiatric disorder changes over time. This is not only because developments in psychiatry and the mental health services lead to changes in the emphasis on particular disorders, as well as bringing new disorders into the psychiatric spectrum and excluding others; it is also because there is nothing necessarily fixed in the relation between gender and particular psychiatric disorders.

Most obviously, as the social expectations shaping male and female behaviour and emotional expression change, often in response to major changes in their situation within society, so the gender differences in psychiatric disorder change. For instance, in as far as women have increasing access to the financial resources and public spaces where alcohol and drugs are available as a result of changing patterns of female labour force participation and greater public freedoms, so their patterns of customary use are changing, and when facing difficulties they may be more likely to handle them by resorting to excessive drug and alcohol use than by becoming depressed.

Changes also arise as a result of the initiatives of mental health professionals and the pharmaceutical industry, who may have an interest in broadening their client group. A striking recent example has been the effort to argue that depression is more common in men than is generally recognised and that much of it goes undetected – activity that may start to change the gender balance in cases of depression. In 1998, the Royal College of Psychiatrists hosted a one-day conference to launch a new pamphlet, *Men Behaving Sadly*, which set out this case and listed the signs of depression to look for in men. A section headed 'How is depression different for men' gives a flavour of the contents:

> The way that men think about themselves can be quite unhelpful. Compared with women, they tend to be far more concerned with being competitive, powerful and successful. Most men don't like to admit that they feel fragile or vulnerable, and so are less likely to talk about their feelings with their friends, loved ones, or their doctors. This may be the reason that they don't ask for help when they become depressed. Men tend to feel that they should rely on themselves and that it is somehow weak to depend on someone else, even for a short time.
>
> (Royal College of Psychiatrists 1998: 3)

Whilst the statements here are probably accurate enough, it is important to note that what is presented as undetected need and suffering that ought to be met is as the same time a potential source of expansion in mental health work. In this context it is significant that both doctors and the pharmaceutical industry stand to benefit if more men are identified as depressed. And although the pamphlet includes a range of practical advice, such as using relaxation techniques, changing one's lifestyle, eating properly, keeping active and not bottling things up, it also emphasises very strongly that the general practitioner is the best place to start in seeking help. It emphasises, too, that depression is an illness and that it is easily treatable – the treatment implied at this point being very clearly drugs: 'Antidepressant tablets are often an important part of getting better – and it's important to remember that this sort of medication is not addictive' (ibid.: 11). What is also of interest is that the psychiatrist who launched the pamphlet argued that the symptoms of depression were not necessarily the same in men as in women (in men they could include aggressiveness and anti-social behaviour), so potentially broad-ening the boundaries of the condition to incorporate more men (*Guardian*, 1 October 1998). With the leaflets being distributed to GP waiting rooms, we can expect to find a shifting gender balance in the levels of depression as a result of changing perceptions.

Given the changing character of gender relations and the situation of men and women, along with the developments in psychiatry and mental health services and practice, which are themselves shaped by a range of factors, we can therefore expect to see some significant changes in the relation between gender and psychiatric disorder. An understanding of the relations between gender and psychiatric disorder requires a very careful unravelling of the complex character of psychiatric ideas and practice as well as of gender re-lations. This chapter, with its focus on the changing categories of psychiatric disorder over time, provides one contribution to that unravelling.

Notes

1 I use the term psychiatric disorder for two reasons. First, it is psychiatrists above all who control the official classifications which set out the terrain of disorder. Second, the terrain so delineated does not focus exclusively on disorders of mind, but increasingly includes behavioural problems, as the ICD title for its own clas-sification, *The ICD-10 Classification of Mental and Behavioural Disorders*, indicates.
2 It might be argued that this approach suggests that clear distinctions can be made in practice between the different disorders. I do not make such an assumption. Rather my claim is that the classificatory schema provides a crucial lens through which a range of problems is refracted.
3 The main functional psychoses are schizophrenia and manic-depression. The latter is discussed further below.
4 The higher proportion of men in this study overall is almost certainly due to factors involved in the selection of individuals for treatment.
5 Such labels are not necessarily alternatives, but in practice action may involve decisions that frames the issues in one way rather than another.
6 In this respect the concept of lunacy can be contrasted with the concept of idiocy, where a judgement of mind was also involved, but in this case the focus was on intellect and its impairment rather than thought processes.
7 The term depression began to appear in discussions of melancholia in the eight-eenth century; it is to be found in the writings of Samuel Johnson who suffered from melancholy (Jackson 1986: 145–6).
8 The paper by Myers and his colleagues reports on data from the US Epidemio-logic Catchment Area study which included a measure of 'cognitive impairment'.
9 The level of schizophrenia identified in the community survey was still raised amongst the Afro-Caribbean group but was far lower than in most surveys (Nazroo 1997: 81–3).
10 A broader definition means that more cases that would have been diagnosed as some form of affective psychosis are included.
11 An element of the retrospective identification of the character of the problems is of course involved in this categorisation.
12 For an excellent account of the conflict and competition between the asylum doctors and those working outside, see Rosenberg 1968.

13 A similar argument can be applied to the term mental disorder which can be taken to suggest disorders with predominantly mental symptoms; equally it can be taken to mean disorders caused by mental processes.
14 One immediate consequence is that anorexia nervosa, which is regarded by many as having a psycho-social causes and could be termed a neurosis, is treated as a behaviour disorder in the ICD-10 classification (it is treated as a disorder of childhood or adolescence in the DSM).
15 Anger management programmes are now quite fashionable.
16 In many cases the location is still hotly contested, as for instance with paedophilia, formulated as a psychiatric disorder yet regarded by the public far more as immoral conduct than as sickness.
17 It is interesting that the Present State Examination (Wing *et al.* 1974) which was developed as an instrument for the detection of psychiatric disorder in the early 1970s did not cover behaviour disorders.
18 The majority of those with a psychiatric disorder are not violent; however, there is evidence that many of those who are violent have some psychological problem (see Busfield, forthcoming).

References

American Psychiatric Association (1994) *Diagnostic and Statistical Manual of Mental Disorders*, 3rd edn, Washington, DC: APA.

Beard, G.M. ([1881] 1972) *American Nervousness: Its Causes and Consequences*, New York: Arno Press.

Beck, U. (1992) *Risk Society: Towards a New Modernity*. London: Sage.

Blum, J. (1978) 'On changes in psychiatric diagnosis over time', *American Psychologist* 33: 1017–31.

Brown, P. (1990) 'The name game: toward a sociology of diagnosis', *Journal of Mind and Behavior* 11: 385–406.

Busfield, J. (1983) 'Gender, mental illness and psychiatry', in M. Evans and C. Umgerson (eds), *Sexual Divisions: Patterns and Processes*, London: Tavistock.

—— (1996) *Men, Women and Madness: Understanding Gender and Mental Disorder*, London: Macmillan.

—— (1999) 'Mental health policy: making gender and ethnicity visible', *Policy and Politics* 27: 57–72.

—— (forthcoming) 'Mental disorder and individual violence: imagined death, risk and mental health policy', in A. Buchanan (ed.), *Care of the Mentally Disordered Offender in the Community*, Oxford: Oxford University Press.

Castel, R., Castel, F. and Lovell, A. (1994) *The Psychiatric Society*, New York: Columbia University Press.

Foucault, M. (1967) *Madness and Civilisation*, London: Tavistock.

Goldberg, D. and Huxley, P. (1980) *Mental Illness in the Community: The Pathway to Psychiatric Care*, London: Tavistock.

—— and —— (1992) *Common Mental Disorders: A Bio-social Model*, London: Routledge.

Goldstein, J.M. (1992) 'Gender and schizophrenia: a summary of findings', *Schizophrenia Monitor* 2: 1–4.

Healy, D. (1998) *The Anti-depressant Era*, Cambridge, MA: Harvard University Press.

Hollingshead, A.B. and Redlich, F.C. (1958) *Social Class and Mental Illness*, New York: John Wiley.

Hunter, R. and MacAlpine, I. (1963) *Three Hundred Years of Pyschiatry, 1535–1860*, Oxford: Oxford University Press.

Jackson, S.W. (1986) *Melancholia and Depression*, New Haven, CT: Yale University Press.

Kessler, R.C. and MacLeod, J.D. (1984) 'Sexual differences in vulnerability to undesirable life events', *American Sociological Review* 49: 620–31.

Loughlin, K. (1996) *Framing Schizophrenia: Gender and Professional Identity in British Psychiatry, c.1890–c.1930*, PhD thesis, Department of Sociology, University of Essex.

MacDonald, M. (1981) *Mystical Bedlam: Madness, Anxiety and Healing in Seventeenth Century England*, Cambridge: Cambridge University Press.

——(1986) 'Women and madness in Tudor and Stuart England', *Social Research* 55: 257–81.

Manning, N. (2000) 'Psychiatric diagnosis under conditions of uncertainty: personality disorder, science and legitimacy', *Sociology of Health and Illness* 22 (5): 621–39.

Meltzer, H., Gill, B., Petticrew, M. and Hinds, K. (1995) *The Prevalence of Psychiatric Morbidity amongst Adults Living in Private Households*, London: Office of Population Censuses and Surveys.

Myers, C.S. (1915) 'A contribution to the study of shell-shock', *Lancet* 13 February: 316–20.

Myers, S.K., Wiseman, M.M., Tichsler, G.L., Holzer, C.E., Leaf, P.J., Orvashiel, H., Anthony, J.C., Boyd, J.H., Burke, J.D., Kramer, M. and Stoltzman, R. (1984) 'Six-month prevalence of psychiatric disorders in three communities', *Archives of General Psychiatry* 41: 9959–67.

Nazroo, J. (1997) *Ethnicity and Mental Health*, London: Policy Studies Institute.

Oppenheim, S. (1991) *'Shattered Nerves': Doctors, Patients and Depression in Victorian England*, New York: Oxford University Press.

Parry-Jones, W. (1972) *The Trade in Lunacy: A Study of Private Madhouses in England in the Eighteenth and Nineteenth Centuries*, London: Routledge and Kegan Paul.

Ramon, S. (1987) 'The category of psychopathy: its professional and social context in Britain', in P. Miller and N. Rose (eds), *The Power of Psychiatry*, Cambridge: Polity Press.

Rosenberg, C.E. (1968) *The Trial of Assassin Guiteau: Psychiatry and Law in the Gilded Age*, Chicago: University of Chicago Press.

——(1992) 'Introduction to framing disease, illness, society and history', in C.E. Rosenberg and J. Gooden (eds), *Framing Diseases: Studies on Cultural History*, New Brunswick, NJ: Rutgers University Press.

Royal College of Psychiatrists (1998) *Men Behaving Sadly*, London: Royal College of Psychiatrists.

Wing, J.K., Cooper, J.E. and Sartorius, N. (1974) *Description and Classification of Psychiatric Symptoms*, Cambridge: Cambridge University Press.

Wootton, B. (1959) *Social Science and Social Pathology*, London: Allen and Unwin.

World Health Organisation (1992) *ICD-10 Classification of Mental and Behavioural Disorders*, Geneva: World Health Organisation.

Young, A. (1995) *The Harmony of Illusions: Inventing Post Traumatic Stress Disorder*, Princeton, NJ: Princeton University Press.

9 Experiences of ADHD

Children, health research and emotion work

Gillian Bendelow and Geraldine Brady

Introduction

This chapter takes as its starting point the challenge to certain well-established sociological conceptualisations about the social order which was begun by Meg Stacey many years ago with the path-breaking paper to the British Sociological Association, 'The division of labour revisited, or over-coming the two Adams' (Stacey 1981). This work questioned the legacy of the founding fathers of such substantially corroborated themes as the division between public and private or definitions of 'work' and labour and has remained a core problematic for feminist academics (and indeed what used to be unproblematically referred to as the 'women's movement') ever since (see, for instance, Garmarnikov *et al.* 1983; Finch and Groves 1983; Graham 1984, 1993; Mayall and Foster 1989; Mayall 1996). Traditionally, the discipline of sociology had shown scant attention to children: located within the private sphere of the family and home; not regarded as rational or competent, so that any investigation or understanding was left largely to the realm of 'scientific' medico-psychological investigation. The approach Stacey and colleagues developed to study the division of labour was distinctive, not just because it was qualitative, but also through its inclusion of the contributions of both lay and professional, paid and unpaid carers, in which each participant was regarded as a social actor and very much part of a social process. Sociology had a role, as the producer of new knowledge, grounded in the experience of real people, which would hopefully be incorporated into the policy and practice of health institutions (Stacey 1988). This approach, appropriated by sociologists of childhood, also meant that children themselves could be seen as viable actors in the social world.

In this chapter, we discuss how two main schools of sociological thought have taken children's role in the social order forward over the intervening period. First, we chart how the development of the sociology of childhood has contributed and widened the debates about the public and the private and the division of labour. Just as second-wave feminism drew attention to the 'otherness' of women, children have been conceptualised as a distinct social group (see, for instance, Oakley 1994), who are all too often spoken for by adults rather than allowed their own voices. In particular we draw upon the substantial body of work by Berry Mayall which has taken Stacey's public/ private dichotomy as a framework in which to bring together sociological concepts of childhood and empirical research in health and illness. Second, we discuss how a sociological approach to emotion and embodiment has further enriched and broadened these themes and allows for unique insights into the links between Mills's (1959) notion of 'personal troubles' and broader 'public issues' of social structure' (Mills). Finally, we use examples of our own research to demonstrate the empirical, as well as the theoretical, development of research strategies which transcend the rigid dichotomisation of public/private divides and which aim to understand and explain children's place in the social order. This dramatic shift in the research paradigm is often described as being about research *for* children rather than *on* them.

Concepts of childhood

Since the end of the twentieth century there has been an upsurge in interest in children and childhood from many spheres. This interest is located within a pattern of broader social change: the need to invest in futures at the begin-ning of a new millennium; changes in the structure of the family; and an ever-increasing ageing population have led to a view of children as precious. A recent Conservative party slogan proclaimed 'Children are 20 per cent of the population, but 100 per cent of the future'. According to the UN Con-vention on the Rights of the Child and the Children Act 1989 children are seen as autonomous individuals, they have a right to be heard and to be protected by the law. Yet, paradoxically, their freedom is being curtailed by increasing use of surveillance techniques – through the police, closed circuit television, parents, teachers, health professionals and the emerging influence of a 'risk' society. Children are no longer just the concern of parents and educators but are now 'popularised, politicised, scrutinised and analysed' (James *et al.* 1998: 3). Sociologists of childhood have employed a largely social constructionist theoretical stance to chart how the concept of 'the child' has changed dramatically from the nineteenth-century discourses (see Jenks 1996; James *et al.* 1998) and, in particular, the '*psy* complex' has been highlighted as a major means of surveillance over the last hundred years, in which children and childhood have become very largely the province of psychology and psychiatry and charting child development has become a major industry in Western industrialised countries. Children have become identified as problems to be solved, as victims and as threats, as vulnerable and as dangerous.

Mayall (1996) and others have accused 'Western' mainstream sociology of an unrelenting and uncritical reliance on the concept of *socialisation*, in which children are essentially the objects of adult work to turn them into adults fit to join society and, theoretically, to render them fit objects or subjects of sociology. Though functionalism has been largely eschewed by sociologists, there is a continued reliance upon it in relation to children and to childhood. The traditional approaches of child psychology, child development and socialisation have served to complement one another.

The discourse of developmental psychology emerged during the early twentieth century, giving 'prominence to biological and psychological explanations of children's every day social experiences' (James and Prout, in Brannen and O'Brien, 1996: 43). Child psychology's body of knowledge has been derived mainly from quantitative research, with a strongly developmental approach; but psychology, unlike sociology, as James *et al.* (1998) have argued, never made the mistake of questioning its own status as a science and, in the guise of developmental psychology, firmly colonised childhood in a pact with medicine, education and government agencies.

The work of Piaget, which characterised childhood as a series of different stages associated with age-spans (Hill and Tisdall 1997: 9), has been criticised for severely underestimating children's abilities and for diminishing the role of emotions. Teacher training has been heavily influenced by Piagetian perspectives of cognitive development; this has led to a situation where 'what children know and how they use knowledge to consider moral and practical issues in their daily lives has been of less interest than what cognitive stage they have reached' (Mayall 1996: 45). Childhood was regarded as 'natural', not social; the notion of developmental stages and a progressive change towards the goal of adult maturity was regarded as universal. Mayall (ibid.) comments that developmental psychology has been individualist in focusing on the child apart from its social context, and universalist in aiming to uncover truths applying to all children, and that socialisation theory fails to acknowledge the agency or intentionality of children and tends to regard them as passive and malleable. Thus, the 'psycho-medical construction of childhood' has proved difficult to challenge, since health professionals, educationalists, welfare workers claim to know the 'truth' about childhood, and use this perspective to justify the treatment of children in Western society as physically, mentally and emotionally immature and subordinate to adults. However, in recent years, routes through symbolic interactionism (e.g., Denzin 1977) and through various versions of social constructionism (e.g., Ingleby 1986) have attempted to rethink childhood; developmental pyschology itself has focused more than before on interactions between context and the child (e.g., Cole 1996). Most importantly, a concerted sociological effort has begun to develop more adequate understandings and there is now, after 15 years of analysis, a substantial body of theoretical work which challenges notions of children as incompetent, immature and under-socialised (e.g., Prout and James 1990; Alanen 1992; Mayall 1996; Jenks 1996). These writers emphasise the competence of children, their abilities within relationships, their wish to participate in decision making and their drive towards social life. As part of the work towards shifting our understandings, research studies have begun to take seriously children's own accounts – their knowledge of the social order, their experiences and their opinions on the childhoods they are asked to live.

The pioneering work carried out in the sixteen-country Childhood as a Social Phenomenon programme (1985–92) established the idea of children as a social group. Indeed, children may have interests in common as a group which differ from and may challenge the interests of adult social groups, notably parents and teachers (see, e.g., Qvortrup 1991, 1994). Like any other social group, children's daily lives, self-appraisal, expectations and opportunities are structured in tension with social policies. More recent research has emphasised the importance of experience, not age or developmental stage (Bluebond-Langner 1991; Alderson 1993).

Although more recent critiques emphasise children's active involvement in constructing their lives and in meaning-making, and emphasise too the agency and intentionality of children, there is also something of a 'backlash' against social constructionism emerging from the findings of the Economic and Social Research Council (ESRC) Research Programme on Children 5–16: Growing into the Twenty-first Century. Recent studies remind us that children are also politically and economically situated, and we must remain aware of the differences of gender, class, ethnicity and disability. An overarching emphasis on children's agency risks becoming a sociology of choice, which fails to recognise the structural freedoms and constraints that the agency of children expresses (Pole *et al.* 1999: 42). Children share 'childhood' but experience childhoods. Traditional accounts are individualistic, and biologically determinist, yet social constructionist accounts eschew the importance of the body. Prout (2000) claims that social constructionists provided a necessary and useful counterpoint to biologically reductionist accounts, but the time now seems right to take embodiment seriously, by incorporating, rather than excluding, biology in the process (Williams and Bendelow 1998). Just as the divisions between public and private have come under challenge, we show how another sociological arena which has developed to a considerable degree over the last 10 years can contribute to understandings of children's lives.

Emotions across the public/private divide

It has often been asserted (see Hochschild 1983; Bendelow and Williams 1998) that emotions lie at the juncture of a number of fundamental dualisms in Western thought, such as mind/body, nature/culture and public/private. The link that emotions provide between a number of traditional divisions and debates within the social sciences, such as the biological versus the social, micro versus macro, public versus private, quantitative versus qualitative, also enables us, again, to question dominant notions of Western rationality; modes of thought which have sought to exclude children, as they have women, from the public world of (male) reason.

As we highlighted earlier, Meg Stacey's conceptualisation of the public/ private divide has shown how the lives of women and children have differed from those of men in socially patterned ways (Ribbens 1994). The notion of a public space dominated by men and a private space occupied by women and children has led to a theoretical rethinking of the social world. Such theoretical movements have led to the development of new and innovative methods in research with children. Research which regards children as active social agents, rather than passive victims, shows that 'Children actively negotiate the diverse contexts of their everyday lives, including the boundaries between home, other household and parenting contexts, institutions, and the external social and physical environment' (www.ESRC.ac.uk: last accessed November 2000). Worldwide, children are active participants in the social order and recent studies have pointed out how children's everyday emotional and bodily lives are constructed by adults (Mayall 1998; Prendergast and Forest 1998). Perhaps children can be better understood as active participants in the management of both their bodies and their minds rather than being merely passive recipients of processes which are imposed upon them in the form of 'civilisation', 'regulation' and 'surveillance' (Mayall 1996, 1998).

In order to understand how emotion is a mediating force between embodiment and the social world, Mayall (1998) suggests we examine how adult models structure children's participation in child–adult transactions; in other words, what children are, how childhood should be lived, and how, since childhood is a relational concept, adults should behave in relation to children. These understandings differ according to setting and, variously, structure how homes, schools, health and welfare agencies operate (Alanen 1994). Most crucially, because of the authority and control adults exercise over all aspects of children's lives, adult models importantly affect children's experience, knowledge and identity; they are critical in constructing the personhood of children (Hockey and James 1993). For example, the requirement that children be happy can lead adults to protect them from knowledge that might sadden them, such as the death of a relative or the cruelty people enact towards each other. Girls learn not to develop their muscles, if they are to be socially acceptable; and to restrict their bodily movements within smaller spaces than boys do (Young 1980). More generally, people, especially in their relationships with their superiors, are required to control and organise their emotions (emotion work) and to use these controls to organise bodily movement in ways approved by their superiors and by more general social legitimation (Hochschild 1979). As Scheper-Hughes and Lock (1987) emphasise, emotions are shaped and given meaning at least in part by social or cultural forces and thus provide links which bridge mind and body, individual, society and the body politic, ideas which we hope to show fit closely with what we know of children's experiences.

In order to understand these processes empirically, we need to access children's own accounts, rather than gathering data from parents, usually mothers or professionals. In this next section, we hope to show how child-centred methods help to access the embodied aspects of children's emotional learning, and their often highly sophisticated grasp of concepts such as health, illness and 'normality'.

Child-centred methods

Recognition of the importance of children and childhood in contemporary social life requires the development of a methodology which is child-centred and appropriate to the needs of children. We have discussed how, in late modernity, the social and political concerns around children's rights (for example, the Children Act 1989 and the United Nations Convention of the Rights of the Child 1991) have been reflected within sociological debates around childhood, but it is important to recognise that this has also happened centrally within health and illness. The voices of children and young people have become an important focus within health research, especially with regard to health education and health promotion. As outlined earlier, sociologists of childhood have argued that, traditionally, much research has been on rather than for children, using adult categories, classifications and taxonomies into which children are expected to fit, and which regards them as incompetent, or at best as immature adults (see Mayall 1996; James and Prout 1996). Subsequently there have been calls to develop 'child-centred' approaches, which incorporate children's own ideas, beliefs and metaphors, and involve children in research in more ethical and humanistic ways (Kalnins *et al.* 1992; Mayall 1994). Given the adult-centred nature of most sociological enterprise, as Pole *et al.* (1999) point out, there will inevitably be difficulties as the process will unavoidably involve adult reflection of the process of childhood itself. However, just as qualitative methodology offered possible ways forward for feminism to challenge malestream/traditional research, and to highlight ethical and social dimensions of research, a number of develpments towards so-called 'child-centred' methods have emerged over the last decade, and we focus here on the 'draw-and-write' technique.

Using children's drawings as data has a long history within social science research encompassing psychology and psychoanalysis (see Pridmore and Bendelow 1995 for a detailed review of the use of children's drawings in research). However, this research history is hardly 'child-centred' as drawings have not always been used to facilitate the so-called 'empowerment' of children; rather the opposite: to 'problematise' and diagnose abnormality and unconformity. Therefore the process of inverting this methodology to 'bottom-up' rather than 'top-down' collection of data needs to be undertaken with care and sensitivity if it is truly aiming to treat children as subjects rather than objects. The Brazilian educator Paulo Freire (1972) developed a method in which pictures were used not to transmit the educators' own messages to the learner but to reflect back to the learners the issues with which they themselves were concerned; this method is now widely used in training programmes throughout Africa and the 'developing' world (Hope and Timmel 1984), drawing on the philosophy and teaching of Freire.

In similar ways, images have been widely used in health education and training to trigger discussion and seek solutions to health issues. Children's pictures, in conjunction with writing or dialogue, can be a powerful method of exploring the health beliefs of young children which inform health behaviours and influence health status (Williams *et al.* 1989; Oakley *et al.* 1995; Barnett *et al.* 1994; Pridmore and Bendelow 1995). The large-scale study by Williams *et al.* (1989) is the UK Health Education Authority's national study of primary school children. In this study 9854 children were asked to draw pictures and write explanatory labels around five key areas of health education: safety, relationships, eating, drugs and exercise/rest. The results provided the insight needed to develop more relevant health learning materials. Occleston and King (1993) used the technique to evaluate school-based Child-to-Child programmes. Bendelow was centrally involved in adapting the 'draw and write' technique (Williams *et al.* 1989) for a study funded by the Women's Nationwide Cancer Control Campaign to investigate children's beliefs about health, illness and cancer (Bendelow and Oakley 1993; Oakley *et al.* 1995) The findings were published in the *British Medical Journal*, achieving some notoriety as it was the first time the journal had used drawings as data. The recent upsurge of interest in the use of this method in health research reflects recognition of the need to develop innovative and participatory approaches which enhance our understanding of children and how they see the world. Draw and write, or 'draw and label' as the technique has more recently been termed as it becomes more refined, has become popular with both researchers and children (Lewis and Lindsay 2000). With colleagues at the University of Warwick, Bendelow has continued to develop the draw and label technique in National Health Service funded research on young people's beliefs about health, risk and lifestyle (Bendelow *et al.* 1998), and there is much interest in the method in the health promotion arena. Also at Warwick, Geraldine Brady has been awarded an ESRC studentship to investigate children's experiences of attention deficit hyperactivity disorder (ADHD), which offers another chance to take this methodology forward. Brady's qualitative doctoral research addresses a gap in the relatively scant literature on perspectives of social order, health and 'normality' held by children who have a diagnosis of ADHD. In the last section of this chapter we look at this research more closely.

Researching children and ADHD

Attention deficit hyperactivity disorder is a diagnosis of the American Psychiatric Association applied to children (and adults) who consistently display certain characteristic behaviours over a long period of time. The three main dimensions of the disorder are inattention, impulsivity and over-activity. ADHD is said to occur in 3–6 per cent of children (Munden and Arcelus 1999), with boys outnumbering girls by three to one (Tannock 1998), along the whole spectrum of the normal range of intellectual development (Barkley 1995). ADHD is indicated to cause difficulties with development, behaviour and performance, as well as family relationships and social interaction. It is not a new disorder, but the name by which it is known has changed often since it was 'discovered' in 1902. Therefore, it is useful to view ADHD as a construct, although debates continue to rage over the cause and 'reality' of the condition. Whatever the label, there is a huge impact on the lives of children and their parents, which makes it all the more important to try and gain an understanding of the condition from the perspective of the child as well as that of the adults.

In many cases, the behaviours associated with ADHD can be helped with the use of medication, preferably combined with psychological, social and educational interventions. In Britain, careful assessment is undertaken by child health professionals before diagnosis and treatment, and regular follow-up appointments help to monitor the child's progress. Psychiatric drugs for children are a relatively new idea; previously, child psychiatrists have been regarded as 'talking doctors', and this new development in their role has been met with criticism from some sources. Media attention has focused on the use of the psychostimulant medication Methylphenidate, more commonly known as Ritalin, often inaccurately referring to it as 'kiddie cocaine'. The demonisation of medication is coupled with a portrayal of 'out of control' children being drugged and socially controlled for the benefit of teachers and parents. Wildly inaccurate claims are made, suggesting that children are being doped up and are more likely to abuse illegal drugs in the future. Insufficient attention is given to the benefits of treatment; no mention is made of those children who, undiagnosed, were sad, under-achieving and often in trouble, but once diagnosed and treated are happier, able to communicate, to make and keep friends and to achieve at school. Children who have always experienced problems of concentration and behaviour often have low self-esteem, which affects every aspect of their life.

Brady's research has developed an in-depth qualitative inquiry into the experiences of children who have been diagnosed with ADHD. Qualitative methods have been used to highlight the meanings which participants give to their actions; the meanings which parents give to their health-seeking behaviour; which professionals give to their practice and delivery of services; and which children give to being diagnosed with a condition known as ADHD. The research focuses on the process of seeking and receiving child health care, and on the subjective experiences of children both before and after receiving a diagnosis of ADHD. It is a particularistic study, which it is hoped could be generalised to a wider population of children, allowing for diversity in background.

Phase I of the research consisted of non-participant observation at a child and adolescent mental health unit, and the gathering of completed questionnaires from forty families. Phase II has involved working with seven children, in their own homes, ranging in age from 6 to 15 years, through three in-depth data-gathering sessions over a period of 6–12 months. Each has a formal clinical diagnosis of ADHD. The research sample consisted of six boys and one girl from diverse socio-economic backgrounds, which is in keeping with what is known about the distribution of ADHD in the UK. The study has tried to develop ways of listening successfully to children in order to discover how they feel about their diagnosis, using a mixture of oral, written and artistic contributions within a sensitive methodology, to allow children to engage fully and express their feelings.

This method allows children to define, both verbally and visually, the meanings which they attach to their lives, and to their health and illness experiences. In this way, a privileged 'insider' view has been allowed, as far as this is possible between an adult and a child, of the children's world. Lay accounts and perspectives on ADHD, especially those of children and young people themselves, are given equal status in this study to the on-going debate between professionals from the fields of medicine, psychology, social work and education, as there has been scarce research which investigates children's own experiences. Drawing is an activity with which children are familiar, and it could also help to unlock feelings and emotions which children may be unable or unwilling to talk about (Johnson 1995). It was thought to be important to give something back to those who took part, so information shared was compiled in an individual book called 'This is Your Life', which the children have been able to keep.

Many parents work with their child as far as possible to make life easier for them, and really try to understand what having ADHD means to them. Yet parents, as adults, cannot fully comprehend their child's world-view, as the following example illustrates.

Case 1: Sean (age 12)

Sean was diagnosed with ADHD aged 10, and has been prescribed Ritalin to be taken morning and lunchtime. Quite often he does not take the prescribed dose, which leads to a deterioration in his behaviour and concentration at school. His mother assumes that the problem is that he forgets to take it:

> He's easily distracted, I suppose he might just think 'Oh, I'll just take my tablet', and then his friend knocks the door to walk to school, all of a sudden he'll think 'Oh, I've got to take my football kit', and go off and look for that and the tablet will fly out of his head! I keep racking my brains thinking of how to get around this, it's the same at school getting him to take it at midday – do I get him a watch that goes 'beep beep' to remind him, but if when it goes 'beep beep' it's not convenient for him to take it, it's not going to beep again in 10 minutes is it?

But by taking time to explore Sean's feelings regarding medication, he eventually tells me: 'I don't like feeling different, it's boring sitting still in class and it doesn't feel right – it's like, it's not the "real me".'

Having cultivated the role of 'class clown', a fun but quite volatile character, Sean associates medication with being 'ordinary'. He acknowledges that he behaves in a more socially acceptable way when he complies, which pleases his mum and teachers, but ultimately it is more important to him to maintain popularity amongst his peers. Cooper and Shea (1999) found that ADHD students in their recent empirical study perceived the 'real me' to be their non-medicated self, and this person was sometimes associated with enjoyment and fun: 'Some students speak of a sense of these effects in terms of their sense of personal identity, often casting their non-Ritalin selves as their authentic selves and the self that is created by the application of Ritalin as a new and different self' (ibid.: 239). This view directly challenges opinions held by some health care workers, who assume that the issue of power and control underlies young people's lack of co-operation regarding medication. It is possible to see it in terms of assertion, challenge to parental authority and decision making, and a battle for control, but preliminary findings suggest that non- or reluctant compliance is far more likely to be connected to the crucial development of identity in this age group.

Case 2: Frank (age 12)

Frank's mother was very concerned about his aggressive, anti-social behaviour, which led to exclusion from school. The medication did not appear to be working, despite Frank's taking it daily for 3 months under her supervision. An excerpt from the clinic consultation follows:

Doctor: How often would you say you skip a tablet?
Frank: Every day. My mum brings it up with a drink, and I swallow it, keep it at the back of my throat, and sick it up out of the window when she's gone.
Doctor: Do you know of anyone else who has ADHD and takes Ritalin?
Frank: Yeah, Tyrone Patrick, he's a psycho, a little firestarter – he comes up behind you if you stand still and sets fire to your trousers – he goes to a special school, and he's tried to kill himself seven times.

Although the medical profession would consider non-compliance to be deviant behaviour, this is based on the assumption that doctors give the orders, provide the information and recommendations, and that patients must duly comply (Sachs 1992: 11). Non-compliance is often associated with irrational behaviour or ignorance, but it can be a rational choice when the social context is taken into consideration; Wirsing and Sommerfield (1992: 17) refer to this as the 'internal rationality of the patient's perspective'. Clearly, Frank would not wish to associate himself with this boy, and if he is the only other child he knows of with ADHD he is going to feel negatively about the diagnosis. Neither does he want to be regarded as 'ill' or 'different'.

Throughout the research, young people's attitudes towards medication have been complex and multi-layered. They acknowledge that medication is a form of control, which can benefit them but is of particular benefit to the significant adults in their lives – parents, grandparents, teachers. They are all desperately seeking social acceptance; above all, they want to identify with their peers, and not be perceived as 'different' or 'mental', and relationships with others are improved when they have taken their tablet. Having said that, Ritalin has been sensationally demonised by the media, and young people would rather not be associated with it; parents, as adults in generational proximity, cannot comprehend their child's world-view. Adult views tend to be 'rational' and sensible, and so if medication is associated with improved behaviour and academic success they may not be able to comprehend why their child is unhappy about taking it.

Children and young people especially felt the benefits of the medication within the context of school; both their academic work and their social relationships improved to a lesser or greater extent with its help.

Case 3: Ross (age 12)

Figures 9.1 and 9.2 show an example of Ross's 'before and after drawings' in which he describes how before he took his medication he was unable to hear or understand his teacher whereas now he depicts himself with his homework ready to hand in. He says his concentration improved, he is calmer, better able to stop and think and better able to communicate.

Case 4: Emma (age 10)

Peer approval is crucial to children's self esteem, as other studies of children's perspectives on health have shown, and the 'Feelings Flag' (see Figure 9.3) which Emma, aged 10, has completed vividly demonstrates the importance of friendship to her emotional health and wellbeing. As she says, 'They all hang out in a gang, if one falls out with me they all do, well they have to really or they're not part of the gang.'

Discussion

Although this study is on-going, several themes are emerging around public/private divisions already between the clinic and the home, between professional/lay perspectives and between adult and child accounts. Dominant definitions of children serve to exclude these particular children: the stereotypes used stigmatise and label them and are exacerbated through unsympathetic media coverage and lack of understanding. At the very least, these children are marginalised and excluded, and at worst pathologised.

This research makes visible the private lives of families, who are known to professionals only via their public personae. By investigating the domestic lives of parents and their children, Brady felt that she learned to appreciate the difficulties they were facing, and that she had a privileged insight to which

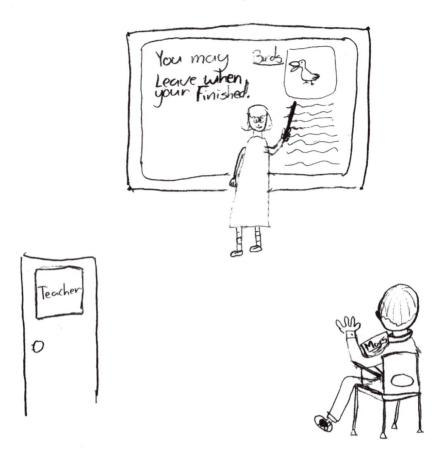

Figure 9.1 Before taking medication Ross could neither concentrate nor comprehend in class.

neither health professionals nor teachers were privy. She also came to respect the tremendous efforts which most parents were making to understand both their child and the condition of ADHD. As Read (2000) notes, when the people who are the subjects of research are members of one of the least powerful groups in society, their understanding often stands in sharp contrast to more dominant views of the world. Parents and children were fully aware that in their encounters with various services their view was not perceived to be as important as that of the 'expert'. Current health service rhetoric says that parents/patients are now in partnership with professionals, yet it is clearly not the case that both are equal in this relationship. As Strong (1979) found through his observations of paediatric consultations, it is simply not a level playing field.

Clearly, there is a power relationship between a professional and a parent, compounded by the professional's other role as gatekeeper to further import-

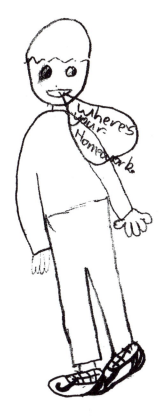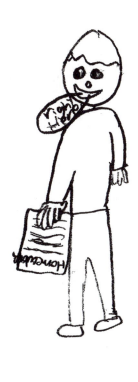

Figure 9.2 Having taken his medication, Ross is pleased to have completed and remembered his homework.

ant resources. The way in which a child's problem is defined, through the process of assessment and possible diagnosis and treatment, may or may not lead to the needs of the child and parents being met. The utilisation of scientific rating scales, physical examination and observation should ensure that outcomes are standardised, but the process is also highly subjective. Parents (of disabled children) have said that it can seem unjust when someone whose involvement is fairly transitory, and may not know the child too well, can have so much of a say (Read 1985).

For mothers in particular, the idea of 'normal' growth and development is not confined to physical or mental health, but incorporates their child's level of social acceptability (Buswell 1980). Mothers, in both Buswell's research and our own, tend not to seek professional help immediately; only after significant 'lay referral' has taken place among family and friends are they likely to enter their child into the structured health care system. Parents had very mixed feelings about their ADHD children: negative in that they were boisterous, rushing around, demanding, self-centred, aggressive, tiring,

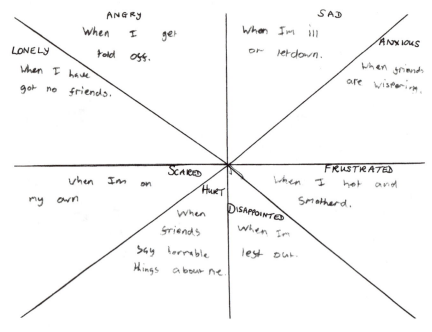

Figure 9.3 Emma's 'Feelings Flag'.

disobedient, often in trouble at school, disruptive of family and school routines. The positive feelings were that they were unique, very loving, caring, made friends easily, were active and lively, noticeable, not likely to be ignored, full of fun.

So contradictions abounded as, despite the so-called negative behaviours, some parents felt they did not want their child's personality to change and therefore either declined medication or restricted its use to weekdays, mainly school times. For children there are also contradictions in that state education promotes cognitive ability above physical ability, yet children do not regard them as separate as they are embodied agents. Children constitute a separate group with interests which cross-cut social settings and often conflict with adult interests, especially as to the importance of friends and peer group in comparison to parents, teachers, other adults. As we have discussed, children's 'best interests' are often defined by adults, and may complement or conflict with children's views of their own rights and needs (Alderson 1994: 49).

Conclusion

This chapter has focused on children's own ability to participate in the construction and reconstruction of the social order of their everyday lives, on the role of emotions in this process, and has used the example of empirical work with children diagnosed with ADHD to illustrate how it is possible to develop research methods to work with children in this way.

Returning to Meg Stacey's work, the emergence of the sociologies of both childhood and emotions over the last two decades can be seen to run parallel with the themes which were formerly 'pigeonholed' and ghettoised as 'micro-studies' and women's studies: namely, gender, healing, the division of labour and the importance of the domestic sphere; in other words, the major themes of this book which Meg has played such a part in establishing as legitimate areas of study in the wider sociological agenda. This chapter shows clearly how central these themes are to children's everyday lives and how they recognise them in various ways. First, children readily understand the role of emotions in sustaining a balanced and 'healthy' lifestyle in relation to their embodied being. Second, children are aware of the hierarchical complexities of everyday life across the public/private divide and the institutional 'order' of the clinic. Third, children understand their subordination to adults and the role of 'emotion work' in the negotiation of these hierarchical relationships, as Mayall (1994: 10) recognises: 'The gloom induced by arm-chair theorizing – which can make childhood look shockingly oppressed, can be offset by hearing children's own perspectives.'

Furthermore, we hope to show that collecting children's own accounts can be shown to challenge prevailing conceptualisations of children as emotionally 'incomplete' or 'immature' in relation to adults.

References

Alanen, L. (1992) 'Modern childhood: exploring the "child question"', in *Sociology, Research Report 50*, University of Jyväskyla, Finland.

—— (1994) 'Gender and generation: the child question', in J. Qvortrup, M. Bardy, G. Sigritta and H. Wintersberger (eds), *Childhood Matters: Social Theory, Practice and Politics*, Aldershot, Hants: Arebury.

Alderson, P. (1993) *Children's Consent to Surgery*, Buckingham: Open University Press.

—— (1994) 'Gender and generation: feminism and the "child question"', in J. Qvortrup, G. Sigritta and H. Wintersberger (eds), *Childhood Matters: Social Theory, Practice and Politics*, Aldershot, Hants.: Avebury Press.

Barkley, R. (1995) *Taking Charge of ADHD*, New York: Guilford Press.

Barnett, E., Francis, V., deKoning, K. and Shover, T. (1994) *Drawing and Dialogue*, Liverpool: Learning Resources Group, Liverpool School of Tropical Medicine.

Bendelow, G. and Oakley, A. (1993) *Young People and Cancer*, London: Social Science Research Unit and Women's Nationwide Cancer Control Campaign.

—— and Williams, S.J. (1998) *Emotions in Social Life*, London: Routledge.

——, France, A. and Williams, S. (1998) *Beliefs of Young People in Relation to Health, 'Risk' and Lifestyles: Final Report to the NHS Executive*, Coventry: University of Warwick.

Bluebond-Langner, M. (1991) 'Living with cystic fibrosis: the well sibling's perspective', *Medical Anthropology Quarterly* 5 (2): 133–52.

Brannen, J. and O'Brien, M. (1996) *Children in Families: Research and Policy*, London: Falmer Press.

Buswell, C. (1980) 'Mothers' perceptions of professionals in child health care', paper given at Paediatric Research Club, Rugby.

Cole, M. (1996) *Cultural Psychology*, Cambridge, MA: Harvard University Press.

Cooper, P. and Bilton, K. (eds) (1999) *ADHD Research, Practice and Opinion*, London: Whurr.

—— and Shea, T. (1999) 'ADHD from the inside: an empirical study of young people's perceptions of the experience of ADHD', in P. Cooper and K. Bilton (eds), *ADHD Research, Practice and Opinion*, London: Whurr.

Denzin, N.K. (1977) *Childhood Socialization*, San Francisco, CA: Jossey Bass.

Economic and Social Research Council (ESRC) *Research Programme on Children 5–16: Growing into the Twenty-first Century*, <http:www.esrc.ac.uk>

Finch, J. and Groves, D. (eds) (1983) *A Labour of Love: Women, Work and Caring*, London: Routledge and Kegan Paul.

Freire, P. (1972) *Pedagogy of the Oppressed*, Harmondsworth, Middx: Penguin.

Gamarnikow, E., Morgan, D., Purvis, J. and Taylorson, D. (1983) *The Public and the Private*, London: Heinemann Educational.

Graham, H. (1984) *Women, Health and the Family*, Brighton, Sussex: Wheatsheaf.

—— (1993) *Hardship and Health in Women's Lives*, Hemel Hempstead, Herts: Harvester Wheatsheaf.

Hill, M. and Tisdall, K. (1997) *Children and Society*, Harlow, Essex: Addison Wesley Longman.

Hochschild, A. (1979) 'Emotion work, feeling rules and social structure', *American Journal of Sociology* 85 (3): 551–75.

—— (1983) *The Managed Heart: The Commercialization of Human Feeling*, Berkeley, CA: University of California Press.

Hockey, J. and James, A. (1993) *Growing Up and Growing Old: Ageing and Dependency in the Life Course*, London: Sage.

Hope, A. and Timmel, S. (1984) *Training for Transformation*, Book 1, Gweru, Zimbabwe: Mambo Press.

Ingleby, D. (1986) 'Development in social context', in M. Richards, and P. Light (eds), *Children of Social Worlds*, Cambridge: Polity Press.

James, A. (1993) *Childhood Identities: Social Relationships and the Self in Children's Experiences*, Edinburgh: Edinburgh University Press.

—— and Prout, A. (1996) 'Strategies and structures: towards a new perspective on children's experiences of family life', in J. Brannen and M. O'Brien (eds), *Children in Families: Research and Policy*, London: Falmer Press.

—— and —— (1995) 'Hierarchy, boundary and agency: towards a theoretical perspective on childhood', *Sociological Studies of Childhood* 7: 77–99.

—— and —— (eds) (1997) *Constructing and Reconstructing Childhood: Contemporary Issues in the Sociological Study of Childhood*, London: Falmer Press.

——, Jenks, C. and Prout, A. (1998) *Theorizing Childhood*, Cambridge: Polity Press.

Jenks, C. (1996) *Childhood*, London: Routledge.

Johnson, P. (1995) *Children Making Books*, Reading and Language Information Centre: University of Reading.

Kalnins, I., MacQueen, D., Backett, K., Curtice, L. and Currie, C. (1992) 'Children, empowerment and health promotion: some new directions in research and practice', *Health Promotion International* 7: 53–9.

Kirk, D. and Tinning, R. (1994) 'Embodied self-identity, healthy life-styles and school physical education', *Sociology of Health and Illness* 16 (5): 600–25.

Lewis, A. and Lindsay, G. (eds) (2000) *Researching Children's Perspectives*, Buckingham: Open University Press.

Mayall, B. (ed.) (1994) *Children's Childhoods Observed and Experienced*, London: Falmer Press.

—— (1996) *Children, Health and the Social Order*, Buckingham: Open University Press.

—— (1998) 'Children, emotions and daily life at home and school', in G.A. Bendelow and S.J. Williams (eds), *Emotions in Social Life*, London: Routledge.

—— and Foster, M.-C.(1989) *Child Health Care: Living with Children, Working for Children*, Oxford: Heinemann Educational.

——, Bendelow, G., Barker, S., Storey, P. and Veltman, M. (1996) *Children's Health in Primary Schools*, London: Falmer Press.

Mills, C.W. (1959) *The Sociological Imagination*, Harmonsdworth, Middx: Penguin.

Morrow, V. (1994) 'Responsible children? Aspects of children's work and employment outside school in contemporary UK', in B. Mayall (ed.), *Children's Childhoods Observed and Experienced*, London, Falmer.

Munden, A. and Arcelus, J. (1999) *The ADHD Handbook: A Guide for Parents and Professionals*, London: Jessica Kingsley.

Oakley, A. (1994) 'Women and children first and last: parallels and differences between children's and women's studies', in B. Mayall (ed.), *Children's Childhoods Observed and Experienced*, London: Falmer Press.

——, Bendelow, G., Barnes, J., Buchanan, M. and Nasseem Hussain, O. (1995) 'Health and cancer prevention: knowledge and beliefs of children and young people', *British Medical Journal* 310: 1029–33.

Occleston, S. and King, P. (1993) 'Innovation in health promotion', *Healthy Cities Newsletter* (Department of Public Health, PO Box 147, Liverpool L69 3BX).

Oldman, D. (1994) 'Childhood as a mode of production', in B. Mayall (ed.), *Children's Childhoods Observed and Experienced*, London, Falmer.

Pole, C., Mizen, P. and Bolton, A. (1999) 'Realising children's agency in research: partners and participants?', *International Journal of Social Research Methodology* 2 (1): 39–54.

Prendergast, S. and Forrest, S. (1998) ' "Shorties, low-lifers, hardnuts and kings": boys, emotions and embodiment in school', in G. Bendelow and S. Williams (eds), *Emotions in Social Life*, London: Routledge.

Pridmore, P. and Bendelow, G. (1995) 'Images of health: explaining beliefs of children using "draw and write" techniques', *Health Education Journal* 54: 473–88.

Prout, A. (1986) ' "Wet children" and "little actresses": going sick in primary school', *Sociology of Health and Illness* 8 (2): 111–36.

—— and James, A. (1990) 'A new paradigm for the sociology of childhood? Provenance, promise and problems', in A. James and A. Prout (eds.), *Constructing and Reconstructing Childhood: Contemporary Issues in the Sociology of Childhood*, London: Falmer Press.

—— (2000) 'Childhood bodies: social construction and translation', in S.J. Williams, J. Gabe and M. Calnan (eds), *Health, Medicine and Society: Key Theories, Future Agendas*, London: Routledge.

Qvortrup, J. (1991) *Childhood as a Social Phenomenon: An Introduction to a Series of National Reports*, Vienna: European Centre.

—— (1994) 'Childhood matters: an introduction', in J. Qvortrup, M. Bardy, G. Sigritta and H. Wintersberger (eds), *Childhood Matters: Social Theory, Practice and Politics*, Aldershot, Hants: Avebury Press.

Read, J. (1985) 'A critical appraisal of the concept of partnership: reflections on the working relationship between professionals and parents who have children with disabilities', unpublished MA thesis, University of Warwick.

—— (2000) *Disability, the Family and Society*, Buckingham: Open University Press.

Ribbens, J. (1994) *Mothers and Their Children: A Feminist Sociology of Child Rearing*, Buckingham: Open University Press.

Sachs, L. (1992) 'Health and illness: theoretical perspectives. Concepts within the anthropology of medicines', in D.J. Trakas and E.J. Sanz (eds), *Studying Childhood and Medicine Use: A Multidisciplinary Approach*, Athens: ZHTA Medical Publications.

Scheper-Hughes, N. and Lock, M. (1987) 'The mindful body: a prolegomenon to future work in medical anthropology', *Medical Anthropology Quarterly* 1 (1): 6–41.

Stacey, M. (1981) 'The division of labour revisited, or overcoming the two Adams', in P. Abrams, R. Deem, J. Finch and P. Roch (eds), *Development and Diversity: British Sociology, 1950–1980*, London: Allen and Unwin.

—— (1988) *The Sociology of Health and Healing*, London: Unwin Hyman.

Strong, P. (1979) *The Ceremonial Order of the Clinic*, London: Routledge and Kegan Paul.

Tannock, R. (1998) 'ADHD: advances in cognitive, neurobiological and genetic research', *Journal of Child Psychology and Psychiatry* 29: 289–300.

Williams, D.T., Wetton, N. and Moon, A. (1989) *A Way In: Five Key Areas of Health Education*, London: Health Education Authority.

Williams, S.J. and Bendelow, G.A. (1998) *The Lived Body*, London: Routledge.

——, Gabe, J. and Calnan, M. (eds) (2000) *Health, Medicine and Society: Key Theories, Future Agendas*, London: Routledge.

Wirsing, R. and Sommerfield, J. (1992) 'Compliance: a medical anthropological re-appraisal', in D.J. Trakas and E.J. Sanz (eds), *Studying Childhood and Medicine Use: A Multidisciplinary Approach*, Athens: ZHTA Medical Publications.

Young, I.M. (1980) 'Throwing like a girl: a phenomenology of feminine body comportment, motility and spatiality', *Human Studies* 3: 137–56.

Part III

Health care in transition

Ferment and change?

10 Gender equity in health*

Debates and dilemmas

Lesley Doyal

Introduction

Gender equity is increasingly identified as one of the goals of health policy at both national and international levels. However, the precise meaning of the term is not always clear. Are there any examples of it in the real world? Would we recognise them if we saw them? In attempting to answer these and other questions this chapter addresses some key policy concerns. It also identifies some of the underlying theoretical and conceptual issues that need resolution if anything resembling gender equity in health is to be realised.

In recent years there has been a shift away from talking about 'women' to talking about 'gender'. Instead of focusing on women as an underprivileged group, the emphasis is now on the social construction of gender identities and on the nature of the relationships between women and men. This shift is evident in academic discourse where 'gender studies' is increasingly replacing 'women's studies' as the framework for generating new knowledge. It is also apparent in many policy settings where the language of gender equity is increasingly heard. However, closer examination reveals a distinct lack of clarity about how such a goal should be defined or about how it might be achieved.

In addressing these conceptual confusions, this chapter follows very clearly in the steps of Meg Stacey, who has done so much to make us all think more clearly about the terms we use both in the sociology of health and illness and in sociology more generally. It also builds on the pioneering work she has done in highlighting the importance of gender in understanding inequalities in patterns of human wellbeing.

Gender equity: the politics of confusion

The essential contestability of the term 'gender equity' can be illustrated through an examination of debates at the UN conferences in Cairo and

* We are grateful to Elsevier Science for permission to reproduce an amended version of this chapter which appeared in Social Science and Medicine (2000) vol 51: 6 pp 931–939.

Beijing. Participants in these debates could be loosely categorised into three major groups. Each would claim to represent the interests of women but all perceive gender equity in very different ways (Baden and Goetz 1998).

First, there is a loose grouping of individuals who could be called traditionalists, many but not all of whom would ground their views on gender in fundamentalist beliefs of a nationalist and/or a religious kind. Members of this group find the notion of 'gender' itself unhelpful on the grounds that it overpoliticises what they see as the 'natural' differences between men and women. These differences they regard as unavoidable and indeed desirable. Hence they argue that public policies should be 'equitable' in meeting what they see as the very different developmental needs of the two sexes in their separate spheres. However, they reject the idea of attempting to achieve some kind of spurious equality.

Members of the second grouping could be called feminist radicals. They would certainly welcome much greater equality between the sexes but do not believe that this can be achieved through the adoption of 'gender equity' as a political goal. Citing a range of examples they argue that policies such as gender mainstreaming are too often used as a technological fix. Once a gender policy has been introduced, they say, it is all too easy for those in power to claim that they have 'done gender' and now it is time to move on to something else. So for these feminist radical sceptics, the best strategy is to retain a single focus and to pursue an agenda based not so much on equality between the sexes but on the rights of women.

The third group could be called the gender radicals. This group holds to the belief that, despite the obvious difficulties, the pursuit of greater gender equity in health is still a worthwhile goal. At a conceptual level they argue that the emphasis on gender relations offers considerable potential for a critical understanding of inequalities in health between men and women. At a more practical level the pursuit of gender equity as a policy goal is seen to offer opportunities for collaborative action between a range of different groups (including both women and men) concerned with wider campaigns for equality and social justice.

It is clear, then, that the definition of gender equity itself, judgements about its desirability and strategies for its achievement are all open to question. Within this context of continuing political and theoretical debate it is the third or 'gender radical' position which provides the underlying rationale for this chapter; that is to say, the arguments presented here are based on the assumption that the pursuit of gender equity in health is a legitimate goal of public policy and that the health of women (and maybe men) could be improved as a result. However, the task will not be an easy one.

Defining the problem

Any attempt to promote gender equity in health must begin with a clear definition of what is being sought. The most obvious goal might seem to be equality in health outcomes between men and women. However, this is clearly unachievable: because individuals (and groups) begin with very different biological constitutions, any attempt to equalise male and female life expectancy or morbidity rates is doomed to failure. Instead, policies in pursuit of gender equity must focus not on health outcomes themselves but on the inputs that provide the basis for human flourishing. The only practicable strategy for reducing unfair and avoidable inequalities in health outcomes between men and women is to ensure that the two groups have equal access to those resources which they need to realise their potential for health (Doyal and Gough 1991; Nussbaum and Glover 1995).

However, this still leaves questions about how such a strategy should be carried out. It is clear that the implementation of equal opportunities in the allocation of resources for health cannot mean treating men and women identically. Both sexes have a range of needs that have to be met if they are to achieve their potential for a healthy life. Most of these will be basic requirements such as food, water, shelter and physical and psychological security; these are the same for both groups and should be equally available to all. However, there are also significant differences in the health needs of men and women, which stem primarily (but not entirely) from biological differences between male and female reproductive systems. These differences need to be clearly identified so that they can be reflected in equitable strategies for resource allocation.

But in order to ensure that such policies are effective, we need to identify not just the needs themselves but also the ways in which current modes of social organisation place differential constraints on the meeting of those needs for men and women. Of course, many of the constraints will again be the same for the two groups. To take an obvious example, poverty can prevent both men and women realising their potential for health. But poverty itself is a gendered phenomenon in its causes and in its effects (Jackson 1998). The next section therefore takes the argument one stage further through identifying both the differences in the health needs of men and women and the variety of obstacles that currently prevent them meeting those needs.

Nature or nurture?

This investigation requires an examination of both the biological (sex) and the social (gender) dimensions of difference as well as the relations between them. There is, of course, a variety of philosophical problems awaiting the unwary who talk in any simple way about separating these two domains. Indeed, much recent work in gender studies has been concerned in one way or another to demonstrate their intrinsic interconnectedness (Butler 1993). Some of this has been extremely valuable in drawing attention to the social construction of much that had previously been taken as purely biological in character. However, there is also a danger that our understanding of the material dimension of human health will be undermined by the spread of radical deconstructionism.

Paradoxically, perhaps, some of the new writing on the body is especially problematic on this score. Far from 'bringing the body back' into social science, too much of this work has conceptualised fundamental bodily processes in an overly theoreticised and abstract way which adds little to the conceptual armoury needed to improve human wellbeing (Davis 1997). In order to avoid the paralysis that sometimes results from these approaches, this chapter explores the biological and the social domains in turn in order to identify those issues central to gender equity strategies. The importance of (re)integrating the two perspectives is addressed later.

The biology of risk

In biomedical theory and practice the analysis of maleness and femaleness starts (and usually ends) with sex differences in reproductive systems. This is also a useful starting point for thinking about equity in public policy since it is an area in which women start off at a considerable disadvantage by comparison with men. If they are to realise their potential for health, most women require access to the resources necessary to control their fertility and also, intermittently, to those which will ensure healthy pregnancy and childbirth. They therefore have what could be called 'special' biological needs and these must be taken into account in any strategy for gender equity (Sen and Snow 1994; Sen *et al.* 1994).

Men do not need reproductive health care in the same way that women do. Of course, every act of intercourse puts them at risk of contracting a sexually transmitted disease (though the biological risk is lower for a man than it is for a woman). But once the initial conception has happened, men need to take no further risks to achieve fatherhood. Hence, they can, in theory, have as many children as they like without damaging their health. But despite what could be seen as a biological advantage, there are now very few societies in which men have a longer life expectancy than women.

This appears to be due, at least in part, to the fact that men are innately the weaker sex and this is reflected in higher numbers of male deaths both *in utero* and around the time of birth (Waldron 1995; Hart 1988). So men could also claim to have 'special needs' in any debate about gender equity in health. However, the situation of men is not like that of women in that modern medicine does not currently have the technology to compensate for their particular disadvantage. While it is theoretically possible for all women to have their need for high-quality reproductive health care met, the technology is not (yet) available to prevent what is seen as 'premature' death among men. Hence, even if we could guarantee both sexes equivalent access to health-related resources, women would still be likely to live longer lives on average than men in the same groups as themselves.

This sex difference in potential longevity alerts us to the fact that biological differences between women and men go beyond the obvious ones related to reproductive systems, to include genetic, hormonal, metabolic and other variations. Sex differences in the causes, the incidence and the prognosis of a number of health problems including HIV/AIDS, tropical infectious diseases, tuberculosis and coronary heart disease are just beginning to emerge (Doyal 1998; Garenne and Lafon 1998; Hudelson 1996; Vlassoff and Bonilla 1994). They reveal complex biological differences in patterns of risk and susceptibility which need to be taken seriously if equity is to be achieved in service delivery.

However, these biological influences can tell only part of the story. Socially constructed inequalities or gender differences between males and females are also important in determining whether individuals are able to realise their potential for a long and a healthy life. And as we shall see, it is generally males who have a significant advantage over females in access to health-related resources.

The hazards of female gender

All societies are divided in two along a male/female axis. This means that those falling on opposite sides of the divide are seen as fundamentally different types of creatures with different duties and responsibilities as well as different entitlements (Charles 1993; Moore 1988). Though the precise formulation of these definitions varies between societies, there is also a surprising degree of consistency, with those who are defined as female having primary responsibility for household and domestic labour. Conversely, males have generally been more closely identified with the public world, with the arena of waged work and the rights and duties of citizenship.

Of course, in most societies there are not just differences but inequalities inherent in the social definitions of femaleness and maleness. Those things defined as male are usually valued more highly than those things defined as female and men and women are rewarded accordingly (Charles 1993; Moore 1988; Papanek 1990). Not surprisingly, these inequalities have a significant effect on the health of both men and women though so far it is only their impact on women that has been explored in any detail.

In recent years women and their advocates have built up a large body of work demonstrating the intimate interrelationship between gender inequalities and both mental and physical health (Annandale and Hunt 2000; Doyal 1995, 1998; Stein 1997). Most importantly, they have looked not just at life expectancy but at more qualitative dimensions of wellbeing. They have shown that many of the health problems women face are not related in any direct way to their specific biological characteristics. Rather they reflect the discrimination and disadvantage that so many continue to experience as they carry out the gendered activities making up their daily lives (Belle 1990; Kitts and Roberts 1996). Anxiety and depression, for instance, are more common among females than among males in most parts of the world (Desjarlais *et al.* 1995). Yet there is no evidence that women are constitutionally more susceptible than men to these problems (Busfield 1996).

Gender inequalities in income and wealth make women especially vulnerable to poverty. Though levels of discrimination vary significantly between societies, millions still find it difficult to acquire the basic necessities for a healthy life (UNDP 1995). Poverty can affect both males and females but women and girls often suffer additional disadvantage as a result of discrimination (Jackson 1998; Dwyer and Bruce 1988; Kabeer 1994: ch. 5). Lack of adequate nourishment and unequal access to health care mean that sometimes their most basic needs are not met (Tinker *et al.* 1994). The gender division of work means that women are often denied the opportunity to meet other basic needs such as time for rest and recuperation (Charles 1993; Moore 1988).

Within the household women often have little support and too many end up being abused by others (Doyal 1995: ch. 2; Heise *et al.* 1995; WHO 1996). Hence their need for physical and psychological security may also be denied. The process of 'growing up female' influences the type of identity girls are able to develop. Being raised as members of the less valuable group can make it more difficult for them to develop the positive sense of themselves that is usually associated with good mental health (Papanek 1990). In many societies this means that women's identities are shaped in ways that encourage them to put the wellbeing of others before their own (Kandiyoti 1998).

So we can see that gender inequalities in access to a wide range of resources have a significant impact on the health of women. Though they have a longer average life expectancy than men, they do not necessarily lead healthier lives. And most importantly, a considerable amount of the illness they experience can be traced back in one way or another to the nature of their daily lives and should therefore be preventable through public policy. Since gender relations affect men as well as women we need to ask whether they face similar risks. Are the health problems experienced by men preventable in the same way?

Male gender: a mixed blessing?

Thus far, relatively little attention has been paid to the impact of gender on the health of men. Indeed, this is part of a much broader pattern whereby men's lives have not usually been seen as gendered at all. This has now begun to change with the creation (mostly in the developed countries) of the sociology of masculinities, men's studies and associated men's movements (Brod and Kaufman 1994; Connell 1995; Hearn and Morgan 1990; Mac an Ghaill 1996). A major focus of many of those working in these new paradigms has been the exploration of male (homo)sexualities and their implications for health promotion in the context of the HIV/AIDS epidemic (Kimmel and Levine 1993). Other aspects of men's health have received less attention but important links are now beginning to emerge between gender, heterosexuality and wellbeing (Huggins and Lamb 1998; Sabo and Gordon 1993).

First, it is evident that in some societies the stereotyped role of provider puts men at greater risk of dying prematurely from occupational accidents. Just as women face hazards in carrying out their domestic tasks, so many men may also be at risk from doing the duties that are socially expected of them (Hart 1988). However, the other risks associated with maleness are of a rather different order from those linked to femaleness. Gender inequalities themselves rarely deprive men of the resources to meet their needs. If anything, they operate in the other direction. But it does appear that constructing and maintaining a male identity often requires the taking of risks that can be seriously hazardous to health.

Many men feel compelled to engage in risky behaviour in order to 'prove' their masculinity and to 'do' gender in the socially approved way (Kimmel and Messner 1993). Their behaviour has been shaped by what Connell (1995) calls the 'hegemonic' version of masculinity, and as a result men are more likely than women to be murdered, to die in a car accident or in dangerous sporting activities (Canaan 1996; Pleck and Sonenstein 1991). In most societies they are also more likely than women to drink to excess and to smoke, which in turn increases their biological predisposition to early heart disease and other health problems (Waldron 1995). They also seem to be more likely than women to desire unsafe sex (Zeidenstein and Moore 1996).

The significance of a male identity in the arena of mental health has also received attention, especially from participants in the new men's movements. It has been argued that growing up male renders many men unable to realise what might be their emotional potential. The desire to be seen as a 'hard' man, for instance, may prevent them from exploring the 'caring' side of their nature while a refusal to admit weakness may prevent them from consulting a doctor when they are ill (though the evidence here is rather inconclusive) (Harrison *et al.* 1992; Kristiansen 1989). Indeed, illness itself may be especially feared because of its capacity to reduce men to what has been called 'marginalised masculinity' (Cameron and Bernardes 1998).

The implications of male gender for health have been highlighted by recent debates about mortality and morbidity in central and eastern Europe (Chenet 2000). In many countries, the health of both men and women has been deteriorating since the 1960s and this trend has accelerated over the past decade. However, the impact has been much greater on men: premature deaths from circulatory diseases and some cancers have risen dramatically. Between 1989 and 1994 life expectancy in Russia declined by more than 6.7 years in men and by 3.4 years in women (Bobak *et al.* 1998). As a result there is now a 14-year gap in life expectancy between the two groups (Chenet 2000). Some of this difference can be explained by gender differences in accidents and in smoking and alcohol consumption (Leon *et al.* 1997; Peto *et al.* 1992). However, more qualitative variations in the lives of men and women may also be involved (Bobak *et al.* 1998; Chenet 2000; Watson 1995, 1997).

Both men and women have been affected by the disruption of civil society which can result in feelings of hopelessness and lack of control (Bobak *et al.* 1998), but there may be significant gender differences in these experiences.

The collapse of state socialism highlighted the importance of the family as a locus for 'getting by'. In this context, women's social support networks and their capacity to generate survival strategies have come to the fore. This has meant that unmarried men may be materially and socially disadvantaged by lack of a family and this is reflected in their higher mortality rates. At the same time, there are now fewer opportunities for men to carry out the economic activities traditionally associated with masculinity. This has generated feelings of helplessness and frustration which have been linked both directly and indirectly to the greater decline in male health (Bobak *et al.* 1998; Watson 1995).

Thus far we have explored the complex ways in which both sex and gender need to be taken into account in thinking about strategies for equity in health. Developing an integrated perspective is not easy but important insights are emerging into how this interdisciplinary work can best be done. In the context of HIV/AIDS, for instance, many biomedical scientists have come to recognise the importance of social and cultural factors in explaining the epidemic. At the same time an increasing number of social scientists have begun to explore the nature of 'material embodiment' and its differential implications for the health of women and men (Davis 1997; Shilling 1993; Scott and Morgan 1993). Further work of this kind is needed if the interrelations between sex and gender in the shaping of human health are to be properly understood.

Sex, gender and diversity

We have now explored the biological and the social commonalities that identify men and women as separate groups. But of course this does not imply homogeneity within each group. Hence socio-economic, cultural and age differences among women and among men also need careful exploration in order to assess their implications for the promotion of gender equity in health.

Despite the fact that they share the same biology, it is clear that women's reproductive health status is profoundly affected by who they are and where they live. The technical means to ensure safe contraception, abortion and childbearing do exist but they are not equally available to all. Half a million women still die each year as a result of pregnancy and virtually all of these avoidable deaths occur in poor countries where there is insufficient access to trained health workers (WHO 1991; Rooney 1992; Royston and Armstrong 1989). It is therefore impossible to understand the impact of sex on health without also taking factors such as class, race and geopolitical status into account.

Shifting to the gender differences between men and women, again we have to take seriously the issue of diversity. The reality of 'maleness' and 'femaleness' varies significantly between cultures and communities. Hence the impact of gender on wellbeing will vary too. The implications for health of being a woman will be very different depending on whether the 'femaleness' in question is mediated through poverty or wealth, through an urban cosmopolitan existence or life in a traditional village. To be a single female lawyer in an affluent London suburb may well be considerably healthier than being a working-class mother of two in a run-down tower block in the same city. However, both will face many fewer social and economic constraints on their health than a landless woman with seven children in a village in Bangladesh.

Age too is crucial. It is increasingly clear that the health needs of men and women and the resources available to meet these needs vary significantly across the life cycle. Nevertheless, these differences are again complex. On the one hand the 'special needs' of women for reproductive care are at their most acute during the childbearing years when they are most dependent on men. In mid-life, levels of need may be reduced, only to rise again in old age. Yet in many societies older women lose what little status they had with the disappearance of childbearing potential and the sexual allure of youth (Owen 1996). This mix of social and biological influences has profound effects on the nature of gender relations at different ages and these need to be included in any planning for gender equity.

It is clear from this analysis that the pursuit of gender equity is likely to be more challenging than is often assumed. A complex matrix of variables still requires clarification both conceptually and also in terms of policy implications. However, some preliminary conclusions can be drawn both about the way forward and also about the questions that remain to be resolved.

Policies for gender equity: a preliminary agenda

It can be argued that universal access to high-quality reproductive health care is the single most important element that must be included in any global strategy for gender equity. In the richer parts of the world this has largely been achieved and its impact on women's capacity to realise their potential for long and healthy lives is very obvious. In the UK the gap between male and female life expectancy is now around 7 years but in India it is less than 2 years while in Bangladesh men live around 1 year longer than women (UNDP 1995). Access to reproductive health care is an essential component in explaining these differences.

However, this can only be part of the strategy. As we have seen, gender relations themselves also create obstacles to the realisation of health. On the one hand they sustain inequalities in the allocation of resources and on the other they shape male and female identities in ways that can have a significant effect on wellbeing. These dimensions of gender also need to be addressed but the resolutions are likely to be complex and highly political, as we can see from a brief exploration of current debates on gender, masculinity and health.

Health and the politics of gender

Concerns about health and masculinity have recently come to the fore both in academic and policy arenas and also in the popular press. While these debates are taking place mainly within the developed countries, they do have a broader significance for the gender equity debate. A number of different positions can be identified and these will be examined in turn.

The first argument could be characterised as 'back to the future'. The supporters of this position claim that in many societies, changes have challenged men's sense of identity, causing a significant decline in wellbeing. The rise of male unemployment, for example, the entry of more women into the labour market and the increase in one-parent families are all said to be the cause of significant mental health problems. In the UK the rise in suicides among young men has been linked to these trends (Charlton *et al.* 1993). These are important concerns, as the example of central and eastern Europe demonstrated, but the policy implications are by no means clear. According to some observers, these trends demonstrate the need for a return to traditional models of masculinity, which they claim would benefit women as well as men. However, it is unlikely that such an approach would be either practicable or justifiable as part of a strategy for achieving gender equity.

The second position has also been developed predominantly by men but it is very different from the one above. Indeed, it has been referred to as a 'women centred' approach to men's health by some of its main proponents (Sabo and Gordon 1993). This approach is based on a recognition that unreconstructed masculinity can be dangerous to the health of both women and men. Thus men who are oppressed or even beaten by other men or feel constrained by social expectations may respond by turning on women. Similarly the failure of some men to realise their emotional potential will also be damaging to the women (or of course the men) with whom they live since it will limit the quality of the relationships of which they are capable.

It follows for the proponents of this view that the road to gender equity in health lies in the reconstruction of masculinity to make it healthier for both men and women. The main aim would be to enable men to change first their sense of themselves and then their behaviour so that they were less self-destructive and also less aggressive towards others (Lloyd and Wood 1996). Paradoxically, perhaps, what this strategy requires is that men behave more like women; that is to say, that they model their behaviour not on what is usually perceived as 'masculinity' but rather on what has stereotypically been regarded as 'femininity'.

This approach also contains a great deal of value. At a conceptual level it reminds us of the importance of not assuming that 'masculine' or 'feminine' behaviour is inextricably linked to either biological sex or female gender (Annandale and Hunt 1990). At a practical level it would help men to achieve their potential for health if it reduced the risk taking that currently constitutes one of the main hazards of maleness. It would also benefit women since these 'new men' would be less likely to be irresponsible or abusive. However, it still leaves a number of important issues unresolved. In particular it places a great deal of emphasis on changes in male identity and masculine subjectivity while leaving largely untouched the material and institutional inequalities between men and women that constitute such major obstacles to gender equity.

This limitation is recognised in the third position on gender equity and health which could be called a broadly feminist approach. While it is not always clearly spelled out, this position does provide the underpinning philosophy for much of the women's health advocacy that is taking place around the world. A large part of the burden of preventable morbidity and mortality experienced by women is related directly or indirectly to the patterning of gender divisions. If this harm is to be avoided there will need to be significant changes in related aspects of social and economic organisation. In particular, strategies will be required to deal with the damage done to women's health by men, masculinities and male institutions.

While men may be exposed to risks because of the need constantly to affirm their gender identities they also derive major benefits from the gender system as a whole. In fact, for most men the social gains of masculinity probably far outweigh the losses. Yet if gender equity is our goal many of these advantages might have to be given up. Hence men and women cannot be assumed to have an automatic identity of interests in the reform of gender relations. Policies will need to be developed to ensure that women receive an equal share of social and economic resources. Some men will certainly co-operate in working for these and other changes in the nature of gender relations. However, many others will be opposed to the removal of privileges which they have come to see as an inalienable right.

We are left then with a schematic policy for gender equity in health that places the greatest emphasis on universal access to reproductive health care followed by the removal of gender inequalities in access to resources. But there is also a need for policies to free up individuals from the constraints of rigidly defined gender roles. Since it is now accepted that gender identities are essentially negotiated, policies are needed which will enable individuals to shape their own identities and actions in healthier ways. These could include a range of educational strategies as well as more flexible employment policies and changes in the structure of state benefits. By this means both women and men would have opportunities to open up their lives in ways that could be beneficial to both physical and mental health.

It is important to acknowledge that the implementation of a strategy of this kind would be of most benefit to women. Indeed, it could even be described as a recipe for reducing gender equity since, in some parts of the world at least, it would increase the gap between male and female life expectancy still further. However, the justification for this approach should be self evident. Since women have the potential for longer life expectancy and also suffer more severe social constraints on that potential, then these conclusions should logically follow. Yet the implementation of a strategy along these lines would not solve all problems related to gender equity in health and might raise new ones in the process. These outstanding concerns are briefly examined in the conclusion.

The way forward: dilemmas and constraints

The first dilemma is whether we can improve the health of women without men losing out. And if we cannot, what implications does this have for the equity debate? If improvements in women's health necessitate their receiving a fairer share of available social resources, then men may have to get less and this will sometimes have a negative impact on their health. Men on the edge of poverty, for example, might be dragged down below subsistence if their income had to be shared equally with their wives. Similarly, the mental health of men whose self-esteem is dependent on feeling superior to female kin might be damaged if the status of women improved. Will trade-offs of this kind be necessary and, if so, how do we conceptualise them within an equity framework?

The second concern is primarily an empirical one and relates to how the transformations necessary to achieve gender equity are actually to be achieved. Many aspects of gender are deeply embedded in individual psyches (both male and female), making them difficult to change. This resistance will be reinforced by the location of many of these inequalities within the private space of the household. This creates problems about how best to balance equity issues with what may be legitimate concerns about privacy. But mostly it raises questions about how successful public policy can ever be in changing some of the more fundamental aspects of human behaviour. This will clearly be especially problematic in the case of those men (and some women) who would be required to make sacrifices without any obvious short-term gain.

Finally, it is important to conclude with what must be a continuing debate about the priority to be given to gender equity in the face of the many different injustices that continue to confront us. Health outcomes for both individuals and populations are profoundly influenced not just by gender but by factors such as race, class, ethnicity and geopolitical status. Indeed, in particular circumstances these may be more powerful than either sex or gender in determining health status. However, it is clear that many women (and some men) will continue to experience avoidable constraints on their well-being until gender issues are taken seriously by all those seeking to achieve equity in health and health care.

References

Annandale, E. and Hunt, K. (1990) 'Masculinity, femininity and sex: an exploration of their relative contribution to explaining gender differences in health', *Sociology of Health and Illness* 12 (1): 24–46.
—— and —— (2000) *Gender Inequalities in Health*, Buckingham: Open University Press.
Baden, S. and Goetz, A.M. (1998) 'Who needs sex when you can have gender? Conflicting discourses on gender at Beijing', in C. Jackson and R. Pearson (eds), *Feminist Visions of Development*, London: Routledge.

Belle, D. (1990) 'Poverty and women's mental health', *American Psychologist* 45: 385–9.

Boback, M., Pikhart, H., Hertzman, C., Rose, R. and Marmot, M. (1998) 'Socio-economic factors, perceived control and self-reported health in Russia: a cross-sectional survey', *Social Science and Medicine* 47 (2): 269–79.

Brod, H. and Kaufman, M. (1994) *Theories of Masculinities*, Thousand Oaks, CA: Sage.

Busfield, J. (1996) *Men, Women and Madness: Understanding Gender and Mental Disorder*, London: Macmillan.

Butler, J. (1993) *Bodies That Matter: On the Discursive Limits of Sex*, New York: Routledge.

Cameron, C. and Bernardes, D. (1998) 'Gender and disadvantage in health: men's health for change', *Sociology of Health and Illness* 18 (3): 673–93.

Canaan, J. (1996) 'One thing leads to another: drinking, fighting and working class masculinities', in M. Mac an Ghaill (ed.), *Understanding Masculinities*, Bucking-ham: Open University Press.

Charles, N. (1993) *Gender Divisions and Social Change*, Hemel Hempstead, Herts: Harvester Wheatsheaf.

Charlton, J. *et al.* (1993) 'Suicide trends in England and Wales: trends in factors associated with suicide deaths', *Population Trends* 71, Spring.

Chenet, L. (2000) 'Gender and socio-economic inequalities in morality in Central and Eastern Europe', *Social Science and Medicine* 40 (10): 1355–66.

Connell R. (1995) *Masculinities*, Oxford: Polity Press.

Davis, K. (1997) *Embodied Practices*, London: Sage.

Desjarlais, R., Eisenberg, L., Good, B. and Kleinman, A. (1995) *World Mental Health: Problems and Priorities in Low Income Countries*, Oxford: Oxford Uni-versity Press.

Doyal, L. (1995) *What Makes Women Sick: Gender and the Political Economy of Health*, London: Macmillan.

—— (1998) *Gender and Health: A Technical Document*, Geneva: World Health Organization.

—— and Gough, I. (1991) *A Theory of Human Need*, London: Macmillan.

Dwyer, D. and Bruce, J. (eds) (1988) *A Home Divided: Women and Income in the Third World*, Stanford, CA: Stanford University Press.

Garenne, M. and Lafon, M. (1998) 'Sexist diseases', *Perspectives in Biology and Medicine* 42 (2): 773–87.

Harrison, J., Chin, J. and Ficarrotto, T. (1992) 'Warning: masculinity may damage your health', in M. Kimmel and M. Messner (eds), *Men's Lives*, New York: Macmillan.

Hart, N. (1988) 'Sex, gender and survival: inequalities of life chances between Euro-pean men and women', in A.J. Fox (ed.), *Inequality in Health within Europe*, Aldershot, Hants: Gower.

Hearn, J. and Morgan, D. (eds) (1990) *Men, Masculinities and Social Theory*, London: Unwin Hyman.

Heise, L., Moore, K. and Toubia N. (1995) *Sexual Coercion and Reproductive Health: A Focus on Research*, New York: Population Control Council.

Hudelson, P. (1996) 'Gender differentials in tuberculosis: the role of socioeconomic factors', *Tubercule and Lung Disease* 77: 391–400.

Huggins, A. and Lamb, B. (1998) *Social Perspectives on Men's Health in Australia*, Melbourne: Maclennan and Petty.

Jackson, C. (1998) 'Rescuing gender from the poverty trap', in C. Jackson and R. Pearson (eds), *Feminist Visions of Development*, London: Routledge.

Kabeer, N. (1994) *Reversed Realities: Gender Hierarchies in Development Thought*, London: Verso.

Kandiyoti, D. (1998) 'Bargaining with patriarchy', *Gender and Society* 2 (3): 274–90.

Kimmel, M. and Levine, M. (1993) 'Men and AIDS', in M. Kimmel and M. Messner (eds), *Men's Lives*, New York: Macmillan.

—— and Messner, M. (eds) (1993) *Men's Lives*, New York: Macmillan.

Kitts, J. and Roberts, J. (1996) *The Health Gap: Beyond Pregnancy and Reproduction*, Ottawa: International Development Research Centre.

Kristiansen, C. (1989) 'Gender differences in the meaning of health', *Social Behaviour* 4 (3).

Leon, D., Chenet, L., Shkolnikov, V., Zakharov, S., Shapiro, S., Rakhmanova, G., Vassin, S. and McKee, M. (1997) 'Huge variations in Russian mortality rates 1984–94: artefact, alcohol or what?', *Lancet* 350: 383–8.

Lloyd, T. and Wood, T. (1996) *What Next for Men?*, London: Working with Men.

Mac an Ghaill, M. (ed.) (1996) *Understanding Masculinities*, Buckingham: Open University Press.

Moore, H. (1988) *Feminism and Anthropology*, Oxford: Polity Press.

Nussbaum, M. and Glover, J. (eds) (1995) *Women, Culture and Development: A Study of Human Capabilities*, Oxford: Clarendon Press.

Owen, M. (1996) *A World of Widows*, London: Zed Books.

Papanek, H. (1990) 'To each less than she needs, from each more than she can do: allocations, entitlements and value', in I. Tinker (ed.), *Persistent Inequalities: Women and World Development*, Oxford: Oxford University Press.

Peto, R., Lopez, A., Boreham, J., Thun, M. and Heath, C. (1992) 'Mortality from tobacco in developed countries: indirect estimation for national vital statistics', *Lancet* 339: 1268–78.

Pleck, J. and Sonenstein, F. (eds) (1991) *Adolescent Problem Behaviors*, Hilldale, NJ: Lawrence Erlbaum.

Rooney, C. (1992) *Antenatal Care and Maternal Health: How Effective Is It? A Review of the Evidence*, Geneva: World Health Organization.

Royston, E. and Armstrong, S. (1989) *Preventing Maternal Deaths*, Geneva: World Health Organization.

Sabo, D. and Gordon, G. (1993) *Men's Health and Illness: Gender, Power and the Body*, London: Sage.

Scott, S. and Morgan, D. (eds) (1993) *Body Matters: Essays on the Sociology of the Body*, London: Falmer Press.

Sen, G., Germain, A. and Chen, L. (1994) *Population Policies Reconsidered: Health, Empowerment and Rights*, Boston, MA: Harvard University Press.

Sen, G. and Snow, R. (1994) *Power and Decision: The Social Control of Reproduction*, Boston, MA: Harvard University Press.

Shilling, C. (1993) *The Body and Social Theory*, London: Sage.

Stein, J. (1997) *Empowerment and Women's Health: Theory, Methods and Practice*, London: Zed Press.

Tinker, A., Daly, P., Green, C., Saxeman, H., Lakshminarayan, R. and Gill, K. (1994) *Women's Health and Nutrition: Making a Difference*, Washington, DC: World Bank.

United Nations Development Programme (1995) *Human Development Report 1995*, New York: UNDP.

Vlassoff, C. and Bonilla, E. (1994) 'Gender related differences in the impact of tropical diseases on women: what do we know?', *Journal of Biosocial Science* 26: 37–53.

Waldron, I. (1995) 'Contributions of changing gender differentials in behaviour to changing gender differences in mortality', in D. Sabo and G. Gordon (eds), *Men's Health and Illness: Gender, Power and the Body*, London: Sage.

Watson, P. (1995) 'Explaining rising mortality among men in Eastern Europe', *Social Science and Medicine* 41 (7): 923–4.

—— (1997) 'Health differences in Eastern Europe: preliminary findings from the Nowa Huta study', *Social Science and Medicine* 46 (4–5): 549–58.

World Health Organization (1991) *Maternal Mortality: A Global Factbook*, Geneva: World Health Organization.

—— (1996) *Violence Against Women: WHO Consultation 5–7 February 1996*, Geneva: World Health Organisation.

Zeidenstein, S. and Moore, K. (1996) *Learning About Sexuality: A Practical Beginning*, Washington, DC: World Bank.

11 Children, healing, suffering and voluntary consent

Priscilla Alderson

[W]e have accorded doctors the right to inflict pain. Our concern therefore has to be to see that health workers do not inflict pain unnecessarily. . . . We believe our skills as social scientists make it possible for us to point out the unintended suffering inflicted, suffering which is unrecognised and which may perhaps be unnecessary or avoidable. . . . Our gaze has been trained to look at the working of the mind and of society . . . to look below the surface of the commonsensical and to see the deeper implications.

(Stacey 1979: 186–7)

Introduction: preventing avoidable suffering

The above words concluded a book about the welfare of children in hospital. In *Beyond Separation* (Hall and Stacey 1979) sociological researchers showed how children in hospital were not suffering simply from the maternal deprivation which the Robertsons (1989) reported. Children also suffered from being lifted from their everyday social contexts into hospital wards where they languished, bored, lonely, frightened, and the 'work objects' of health professionals. The book reported years of team research which was indirectly initiated by the government's expert report *The Welfare of Children in Hospital* (DHSS 1959). Most hospitals took no notice of the new government policies that mothers should be encouraged to care for their children in hospital and continued to ban parents from children's wards. Struck by the contrast between official policy and her own experience of local hospitals, Meg Stacey started the Welsh Association for the Welfare of Children in Hospital (AWCH) to campaign for change; she also organised related research. An English version started, eventually being named the National Association for the Welfare of Children in Hospital (NAWCH).

By the mid 1970s, hospitals varied. Some welcomed and supported parents in children's wards, others continued to limit access, as I found when my children became patients, and I joined NAWCH to help to change hospitals. Practical and policy experience developed into theoretical interest and 10 years later I began work on a PhD about parents' consent to children's heart surgery.[1] The paediatric cardiac centres were sites of intense suffering as well as of joy and relief. One in ten of the children who had surgery died. The units still had ambiguous policies about welcoming or excluding parents, which exacerbated the unintended suffering of families who were often far from their homes and support networks. Later, I researched children's consent, mainly to orthopaedic surgery.[2]

This chapter reviews research about informed and voluntary consent, and how suffering and moral feelings can expand the awareness which informs consent. Legal and ethical meanings of consent are contrasted. The opportunities for consent to prevent and reduce suffering are reviewed, and contributions from social science which look below the surface of the commonsensical, towards understanding these links and opportunities, are discussed, mainly in relation to parents' and children's consent.

Informed and voluntary consent

The law treats consent in terms of precise verifiable facts, requiring that patients be told the purpose and nature of proposed treatment, the risks and hoped-for benefits, short- and longer-term effects and any alternative treatments (Montgomery 1997: 227–48). People should know that they can ask questions, discuss and possibly negotiate proposals, have time to reflect, and are free to make an unpressured decision, which may be to withhold consent.[3] Most research about consent consists of psychological surveys of how patients can recall and recount medical information (though often without detailing what they were told) and tends to find that patients' understanding is inadequate (see, for example, Kaufman 1983). Psychometric research assesses patients' anxiety levels on being informed, implicitly assuming that anxiety is a negative reaction to be reduced and avoided (Fallowfield 1990). Analyses of decision making in medicine (Thornton 1993) and bioethics (Beauchamp and Childress 1989) examine how patients use expert clinical information to make rational cost-benefit and risk calculations. Much of this literature seems to regard the patient as a philosopher in pyjamas, giving consent to his (*sic*) own treatment as the calm, intellectual equal of the doctor (Gillon 1994).

Medico-legal consent combines partial contradictions between Kantian autonomy which makes correct personal decisions without interference or constraint (Kant [1796] 1972), and Mill's respect for liberty, which is so precious that people must be free to make personal choices, including foolish ones and best guesses (Mill [1858] 1982). The correct choice and the best guess meet in cases of high-risk surgery, when people strive to make the wisest possible decision while accepting danger and uncertainty. Until recently, minors were excluded as being too immature to make either correct decisions or best guesses, lacking courage to stand by their mistakes, and needing their 'best interests' to be protected until they develop adult autonomy.

In the mid 1980s, Mrs Victoria Gillick sought to ensure that the courts would close the legal gap left by the Family Law Reform Act 1969, which allowed minors aged over 16 to give valid consent to treatment but said nothing about people aged under 16 years. Eventually the Law Lords ruled that a competent child is one who 'achieves a sufficient understanding and intelligence to enable him or her to understand fully what is proposed' and 'has sufficient discretion to enable him or her to make a wise choice in his or her own best interests' (*Gillick* v. *Wisbech and W Norfolk AHA* [1985] 3 All ER 423). Doctors who decide that in their clinical judgement a child is competent can legally accept that child's consent (Age of Legal Capacity (Scotland) Act 1991, s. 4, 2). Later court cases, however, complicated the law, as reviewed later.

All the aspects of consent considered so far are very important, but they concentrate on the reasoning 'informed' side of consent to the exclusion of the equally important 'voluntary' side. Medical research is regulated by the Declaration of Helsinki (WMA 1964/2000) which emphasises the value of research to 'help suffering humanity' (this phrase is deleted from the 2000 version). Not until clause 9 is 'the subject's freely given informed consent' mentioned. The Declaration, written by doctors, differs from the first international guidance on consent (Nuremberg Code 1947). The Code was written by lawyers mindful of human rights and the crucial respect for physical and mental integrity which was violated during the 1940s, as illustrated during the Nuremberg trials. The Code begins: '1. The voluntary consent of the human subject is absolutely essential.' It sets voluntariness, an emotional experience, act and state of mind, first: 'the exercise of free power of choice, without the intervention of any element of force, fraud, deceit, duress, overreaching, or other ulterior form of constraint or coercion'. These phrases come well before 'having the knowledge . . . to make an understanding and enlightened decision' which the Code assumes that ordinary adults can do, whereas Helsinki contrasts scientists' expertise and ultimate responsibility versus lay people's much less informed views.

Voluntariness has also become rather lost in positivistic research and bioethics. For example, this leading bioethics text on consent concludes:

> These many confusing terms surrounding the term 'voluntariness' are too much, we believe, to combat successfully through a conceptual analysis that attempts to tidy up its meaning, and hence we avoid the word entirely. We substitute a conception of noncontrol that does not have the history and connotation that burdens [*sic*] the terms 'freedom', 'voluntariness' and 'independence'.
>
> (Faden and Beauchamp 1986: 257)

This 'tidy' solution of 'noncontrol' paradoxically denies the essence of voluntariness which concerns patients' agency, power and control to give or withhold consent. The quotation reveals the underlying notions in much functionalist bioethics of eschewing emotion, and of the expert, correct and active doctor and the relatively ignorant, fallible and passive patient, so that 'noncontrol' is seen as avoidable coercions which health staff refrain from exerting. This approach reflects the current trend away from remembering Nuremberg, and consent as an essential defence against the violation of human integrity, towards preoccupation with 'informed choice', which implies that life and death decisions are as mundane as shopping. Consent then dwindles into a polite formality which tolerates patients' idiosyncratic preferences abstracted from those issues in their daily lives which make their hopes and fears significant.

Consent thus tends to be seen mainly as the medico-legal device which transfers responsibility for risk and injury from the doctor to the patient. Consent can also protect patients from unnecessary suffering, make doctors be accountable, and help patients to become informed and prepared for interventions; although the law prevents bad practice rather than promoting best practice. In contrast, an ethical approach sees consent as the formal means of promoting mutually respectful partnership between doctors and patients throughout the treatment. Yet how can bewildered and extremely distressed parents and children who are considering major treatment possibly achieve Kantian wisdom and Millean courage? And even if people are accepted as having some voluntary power, despite being unavoidably constrained by illness, fear and pain as they struggle to resolve dilemmas and arrive at a firm decision, how can such elusive invisible issues as voluntariness, wisdom, respect and trust be researched?

My PhD research (Alderson 1990) involved learning about sociology, cardiology, bioethics and law, which, with evidence about parents' experiences, seemed to stretch the topic of parents' consent into conflicting directions and a mass of irreconcilable contradictions. Gradually, they merged into some coherence with help from theories about the following: moral emotions which inform, rather than undermine, moral reasoning (Gilligan 1982); respect which includes care (Seidler 1986); contradictions which are also complementary and can be held in tension together (Ramazanoglu 1989); and philosophy which sees everyday experiences and settings as constituting moral problems instead of cluttering up and obscuring abstract moral principles (Grimshaw 1986).

The social context and knowledge

The work of AWCH and NAWCH set a practical background to my research on consent by emphasising the importance of the social context. How can parents give valid, informed consent if they are not allowed into the wards and intensive care units, or if there is no chair for them beside the cot, or if they have little idea about what is going on? Ethnographic research showed how parents' consent to complex treatment plans is a process, not an event, grounded in hours spent sitting with their child, watching and talking with the staff, gradually learning and emotionally coming to terms with new knowledge. In turn, these opportunities are influenced by hospital funding and policies, staff training and support, whether there are quiet times and spaces for practitioners and families to exchange knowledge, and whether parents have sufficient help with high transport costs, care of their other children, and their other severe anxieties. Such support respects their priorities and responsibilities.

Clinicians who respect parents and children accept their knowledge as valid when, for example, a mother considers that regular injections are less distressing to her baby than numerous attempts to insert a line into her veins. Orthopaedic surgery aims to relieve pain or to improve mobility or appearance. In all three areas, the patients are the experts in knowing how much pain, difficulty or difference in appearance they can accept before they are willing to undergo surgery which might not work and might make matters worse. Some surgeons respect children's knowledge and wishes, correcting a 'minor' spinal curve if a child is very unhappy, but leaving some more serious curves untreated or waiting until a child is ready to consent. Decisions about the timing of extremely risky heart surgery, as children become progressively weaker, involve clinical tests and also social evaluations: is it better to wait another year or two, or to try earlier surgery when the child has more strength to survive it, and it might lead a much fuller life afterwards? Consent as a process of exchanging personal and medical knowledge and discussing options can prevent the suffering of feeling coerced or deceived, and the fear and possibly increased pain of unwanted treatment.

Consent works in cycles. Continuing discussion informs staff about the processes and outcomes of their care, they can monitor and raise standards, and also give more accurate information to future patients. One example is how the staff gradually gave in to pressure from parents who wanted to accompany their children into the anaesthetic room and stay until they were asleep, instead of having to watch a crying child being taken from the ward, especially when the operation might be fatal.

The working of the mind

Besides the external, observable processes there are inner, psychological ones. Knowledge as factual information differs from knowledge as deeply absorbed and experienced awareness of the personal implications. People need time to acquire the latter, if their consent is to be informed and committed. Parents and children described their emotional and intellectual journey, initial fear and horror on hearing the diagnosis and treatment proposals, gradually growing trust in the hospital staff and confidence in their skills, slow acceptance that the untreated illness would be worse than the high-risk heart surgery and its hoped-for benefits, and increasing faith and courage. Their moral feelings of trust and hope and parents' pity and concern for their child gained strength and meaning through their experiences and relationships. Anxiety was not wholly negative and could bring insight and courage.

Families described how doctors who seriously informed and consulted with them relieved their anxiety and misunderstandings and increased their courage and mutual respect. This also encouraged their informed co-operation on which the success of treatment might depend, such as with exercises, diet or medications. Alison, aged 14, fainted on first learning that her curved spine would be straightened during two risky operations but added that she would much rather be told. Kerry, aged 12, agreed to the proposed surgery but was extremely distressed when plans were changed at the last minute to another procedure, and later she wanted to refuse all further treatment; this gives one of many instances of the advantages of respecting patients' voluntary consent if possible, and the suffering that can ensue when it is bypassed (Alderson 1993: 123–9).

During emergencies, this emotional journey cannot be experienced, yet 'emergency' is an elastic term, stretching sometimes into days when there may be time to consider consent, albeit less thoroughly. Shock and grief do not necessarily inhibit thought; people are shocked because they understand, and if parents were not shocked when considering their baby's heart surgery they would be insufficiently aware. Years later, parents recalled neonatal emergencies in intense detail, indicating that they were highly aware at the time: 'After the Caesarean, the nurse put her head round the door and asked my religion, and I thought my baby was dying.' Children also remembered times when they might have seemed scarcely aware. An anaesthetist came to see Brenda and, remembering surgery three years earlier when she was aged 6, Brenda said: 'Please can I have gas? I don't like the injection and please can I have the mint flavoured gas like I had last time?'

People especially remember any hints of good or bad news. Observations in the wards showed how they sifted information into these categories, and showed the difficulties for the staff in managing the import of any news they gave to parents, trying to sustain reasonable but not undue optimism, trying to help parents to lose hope if their child was dying. The large busy medical, surgical and nursing teams also had to attempt to sustain some uniformity in their accounts to families, and inevitably there were discrepancies in tone and language when even simple phrases could be confusing. Heart valves were referred to by one doctor as thicker and by another as narrow, both meaning that the thicker valve walls narrowed the space between them.

Perhaps most importantly, the consent process helps people to make sense of painful and alarming experiences, to see the context and the 'story' of how they might recover, to help them to cope during stressful times and come to terms with the outcomes, successful or not. This means making a decision they can live with in future. During my research in the 1980s, many parents said they attached exceptional importance to being informed, respected and consulted about the child for whose life they were responsible – 'we have to sign the consent form' – while having to make what they said was the hardest decision in their life. During 1999–2000, major inquiries were being conducted in England into parents' consent: to heart surgery; to the removal of deceased babies' organs; to surveillance of suspected Munchausen-by-proxy;

and research about ventilation. Some parents express gratitude after their child has died, when they feel that everything reasonable has been attempted with care and respect. Other still express grief and anger, 12 or 20 years later, about being misinformed or excluded from decision making about their child (Power 1998).

Beyond the commonsensical

The ethnographic research revealed intense emotions which the families and staff discussed during interviews. But how can valid social research interpret such data? The following reservations about interviews will be reviewed.

> Humanistic interviewing methods which try to elicit intimate data are superficially seductive . . . Just as we are suspicious of the media's claim to access personal experience through interviews with celebrities, we should be wary of the claim that research interviews have uncovered authentic human experience . . . we may have done nothing more than elicit familiar and socially acceptable ways of accounting for success or failure.
>
> (Silverman 1993: 95).

Yes, indeed we may have, although assuring confidentiality and concealing people's identity in reports, besides addressing issues other than self-promotion, may make research interviews very different from media celebrity interviews.

> Interviews are like a dance of expectations, opportunities for impression management (Goffman 1959). I produce my actions in the expectation that you will understand them in a particular way. Your understanding reflects your expectations of what would be a proper action for me in these particular circumstances which, in turn, becomes the basis of your response which, itself, reflects your expectations of how I will respond, and so on.
>
> (Dingwall 1997: 56)

Reflexive research can also analyse how people step out of the dance of expectation, such as when young children show profound understanding and competence, or challenge how researchers infantilise them, leading to re-examination of how childhood is socially constructed (Alderson 1993; Mayall 1994).

> It may be dressed up like a conversation between friends. But an interview is not [that]. It is a deliberately created opportunity to talk about something which the interviewer is interested in and which may or may not interest the respondent.
>
> (Dingwall 1997)

Conversations between friends are not always mutually interesting. When the interview is about topics of central importance to interviewees, if they are not interested this may be a failure of the interviewer rather than of the interview medium:

'A meeting between strangers, unfamiliar with each others' "socially organised contexts" does not provide the necessary contextual basis for adequate interpretations' (Mischler 1979). Many meetings between strangers depend on rapidly established 'bases for adequate interpretations' – in health care, business or parties. Society could not exist without strangers' abilities to establish these at some adequate level, and neither could informed consent. Rather than assuming that an ideal level should, but cannot, be reached, sociological interpretations can take account of the limitations of brief encounters and of all other research methods.

> Rather than evaluating interview data as more or less accurate reports of external reality, we are obliged to view them as occasions when individuals feel called upon to give accounts of their actions, feelings, opinions etc., in such a way as to present themselves as competent, and indeed moral, members of particular communities.
>
> (Murphy *et al.* 1998: 120)

This method, of treating interviews not as topics (sources of overt information) but as a resource (through examining underlying structures, such as the moral account, generating findings, and constructing meaning), is, however, suspended when researchers select which data to treat as topics, and when they assume that readers will treat their reports as topic not as resource. When researchers examine how, for example, parents of children with a heart condition structure their accounts to present themselves as moral people (Baruch 1981), rather than taking accounts 'as more or less accurate reports of external reality' this can be covert and deceptive research. Interviewees may sense this and be more defensive. Gaining their informed consent would involve saying something such as: 'My main interest is not your experiences of your child's illness, but how you structure your account to rationalise your reactions morally. It is irrelevant whether your account is "true" except for what you unconsciously reveal in structuring your replies.' Few people would, perhaps, then agree to be interviewed, and if they knew the research was about moral accounts, this could affect their responses and jeopardise the research. Interviews with parents and children about consent and their competence to understand the plans have some 'internal reality' in that they partly repeat their observed 'real' conversations with hospital staff.

In contrast to these commentaries, Oakley (1981), Cornwell (1984), West (1990), Pill (1995), and many other researchers describe breaking through formalities into 'private', frank and mutually absorbing discussions, and into unanticipated areas (Britten 1996), such as discussions about 'non-compliance' with prescribed health care (Morgan and Watkins 1988), sometimes so successfully that some researchers are concerned that this shared intimacy risks over-exposing and exploiting people (Finch 1984).

If we cannot know whether we can elicit private accounts about 'deep' feelings and experiences, we cannot be certain that we are not doing so. Gender differences between the sceptics, mainly men, and those generally convinced by interviews, mainly women, suggest psychological bases for their differing views, such as that women tend to welcome intimacy and men tend to fear it (Gilligan 1982); women tend to use communication to make connections and men tend to use it to take control; one to become engaged the other to remain detached (Tannen 1991). The 'radical critique' of interviews (Murphy *et al.* 1998: 120) may be influenced by the sceptics' own research interests in such 'public' topics as professionalism, organisation, management, and the professional presentation of self (Atkinson 1981; Dingwall 1977; Silverman 1984, 1989), in preference to more intimate topics. Trust is unlikely to develop when people describe their most intense, painful experiences to a researcher who 'brackets off' the 'truth' of their account. This reservation is not simply neutral. By bracketing off,

> and trying to ignore questions about the content of a [religious] belief, [sociology] fails to take seriously the fact that to the person holding it, the most important aspect is that *it is true* . . . Any sociological interpretation which undercuts this, falsifies what it is interpreting . . . By sidestepping issues of truth and falsity, sociology has often forgotten the importance of claims to truth. Ignoring that can appear tantamount to assuming their falsity.
>
> (Trigg 1985: 36)

There appears to be an implicit model of people as empty vessels through which shared public discourses swish. 'Familiar and socially acceptable ways of accounting for success or failure' (Silverman 1993) are voiced like empty clichés with no way of telling how true or relevant each comment is. Yet as, for example, Hochschild (1976: 281–3) asked about Goffman's (1959) theory of the person's presentation of many selves like costumes hung on a peg, where is the core self that they are all hung on to? If parents and cardiologists cannot be regarded as telling what they see as the truth, or if there are no such truths, how can any statement have any validity, including statements which deny truth in interviewees' accounts, and so on in endless regress? Then, why should anyone care to say anything, without some way of ordering priorities of meaning, relevance and importance? How can sociologists claim that their own reports are valid and more than moral presentations? It is also unclear why parents' and doctors' concern with self-presentation should predominate over concern for the sick child.

Morality seems to be reduced to manners, to an etiquette of being seen to do the correct thing, rather than of wanting and trying to do so. Presenting oneself as a moral person is an important part of much of our discourse, but it is not the whole or always the main part. Murphy *et al.* (1998) make many valuable points about conducting qualitative research. But they dismiss patients' views about health technology assessments (though not professionals' views) although patients' unique and essential knowledge of the processes and effects of health technologies is among the richest resources and findings of social research. The practical value of research about moral accounts is usually illustrated with the sole example of a new support clinic being organised for parents in a heart surgery centre (Baruch 1981; Silverman 1985: 171; Murphy *et al.* 1998: 122). Yet the clinic was soon discontinued as impractical. Many more useful policy and practice changes have been effected through taking users' directly expressed concerns seriously, while also taking account of the sociological reservations listed above, and treating interviews as topic and resource.

The working of society

Our research about children's consent (see note 2) began in the year of the Children Act 1989 and the UN Convention on the Rights of the Child, which both enshrine Gillick-like precepts about listening to children. The research ended in 1991 when Lord Donaldson in the Court of Appeal began the 'backlash against Gillick'. He ruled that R, aged almost 16 and refusing mental health treatment, could be forced to have medication (*RE R* [1991] 3 WLR 592), and that W, aged 16, who had anorexia, could be force-fed (*RE W* [1992] WLR 33: 758–82). This overturned the 1969 Act mentioned earlier which respected 16-year-olds as having adults' rights of consent. The 1989 Children Act increased the potential number of people with 'parental responsibility', and Lord Donaldson further ruled that if any one of these adults gave consent, this could override the refusal of everyone else concerned, including the 'Gillick competent child' aged up to 18 (reviewed in Alderson and Montgomery 1996).

Lawyers criticised both rulings on several grounds, including the point that the cases concerned mental illness rather than children's (in)competence, and so should not be generalised to all minors, although this has happened. Doctors often mention that 'the law does not allow children to refuse'. Of course children can refuse, no law can stop them. The question is whether doctors should or must override refusal. They can respect the informed decision of a child they deem to be competent as mentioned earlier, and they may feel ethically obliged to do so. There are probably many unreported cases of doctors and parents accepting the informed refusal of terminally ill young children (Alderson 1993), such as Samantha, aged 6, who refused a third liver transplant (Irwin 1996). Yet debate is dominated by the reported court cases which all authorise doctors to treat or not treat as they originally intended and rule against children's and parents' wishes. The sole exception was the young boy whose parents refused a proposed liver transplant. They were intensive care nurses and may have been seen as experts counterbalancing the expert medical views which the courts usually favour against the families' lay views.

Medical authority was taken still further when doctors were authorised to transplant a new heart into M, aged almost 16, despite her refusal. Previously healthy, she had developed heart disease a few weeks earlier and a transplant was proposed two days before the court hearing (Dyer 1999a). M was quoted as saying that she did not want to die but that she did not want a new heart either, and the judge concluded that she was too overwhelmed to make a competent decision. Yet M's reactions are typical of the initial stages of parents' consent to heart surgery as they begin to address dilemmas between mutually incompatible ends, such as gaining health and avoiding surgery, and gradually think and feel their way towards a resolution.

The desperate urgency felt by M's parents and doctors and the judge is understandable, but it is unfortunate when such extreme cases encourage beliefs that almost any procedure can be enforced on minors. Adults' own refusal has to be respected in English law, to the extent of respecting women's refusal of Caesarean section even if the baby might die. Newspapers compared M's case with cases of force-feeding girls with anorexia (London *Metro*, *Daily Mail* 17 July 1999), ignoring the great differences between administering food and implanting a heart. Most seriously, these rulings undermine the respect for informed, willing consent which, to many practitioners, is an integral part of therapy. Shortly after, M was reported to have agreed to surgery.

The judge said he considered M's views, but these had little influence in the inevitable precedents-based legal outcome of supporting medical opinion, demonstrated in two further cases that month. David Glass's mother failed to obtain a court ruling that treatment should not be withheld from her severely disabled son, aged 13 (Dyer 1999b). The courts also upheld consultants' refusal to refer Katie Atkinson, aged 9, who has Down's syndrome, to be assessed for a possible heart transplantation. The cases should be understood as enforcing the 'medieval power of the courts' and not as rulings on children's rights or competence (Bynoe 1993), despite their powerful influence over society's views on these issues.

Sociological study of consent can bring together seemingly conflicting views into some coherence: medico-legal concepts of consent as precise knowledge, and the key which gives doctors the right to inflict pain but can prevent avoidable suffering; ethical concepts of respect for the wise choice or the best guess; evidence of complex experiences which challenge popular dichotomies such as reason/emotion, medical/lay knowledge, competent adult/incompetent child, inner feelings/public policies, showing how they overlap. A minority want to decide for themselves or to leave others to decide for them, but most adults and children want to have more or less share in deciding about their consent, partly depending on the information, respect and support they receive over time. Like the nurse who described gently 'nudging' girls into talking about their fears and misunderstandings before their operations, clinical staff who use open questions, conversational exchanges and narratives appear to encourage consent that is more informed and voluntary.

Notes

1 Parents' consent to paediatric cardiac surgery, 1984–7, funded by the ESRC; ethnographic research in two London hospitals in all related hospital departments; interviews with parents and staff; surveys of parents' and nurses' experiences (Alderson 1990).
2 Children's consent to surgery, conducted with Jill Siddle in three London hospitals and one in Liverpool, 1989–91, funded by the Leverhulme Trust; observations and interviews with 120 patients aged 8 to 16, their parents and 70 staff (see Alderson 1993).
3 In the absence of statute law in Britain, standards of consent to medical treatment and research have evolved through case law and guidance, for example, from the Department of Health (1991), the Royal College of Paediatrics and Child Health (2000), and the British Medical Association (Romano-Critchley and Somerville 2000).

References

Alderson, P. (1990) *Choosing for Children: Parents' Consent to Surgery*, Oxford: Oxford University Press.
—— (1993) *Children's Consent to Surgery*, Buckingham: Open University Press.
—— and Montgomery, J. (1996) *Health Care Choices: Making Decisions with Children*, London: Institute for Public Policy Research.
Atkinson, P. (1981) *The Clinical Experience*, Farnborough, Hants.: Gower.
Baruch, G. (1981) 'Moral tales: parents' stories of encounters with the health profession', *Sociology of Health and Illness* 3: 275–7.
Beauchamp, T., and Childress, J. (1989) *Principles of Biomedical Ethics*, New York: Oxford University Press.
Britten, N. (1996) 'Qualitative interviews in medical research', in C. Pope and N. Mays (eds), *Qualitative Research in Health Care*, London: BMJ Publishing Group.
Bynoe, I. (1993) 'Consent and the law', in P. Alderson (ed.), *Young People, Psychiatric Treatment and Consent*, London: Institute of Eduction.
Cornwell, J. (1984) *Hard-earned Lives*, London: Tavistock.
Department of Health (1991) *Local Research Ethics Committees*, London: Department of Health.
Department of Health and Social Security (DHSS) (1959) *The Welfare of Children in Hospital*, London: HMSO.
Dingwall, R. (1977) *The Social Organisation of Health Visitor Training*, London: Croom Helm.
Dingwall, R. (1997) 'Accounts, interviews and observations', in G. Miller and R. Dingwall (eds), *Context and Method in Qualitative Research*, London: Sage.
Dyer, C. (1999a) 'English teenager given heart transplant against her will', *British Medical Journal* 319: 209.

—— (1999b) 'Mother fails to win right to control treatment for son', *British Medical Journal* 319: 278.

Faden, R. and Beauchamp, T. (1986) *A History and Theory of Informed Consent*, New York: Oxford University Press.

Fallowfield, L. (1990) *The Quality of Life*, London: Souvenir Press.

Finch, J. (1984) ' "It's great to have someone to talk to": ethics and politics of inter-viewing women', in C. Bell and H. Roberts (eds), *Social Researching: Politics, Problems, Practice*, London: Routledge.

Gilligan, C. (1982) *In a Different Voice*, Cambridge, MA: Harvard University Press.

Gillon, R. (ed.) (1994) *Principles of Biomedical Ethics*, Chichester, Sussex: John Wiley.

Goffman, E, (1959) *The Presentation of Self in Everyday Life*, Harmondsworth, Middx: Penguin.

Grimshaw, J. (1986) *Feminism and Philosophy*, Brighton, Sussex: Wheatsheaf.

Hall, D. and Stacey, M. (eds) (1979) *Beyond Separation*, London: Routledge and Kegan Paul.

Hochschild, A. (1976) 'The sociology of feeling and emotion: selected possibilities', in M. Millman and R. Kanter (eds), *Another Voice*, New York: Octagon Books.

Irwin, C. (1996) 'Samantha's wish', *Nursing Times* 92 (36): 29–30.

Kant, I. ([1796] 1972) *The Moral Law*, trans. and ed. H. Paton, London: Hutchinson.

Kaufman, C. (1983) 'Informed consent and patient decision making: two decades of research', *Social Science and Medicine* 17 (22): 1657–64.

Mayall, B. (ed.) (1994) *Children's Childhoods: Observed and Experienced*, London: Falmer Press.

Mill, J. ([1858] 1982) *On Liberty*, Harmondsworth, Middx: Penguin.

Mischler, E. (1979) 'Meeting in context: is there any other kind?', *Harvard Educational Review* 49: 1–19.

Montgomery, J. (1997) *Health Care Law*, Oxford: Oxford University Press.

Morgan, M. and Watkins, C. (1988) 'Managing hypertension: beliefs and responses to medication among cultural groups', *Sociology of Health and Illness* 10: 561–78.

Murphy, E., Dingwall, R., Greatbatch, D., Parker, S. and Watson, P. (1998) 'Qualita-tive research methods in health technology assessment: a review of the literature', *Health Technology Assessment* 2: 16.

Nuremberg Code (1947) in A. Duncan, G. Dunstan and R. Wellbourn (eds), *Dictionary of Medical Ethics*, London: Darton, Longman & Todd.

Oakley, A. (1981) 'Interviewing women: a contradiction in terms?', in H. Roberts (ed.), *Doing Feminist Research*, London: Routledge.

Pill, R. (1995) 'Fitting the method to the question: the quantitative or qualitative approach?', in R. Jones and A. Kinmouth (eds), *Critical Reading for Primary Care*, Oxford: Oxford University Press.

Power, C. (1998) 'When things go wrong what should be said?', *Bulletin of Medical Ethics* 141: 13–21.

Ramazanoglu, C. (1989) *Feminism and the Contradictions of Oppression*, London: Routledge.

Robertson, J. and Robertson, J. (1989) *Separation and the Very Young*, London: Free Association Books.

Romano-Critchley, G. and Somerville, A. (2000) *Consent, Rights and Choices in Health Care for Children and Young People*, London: British Medical Association.

Royal College of Paediatrics and Child Health (2000) 'Guidelines on the ethical conduct of medical research involving children', *Archives of Disease in Childhood* 82: 177–82.

Seidler, V. (1986) *Kant, Respect and Injustice*, London: Routledge.

Silverman, D. (1984) 'Going private: ceremonial forms in a private oncology clinic', *Sociology* 18: 191–204.

—— (1985) *Qualitative Methodology and Sociology*, London: Gower.

—— (1989) 'Telling convincing stories: a plea for cautious positivism in case studies', reprinted in D. Silverman, *Interpreting Qualitative Data: Methods for Analysing Talk, Texts and Interaction*, London: Sage, 1993.

—— (1993) *Interpreting Qualitative Data: Methods for Analysing Talk, Texts and Interaction*, London: Sage.

Stacey, M. (1979) 'The practical implications of our conclusions', in D. Hall and M. Stacey (eds), *Beyond Separation*, London: Routledge and Kegan Paul.

Tannen, D. (1991) *You Just Don't Understand: Women and Men in Conversation*, London: Virago.

Thornton, J. (1993) 'Genetics, information and choice', in P. Alderson (ed.), *Consent and the Reproductive Technologies*, London: Institute of Education.

Trigg, R. (1985) *Understanding Social Science: A Philosophical Introduction to the Social Sciences*, Oxford: Basil Blackwell.

West, P. (1990) 'The status and validity of accounts obtained at interview', *Social Science and Medicine* 30: 1229–39.

World Medical Association (1964/2000) *Declaration of Helsinki*, Fernay-Voltaire: WMA.

12 Integrated medicine

An examination of GP–complementary practitioner collaboration

Ursula Sharma

Introduction

'Integrated medicine' is a term which has wide currency in Europe and the US. It is used to refer to collaboration of various kinds between orthodox and non-biomedical practitioners. 'Integration', however, implies a whole. Either some thing is 'integrated' into some other thing through a process of absorption or assimilation, or two pre-existing things are 'integrated' to form a new whole. The term itself can apply to either process, an ambiguity which is capable of political exploitation, as for example when the 'integration' of ethnic minorities or asylum seekers into British society is debated. In the case of 'integrated medicine' (or 'integrative' medicine as it is also called), are complementary medicines simply being absorbed into biomedicine in some way – or are biomedicine and other modes coming together to make a new kind of health care system? Could 'integrated medicine' constitute a radically new kind of medicine, or is it just a benign buzzword, another term for the co-option of complementary forms by the biomedical establishment?

Certainly its most enthusiastic proponents are aware that 'integration' cannot be a simple matter. Reporting on a workshop on 'integrated medicine' held at a Danish conference on complementary medicine, Hoffman-Dorninger (1995) records that three levels of integration were identified. At the *systems* level there has to be some integration in terms of research and training; doctors need to understand more about complementary therapies, but complementary therapists need to have a basic knowledge of biomedical models of disease. At the *professional* level groups of practitioners must have the means and opportunities to work together. At the *treatment* level the care that the patient receives must be integrated: biomedical and/or non-biomedical treatments should be given with due care to the patient's individual needs and to the ways in which these treatments might complement or interact with each other.

In Britain the ideal of 'integrated medicine' has been enthusiastically promoted by the Foundation for Integrated Medicine, a charitable organisation whose patron is the Prince of Wales. The Foundation aims to make complementary forms of treatment accessible, that is, 'available to those who need them' through an 'integrated model of delivery' which, in the British context, must be primarily through the National Health Service (NHS). But for this to happen, according to the Foundation, there needs to be a common educational basis for all who work in health care, that is, an integration of knowledge. This in turn requires more research into the effectiveness of non-biomedical treatments and the proper regulation of those who deliver them.

There is recognition therefore that even the least radical interpretation of 'integration' would require far-reaching changes in present training and practice. In Britain, however, practical collaborations between doctors and practitioners of certain kinds of complementary medicine have galloped ahead of such changes, especially in the context of primary health care. There may be many reasons for this. GPs are increasingly faced with chronic and/or diffuse conditions which cannot easily be resolved through the use of biomedical drugs. Complementary medicines are increasingly used and trusted by the public as adjuncts to (and sometimes instead of) biomedical treatments (for a full discussion of these issues, see Cant and Sharma 1999).

In this chapter, I concentrate on the practical collaboration between GPs and the practitioners of complementary medicine. I review some recent literature on 'integration' in primary health care with a view to working out what such collaboration represents. Does it represent any real modification of biomedical dominance? Does it constitute 'integrated treatment' for the patients? Could it be the point of entry into the NHS for new forms of knowledge about health and illness, a more holistic understanding? Or does it, as some complementary practitioners have feared, represent a co-option of non-biomedical healing, its practical subordination to the control of the medical profession?

The development of 'integrated medicine': background

Biomedicine's capacity to marginalise and delegitimise complementary medicines can be cited as an egregious example of biomedical dominance. When osteopaths sought state registration as long ago as 1935 the British Medical Association (BMA) was instrumental in blocking the progress of the Bill, and 800 medical and biological scientists signed a petition opposing it and arguing that osteopathy was unscientific. This was submitted to the Parliamentary Select Committee set up to consider the issue (Larkin 1992). The attempts of herbalists to achieve state registration had met with similar medical opposition in 1923. The close relationship between the medical profession and the Ministry of Health privileged medical views and proved more effective than the alliances which the osteopaths had managed to forge with sympathetic members of the House of Lords. As Larkin (ibid.: 123) remarks: '[Osteopathy's] pursuit of aristocratic patronage . . . may well have rested on a confusion between symbolic and the real authority in the modern British state.'

The failure of the osteopaths' and the herbalists' early attempts to secure state registration facilitated the exclusion of most forms of complementary medicine from the NHS in 1947 and marked the start of a period of political quiescence on the part of complementary therapy groups. This lasted until the popular resurgence of complementary medicine, which occurred in most Western countries in the late 1960s and early 1970s. Faced with this new challenge, national medical associations have generally expressed public hostility to complementary medicines (albeit some more than others) in spite of the sympathetic interest many individual doctors have evidently taken in certain forms. In Britain the first public pronouncement on the part of the BMA was a report prepared by a special Working Party in 1986 (BMA 1986). This report considered the claims and methods of various well-known forms of complementary medicine and concluded that they were, on the whole, based on unscientific ideas; any benefits they might bring to patients were unproven in the absence of proper controlled trials and were unlikely to be more than 'placebo' effects of some kind.

In Britain, as in many other Western countries, complementary medicines have grown in popularity despite this official negativity on the part of the medical profession. Various opinion polls and national surveys conducted in the 1980s (MORI 1989; RSGB 1984) suggested that around 30 per cent of the population had used some forms of complementary medicine at some time or other, a figure comparable to levels of usage discovered in other Western countries (see, for example, Eisenberg *et al.* 1993). That complementary medicine had achieved an increased legitimacy in the eyes of the British public was indicated by a MORI poll in 1989, according to which only 23 per cent of respondents said that they would not consider using *any* form of complementary medicine (MORI 1989). Another national opinion poll found that 74 per cent of respondents supported the inclusion of certain complementary therapies in the NHS (RSBG 1989).

It was also becoming increasingly evident that there was a degree of division within the medical camp. Whilst the BMA view was that complementary medicines had yet to prove that they brought any benefit to patients, many individual doctors (mainly GPs) clearly thought that certain forms had considerable value and expressed interest either in training in these or in co-operation with their practitioners. A study by Wharton and Lewith (1986), conducted in Avon and published in the same year as the first BMA report, revealed that 38 per cent of respondents claimed to have trained in some form of complementary medicine, 15 per cent wanted to have such training and 76 per cent claimed to have actually referred patients to complementary practitioners (CPs) of certain kinds during the past year. This period also saw a softening of governmental attitudes to complementary medicines. In Britain, unlike many other European countries, there was no law banning practice on the part of non-medical practitioners so it was not a question of replacing existing legislation so much as introducing explicit state recognition of the therapies. During the late 1980s the British government encouraged therapy groups to develop the degree of professional unity and self-regulation that would be required for state registration, although to date only the osteopaths and the chiropractors have achieved this. In 1991 Stephen Dorrell, then Secretary of State for Health, issued a statement clarifying the role of complementary medicines in relation to the NHS subsequent to the introduction of the NHS internal market. He pointed out that under the new arrangements it was open to a fund-holding GP to employ a complementary therapist in his or her practice, subject to the proviso that the GP retain overall clinical responsibility for the patient. This statement did not in itself state anything more than what was already possible, but it was generally interpreted as significant since it represented an explicitly permissive stance. Whilst recent British governments cannot be said to have had any positive policy towards complementary medicines (they have not, for instance, directly funded research into efficacy, as the US government has done), they have clearly had to take into account the popularity with the public and a substantial number of GPs of certain complementary therapies (see Cant and Sharma 1999: 127ff).

In view of this situation it was probably not surprising that the second BMA report on complementary medicines, published in 1993 and entitled *Complementary Medicine: New Approaches to Good Practice*, took a completely different approach from the first report. This document urged the complementary therapy groups to agree standards of training so as to ensure a safe and professional service to the public. It emphasised the need for proper self-regulation, for which each therapy group ought to prepare itself. The need for research and scientific trials was also reiterated but was less prominent than the call for professional regulation.

By the early 1990s it was evident that complementary medicine was already very much present in the NHS. This was not the result of any national-level policy decision though it was certainly facilitated by aspects of the 1991 NHS 'reforms'. But GPs could practise complementary therapies themselves or refer patients to complementary practitioners without these institutional opportunities and probably had been doing so for some time. A study commissioned by the Department of Health and conducted by researchers at the University of Sheffield found that an estimated 40 per cent of GP partnerships in England now provided some form of complementary medicine for NHS patients, 21 per cent providing treatment by a member of the partnership team, 6 per cent employing an independent CP and 25 per cent making NHS referrals for complementary therapy. The authors pointed out, however, that the actual number of patients accessing complementary medicine via the NHS was still relatively small. On the other hand, about 60 per cent of health authorities were commissioning it in one way or another (Thomas *et al.* 1995) and the need to develop proper guidelines for such commissioning was the subject of much debate and at least one national conference (NAHAT 1993; Worth 1995). As a result of the National Association of Health Authorities and Trusts (NAHAT) conference several new pilot projects were set up across the country, such as the referral services piloted by West Yorkshire Health Authority at Kirklees (Worth 1995: 10ff).

In short, it was clear by the mid 1990s that some forms of complementary medicine were being provided through the NHS without any policy decision at national level having been made to this effect, or any but piecemeal sharing of information (ibid.: 12). Health authorities began to attempt (individually) to define the circumstances under which complementary medicine could be incorporated into their NHS services. They started to develop guidelines for its use and evaluation and to identify the issues which needed to be resolved (evidence of efficacy, cost effectiveness, proper training of those who delivered it). A further contribution to the general debate was provided by the Foundation for Integrated Medicine, which convened a national conference in 1998. It was evident at this conference (which I attended) that there was considerable enthusiasm for integrating forms of complementary medicine into NHS provision in a more systematic way, but also that there was still considerable medical scepticism, especially on the part of medical researchers and consultants. If medicine was now to be 'evidence-based', they argued, the paucity of scientific evidence for the efficacy of complementary medicines was a major obstacle to its integration with biomedicine.

'Integrated medicine' in Britain has generally meant integration of complementary medicines into the NHS, the NHS being the chief provider of biomedicine. However, this interest is but the local manifestation of a widespread movement. Integrated clinics of various kinds were being established in European countries and elsewhere (Hernesniemi; 1994; Launsø 1989) and there are instances of integrated medical training and research programmes in Europe and the US (see, for example, Melchart 1996).

In what follows I concentrate on primary care because it is in this area that collaboration is usually most direct in Britain. Moreover, it is with reference to primary care that a body of literature has developed which describes and evaluates the ways in which such collaboration actually works in practice. I am mainly concerned with situations where GPs co-operate with practitioners trained in other therapeutic traditions (i.e. I am excluding the situation where some form of complementary therapy is practised by the GPs themselves, although this raises some equally interesting questions – see May and Sirur 1998).

Delivering 'integrated medicine': the institutional context

Dr Patrick Pietroni, a major pioneer of 'integrated' health care in Britain, enumerated the possibilities for integrating complementary medicine into general practice as they existed in 1992. He includes the following:

> Employment of ancillary staff funded by the FHSA, operating within a health centre in much the same way as counsellors and physiotherapists, supported in part by health promotion reimbursement.

Privately funded; GPs refer patients to complementary practitioners (CPs) who recover fees from the patients themselves. In some cases practitioners share premises with the primary care team. (My research on complementary practitioners suggests that in the late 1980s there was a good deal of informal local networking both among CPs and between GPs and CPs which might have provided the basis for such co-operative arrangements.)

Research studies; trial arrangements funded by regional or district authorities or other medical funding sources.

Local fundraising activities; a GP team employs CPs supported by charitable or voluntary sector funds.

CPs are seconded to GP practices, directly funded by the DHA or FHSA, or fund holding practices employ such practitioners directly.

Practice placements; student CPs provide their services free of charge.

Primary health care referral centres take patients sent from several practices, funded by health authorities.

(Pietroni 1992)

Appendix 1 gives a fuller list of 'outlets' for complementary medicine in general compiled by the Foundation for Integrated Medicine.

As we can see, there are various institutional arrangements for GP–CP collaboration. In all of them the GP retains a degree of therapeutic responsibility for registered patients, but in practice the closeness of co-operation or the degree of supervision on the part of the GP varies considerably. What does the literature on 'integrated' health care at the primary level tell us about the way in which such co-operation works? The following account is based on a number of studies produced by independent researchers contracted to evaluate services (see Appendix 2 for a list of the projects and centres described in these studies) as well as accounts provided by CPs and GPs themselves in the medical and complementary medical press.

Knowledge and language

One issue that emerges very clearly is the problem of relating different systems of knowledge. Whilst some medical schools in Britain have begun to introduce undergraduate courses on complementary medicines (Reilly and Taylor 1993) most GPs' knowledge of them will depend on what they have managed to find out as a result of their own interest. If they have actually trained in some form of complementary therapy it will probably be through short courses designed specifically for medical personnel rather than through the longer courses mounted for non-medically-qualified (NMQ) practitioners. Whatever mutual respect and appreciation exists among a team of

GPs and CPs in general practice, it is unlikely that GPs will have an in-depth grasp of the knowledge bases of their colleagues' therapies. They will already have been socialised into a professional culture in which scientificity is a prime value and in which healing activity is described in the language of science. Yet a common language is desirable if there is to be genuine collaboration. To some extent this is only the kind of problem which faces any interdisciplinary team of health care professionals. Yet although many CPs will have encountered medical notions of anatomy and pathology in the course of their training, mutual acquaintance is not the same as common understanding. David Peters (1994) has described the Marylebone Health Centre in which there was a concerted effort on the part of professionals to achieve in-depth knowledge of each other's knowledge bases. He notes that there was a tendency to rely on acceptable metaphors such as 'energy' without deconstructing the woolliness of such concepts or clarifying exactly what they meant for each kind of practitioner:

> CP–doctor working groups are an intense microcosm of a culture struggling with an emergent paradigm and they probably generate even more difficult dynamics than other interdisciplinary working groups.
>
> (Ibid.: 189).

Consequently such discrepancies represent a greater challenge to the GP than meetings at other interprofessional boundaries and may give rise to feelings of disempowerment on both sides. Another solution to the problem of common language was to discuss patients primarily in terms of 'psychosocial predicament':

> As one of these [complementary] practitioners reflected towards the end of the inquiry, the implication was that their approach could not have any *medical* validity, but what it could have was psychosocial validity.
>
> (Reason *et al.* 1992: 162)

In the case of the Marylebone project, strenuous efforts were made to achieve a mutual learning so that both medical and CP staff understood each other's therapeutic methods better. The benefits derived from this approach and a commitment to patient empowerment has led the Marylebone team to consider a model that would reduce interprofessional conflict and problems about power by handing more discretion to the patient:

> We are currently experimenting with a model where the patient is given the option to choose whether he or she sees the general practitioner or goes straight to the complementary practitioner. A further experiment is that of the discussion of the general practitioner partnership as the core of the health care team.
>
> (Pietroni 1992: 305)

To do away with the gate-keeper role of the GP within NHS practice would be a very radical step indeed and does not seem to have been considered in other general practice collaborations.

Where co-operative groups of CPs cross-refer or collaborate in other ways, comparable problems may arise. In the Hoxton Health Group, for instance, the CPs took tutorials together in anatomy and physiology and developed a joint diagnostic questionnaire (Kettle 1993: 150). Where practitioners make active efforts to inform themselves about each other's clinical practice the results seem to be encouraging, though in the case of the Warwick House Medical Centre at Taunton the CPs were less satisfied with the rate of change than were the GPs (Paterson and Peacock 1995: 257). In the Glastonbury Health Centre, CPs became somewhat frustrated when interprofessional practice meetings tended to get taken up with administrative matters (Hills and Welford 1998: 21). An additional problem arises where CPs are paid strictly by the session and their NHS payment does not cover time taken for practice meetings with other professionals or time spent in mutual information and education sessions. Any time spent on such meetings is therefore voluntary on their part, even assuming that medical colleagues see the necessity for such work. Dialogue groups, such as have been established in some other European countries (see Christie's 1991 account of such groups in Norway), might prove useful if funding could be found to support the attendance of CPs who are not permanent employees of the NHS. In referral schemes where the CPs were not actually housed in the same building as the GPs, any kind of mutual education was difficult and could lead to a feeling of isolation and marginalisation on the part of the CPs (Donnelly 1993: 4). None the less some CPs felt that a referral system did enable them to find out more about how GPs work, the range of problems they treat and the dimensions of their workloads (Emanuel *et al.* 1996: 25).

Whilst a common language is desirable if GPs and CPs are to exchange information on specific patients in a meaningful way, it is perhaps less clear whether an in-depth understanding of each other's knowledge base is truly a *sine qua non* for fruitful co-operation. Doubtless it is essential for GPs to have an adequate understanding of what particular therapies or therapists can do if they are to refer patients in a way that is productive, and some of the frustrations referred to in this chapter are to be avoided. On the other hand, as Maretzki (1987: 1066) shows in the case of the Kur[1] in Germany, it is possible for the institutionalised biomedical health care system to embrace a system of healing with a quite different knowledge base, albeit at the cost of 'a considerable amount of cognitive discrepancy' for both physicians and patients.

Referral criteria and diagnostic categories

In practical terms, the problem of discrepant perspectives on health and illness can manifest itself in problems around referral. In most of the collaborative projects described, the GPs still acted as gate-keepers to the CPs' services to a large extent. If GPs are unclear about what CPs can do and how they work there is a high chance of referrals that CPs will regard as inappropriate. At the Glastonbury Health Centre GP referrals to CPs were predominantly for chronic problems, mainly musculo-skeletal problems, psycho-social problems, multi-system problems (Hills and Welford 1998: 5) and the authors of the report speculate that more patients might have bene-fited had GPs been more prepared to refer acute cases. In any case, the CPs were allowed only six NHS sessions per referral, after which the patient had to go to the back of the waiting-list queue if more sessions were thought desirable. Budd *et al.* (1990) report the same problem in the Wells Park prac-tice, that is, GPs tended to refer mainly chronic patients, elderly patients needing pain relief, and 'fat envelope' cases. However, in this case 'the prob-lem diminished as the general practitioners became more familiar with the boundaries of the alternative therapies through liaison with the therapists, though they admitted to a tendency to refer "difficult" patients' (ibid.: 378).

At the Liverpool Centre for Health CPs resented being 'dumped' with intractable chronic cases and seeing very few acute cases (Donnelly 1993: 4–5). Furthermore, they found that few GPs provided adequate clinical data on the patients they referred, so CPs felt that they wasted time taking basic case histories all over again (ibid.: 2). At the Wigan and Bolton referral scheme, some CPs felt that they were seeing people whose problems had been mismanaged for years and years with inappropriate drug regimes that did not address the basic causes. They felt that they were expected to do something for such patients 'with a bit of manipulation in a few sessions' (Emanuel *et al.* 1996: 26).

These problems notwithstanding, in several cases CPs noted with satisfac-tion that they were seeing a wider range of patients than they encountered in private practice. In particular they were liable to encounter more elderly patients and more working-class patients, a situation beneficial to patients in terms of greater therapeutic choice and to CPs in terms of opportunities for professional development. It did, however, mean that CPs might have to spend more time on the educational aspects of their work, encouraging patients who were not at all familiar with complementary medicines (and who might never have thought of using them had they not been available on the NHS) to take more responsibility for their health (Donnelly 1993: 7).[2]

In some cases, referral systems began to operate really effectively once a satisfactory protocol for referral was worked on. For example, at the Warwick House practice a standard referral form was filled out by the GP. In Kirklees too a proper referral protocol was devised, though Worth (1995: 11) notes that there were initial problems due to (mutual) unrealistic expectations and a need for structured sharing of information. Reason (1995) notes that in the Wells Park practice CPs valued general information about why the patient was being referred as much as strictly clinical data. It was useful to know, for example, if the GP had tried a number of medical treatments that had not worked. Equally, GPs valued information about what CPs had done with the patients. This represents a significant advance in view of fact that earlier research had suggested a general fear on the part of self-referring patients to confide in GPs about complementary treatment they have had (Sharma 1995: 55). Such mutual information must be a major advantage. However, pressure of time often militated against such detailed communication (Reason 1995: 39). Too often GPs provided only limited clinical data, although some GPs noted that their longer treatment times and more sympathetic approach allowed patients themselves to give information to CPs which they had not felt able to confide to GPs.

Complementary practitioners' knowledge of disease and of particular patients is 'inserted' into the structure of general practice rather than integrated into it. By this I do not mean that individual GPs fail to respect the knowledge of their CP colleagues or do not learn from them; rather, practice in primary health care is already organised around the typical diagnostic categories and treatment regimes of biomedicine. These practices are derived from the knowledge system of biomedicine and its typical understandings of the body and of disease, but also from the bureaucratic context in which biomedicine has long been practised.

As we shall see in the next section, these bureaucratic imperatives, especially those which relate to the organisation and allocation of resources, constitute a major obstacle to 'integration' if 'integration' is to mean more than 'subordination to medical control'. Complementary medicines developed and flourished in the private health care sector because that was the only place for them for many years. CPs have worked chiefly as independent practitioners, operating alone or in small, loosely organised groups, and the main resource determinant for their practice has been the market.

Whose time? Whose resources?

Resource constraints in the NHS manifest themselves largely as scarcities of time. Where CPs are employed in general practice, differences in therapeutic time cycles emerge as a major issue, expressed in terms of problems around waiting lists. A preponderance of chronic patients referred by GPs has often meant that CPs are dealing with patients for whom any improvement at all would depend on very long-term treatment strategies, as Budd *et al.* (1990: 378) found at Wells Park. But this would lead to a build-up of waiting lists and delayed treatment for other patients. Demand has also been fuelled when self-referral is permitted or where patients hear about the service and ask GPs for referral. Chris Worth, Director of Public Health for West Yorkshire, where there has been some experimentation with referral services, suggested that if demand is excessive it might be more efficient to provide complementary medicine through the services of existing NHS personnel who have some practical knowledge of them (Worth 1995: 11). This would, he argues, obviate problems involved in integrating independent practitioners into the bureaucratic structures and culture of the NHS. However, many CPs would no doubt regard a complementary therapy service delivered by doctors as less genuinely holistic than their own. Even the BMA has been concerned about the potential dangers of doctors with a little superficial training in an alternative therapy practising such therapies themselves (BMA 1993: 42).

For many CPs, used to practising in the private sector, waiting lists were certainly an unfamiliar problem. They fuelled anxiety stemming from a feeling that the CPs were under pressure for quick results in order to justify their funding (Donnelly 1993: 4). This anxiety is further exacerbated when CPs are unclear as to exactly how their services are liable to be evaluated; in some cases they reported a tendency to 'play safe' in their treatment of patients (ibid. 1993: 5). In the case of Phoenix Surgery, Reason (1995: 39) reports that the pressure of NHS general practice (as opposed to private practice) was experienced, as one CP put it, in terms of 'a sense of going towards that bigger result and shorter treatments'.

This feeling that their therapies were 'on trial' and had to prove themselves – moreover, prove themselves in *medical* terms – meant that in Phoenix Surgery CPs thought that they were concentrating on cases where some rapid improvement might be expected. This was at the expense of cases where perhaps very little could be done for the patient in medical terms, but where the support and empathy of the practitioner might have been of much value (Reason 1995: 40). Where such therapeutic support produces a striking subjective improvement (the patient felt much better in him/herself) this would be regarded as significant progress in healing for a CP, even though the pathological condition is only slightly alleviated in objective medical terms (Reason 1995).

Other problems attend the move from private practice to the bureaucratic ethos of the NHS. CPs may be unfamiliar with the need to audit their practice and to manage and account for resources in ways quite different from those which are required in private practice (Chevallier 1994: 4). The CPs had to educate themselves about the 'contract culture' of the NHS and, as Chevallier notes in respect of the Hoxton Health Group, it was a matter of 'balancing the qualitative needs of good patient care with the quantitative needs of using resources well and seeing as many patients as possible without sacrificing quality of care' (ibid.: 4).

Some CPs practising in NHS health centres felt that in matters regarding the running of the practice they were very much junior partners, having less of a say in general issues than did the GPs. This was the case in the Taunton practice, although the GPs themselves claimed that they saw CPs as 'professionals on an equal footing with themselves' (Paterson and Peacock 1995: 257). In general, CPs learnt much about team work (ibid.), albeit being brought up against professional boundary issues which they did not have to face in private practice. To what extent should they provide for each patient's benefit the full range of therapeutic possibilities in which they have been trained (as they would normally do in private practice)? Or should they simply restrict themselves to treating to the best of their capability the particular condition for which the GP has referred the patient (Donnelly 1993: 6)?

The patient perspective

At the beginning of this chapter I cited Hoffman-Dorninger's (1995) observation that a fully integrated medicine would be integrated from the point of view of the patient. The literature I have considered here does not provide the kind of information on individual patient profiles or treatment regimes that would enable us to say how far this has occurred. However, it would be unfortunate if a focus on professional perspectives were to obscure some of the enormous benefits the literature reports.

First of all, there is no doubt that many referral schemes have widened access to complementary medicines for working-class and elderly patients who did not access it before because they could not afford it, they did not know about it or it was not available in their immediate locality. Large-scale surveys suggest that usage of complementary medicine is no longer (if it ever was) confined to a middle-class, middle-aged, educated clientele. However, it is still less used by the poor, a situation which must persist so long as complementary medicine is still mainly private medicine. Private complementary practitioners do not (typically) set up their practices on council estates or in localities inhabited by the victims of long-term industrial decline. If we feel that complementary medicine in general, or any kind of complementary medicine in particular, has any potential benefit at all for patients, then we must be worried by this lack of provision and cheered by anything that widens access. This can also be satisfying and instructive for CPs, as it extends their experience and fosters professional development.

Where the results of evaluation measures have been published, they are generally very positive. CP services have been much appreciated by patients who would not have had access to them before (Ritchie and Ritchie 1991: 161) and have generally been very popular. In a few cases the incorporation of CPs' services has been associated with specific attempts to increase patient involvement in their treatment and other measures directed to increasing patient empowerment. A notable example of this has been the Marylebone Health Centre, where the team of GPs set up schemes to involve patient-volunteers in the running of the practice (Pietroni and Chase 1993). This kind of patient involvement, however, was more characteristic of collaborative schemes developed on the community project model (such as Hoxton Health Group and Craigmillar), where community participation is an acknowledged aim. It is less true of NHS general practice. In general, if patients felt personally empowered it was because the CPs had encouraged them to take more responsibility for their own health and had increased their understanding of their health problems.

In some cases the provision of CPs' services was associated with a reduction in the prescription of drugs, especially painkillers (Budd *et al.* 1990: 370; Hills and Welford 1998: 22), reductions in referrals to secondary care (Hills and Welford 1998: 22) and a general reduction of pressure on GPs from chronic patients. Where measures of clinical effectiveness have been applied and published, the outcomes seem to be positive. At Glastonbury and at Liverpool the SF36 instrument was used to measure patient improvement and in both cases the results suggest statistically significant improvement on most dimensions of health (ibid.: 12–13; Whelan 1995). Similar results were obtained with a Nottingham Health Project instrument Hoxton (Kettle 1993: 151) where a high level of patient satisfaction increased demand for complementary medicines. An evaluation of the Glastonbury Health Centre also found its service cost-effective in terms of the patient improvement and cost savings in a number of areas (Hills and Welford 1998). However, we cannot assume that complementary medicines will always be judged cost-effective by those who fund them, even where they are popular among patients. There is much debate about how they should be assessed, in particular whether randomised controlled trials (RCTs) are appropriate (see, for example, Resch and Ernst 1996; Kaptchuck *et al.* 1996), and (if RCTs are appropriate) whether it is realistic to demand them when there is little or no funding for such trials.

But in the end, where complementary medicines are funded through the NHS, NHS criteria will be applied. In 1997 there was much consternation in the complementary medicines press when the Lambeth, Southwark and Lewisham Health Authority ceased to pay for GP referrals to the Royal London Homeopathic Hospital on the grounds that there was insufficient evidence that patients had received clinical benefits from homeopathy. A researcher argued that 'the £250,000 spent each year on treatment for patients at the hospital would provide enough for an intensive care unit or 100 hip replacements' (*Natural Medicines Society News* no. 40 (1997): 3).

GP perceptions of efficacy will be most influential where fund-holding GPs buy in the services of CPs, but the patient voice is least likely to be heard in such matters. Donelly reminds CPs that under present arrangements and with the growth of a 'business' culture in NHS, CPs have to impress *managers* with information about 'value for money' as much as (or rather than) *doctors* with evidence of clinical efficacy (Donnelly 1995: 80).

> Value for money is not synonymous with cost effectiveness . . . [and] is driven by more urgent considerations than individual health outcomes. It is shorter term in its thinking, considers time as costly, and as something that can and must be cut (and so on).
>
> (Ibid.: 81)

Discussion: 'integration' and the bureaucratic 'taming' of complementary medicines

From the point of view of the NHS, CPs have generally been found to provide a cost-effective service (albeit still a rather marginal one in most areas) which reduces drug prescriptions and referrals to secondary care. But is it just providing primary health care on the cheap? Possibly, although rates of remuneration for patient care are not reported as a major issue for CPs in the literature I have reviewed. The range of funding and institutional arrangements for delivery of complementary medicines in primary health care is large, and this chapter has no more than touched on the implications of the different models in use. Nor have I dealt with the issue from the perspective of particular therapies. The issues involved in integration for, say, homeopaths might not be the same as those for chiropractors or osteopaths. However, the issue reported most consistently by CPs and to some extent by GPs is that of the discrepancy between clinical modes used by GPs and CPs. This leads to further confusion as to the aim of treatment when referrals gain momentum: different kinds of practitioner have different therapeutic goals and their characteristic time cycles for treatment vary.

The finding that emerges again and again is that where time and care are devoted to mutual education and efficient communication, this is instructive to both CPs and GPs and leads to more effective referral and co-operation. In several cases the participants note changes in outlook over time as different professions gain a better understanding of what the others can do and how they operate (see, for example, Emanuel *et al.* 1996: 27). This applies to CPs gaining understanding of what GP practice is all about just as much as it does to GPs gaining insight into different forms of complementary medicine. Many of the frustrations reported in the studies cited here stem from the fact that time for such beneficial mutual education is hard to find in the NHS. Mutual education, however devised, can be the one thing that goes by the board when the pressure on services is enormous. The centre in which this issue has been tackled most thoroughly is the Marylebone clinic. The participants experienced this as an uncomfortable process in the course of which they had at times been challenged and felt temporarily disempowered. But if it is pursued it can yield genuine mutual understanding and respect.

From some points of view we could describe the CP as a valued but subordinate ally to the GP, something like the practice nurse, counsellor or physiotherapist. However, the complementary medical professions have resisted moves to position themselves as 'professions supplementary to medicine' because of the subordinate status this implies. Indeed, as Reason and others point out, complementary medicines are not 'professions supplementary to medicine' in as much as their knowledge bases present a potential challenge to the GP. They are often based on ideas which, on the face of it at least, are not *supplementary to* but *incompatible with* medical categories – even if the practitioners concerned believe that they are all aiming for the same goals. However, complementary modalities vary a great deal in their claims and the degree to which they wish to be regarded as complete and comprehensive systems of healing (see Pietroni 1992). Osteopathy is now much more assimilated to the medical model, whereas homeopathy and acupuncture, as practised by NMQ therapists, are based on very different assumptions about the human body and person.

Complementary medicines are not inserted into the NHS in such a way as to produce a genuine pluralism, in which different modes of healing have equal weight and status. Indeed, even GPs with positive attitudes to most forms of complementary medicine may discriminate between those that are 'NHS material' and those that are not. As one GP said in a study of GP attitudes:

> When you are talking about remedial massage, aromotherapy, reflexology, those sort of therapies, people wish to exert their freedom to choose. I think it's good because it maintains those particular therapies . . . definitely outwith the medical sphere in the restricted sense of that word. I think it's an acceptance that in many cases we are not dealing with a disease process.
>
> (Redmond-Pyle 1996: 67)

On the whole, the studies which I have reviewed in this chapter demonstrate that whatever 'integration' is achieved in primary care, the relationship between GPs and CPs remains asymmetrical. GPs largely retain their gatekeeping role. Hence their view of what complementary practitioners can do or which patients are appropriately referred to them has more weight than CPs' understanding of what GPs can do. There is a sense in which complementary medicines still enter the biomedical clinic 'on sufferance'; that is, they must demonstrate their effectiveness in a way that is not demanded (or at least not demanded in the same way) from GPs. The asymmetry is more palpably felt when CPs practise on GP 'territory', although inclusion in the physical space of the GP clinic may bring compensatory benefits.

This is perhaps unsurprising; why should we expect the CP to have a more privileged position *vis-à-vis* medical power than that of other professional groups to whom GPs make referrals (for example, physiotherapists)? So long as doctors are expected to retain overall clinical responsibility for patients whom they refer to others, then they are hardly likely to agree to any institutional arrangement that does not give them the upper hand. However, biomedical power is not a zero sum game. First, if doctors have not ceded control or power to CPs with whom they co-operate, this does not mean that the CPs have not made important gains from the collaboration. If such collaboration is more than a passing fashion it will have contributed to the general social legitimisation of certain forms of complementary medicine, as well as advantaging individual practitioners in the pursuit of their livelihood. Second, doctors themselves are subject to more and more budgetary control. Where they have been fund-holders, GPs have had (and under new arrangements GPs may still have) considerable discretion to commission CP services themselves. But under both these and other institutional arrangements within which CPs' services are brought in, considerations of cost-effectiveness are as important as purely clinical efficacy.

The criteria by which complementary medicines will be judged in the end will very largely be those which satisfy NHS managers. At the moment this issue is not really resolved. Will there be a demand in future for 'evidence-based' complementary medicines or will savings on GPs' time and drugs expenditure be sufficient to secure approval of some forms of complementary medicine on the part of the health authorities? Perhaps the popularity of complementary medicines among patients could be a crucial if unacknowledged factor.

Conclusion

This discussion of collaboration between GPs and CPs suggests that the knowledge and practice of complementary practitioners cannot simply be 'inserted' into primary health care in the NHS, or at least that such 'insertion' obliges CPs to accept more modifications to their preferred ways of doing things than it does doctors. Given the amount of attention sociologists have paid to medical dominance and its sources we ought not to be surprised at this. But medical dominance is a very broad concept and does not take us very far in itself: we need to identify the particular aspects of medical dominance that operate in the context in which we are interested.

One such aspect is the organisation of therapeutic responsibility which results from the edicts of the General Medical Council (GMC) and the ways in which these are embedded in the NHS. A GP may delegate treatment to other kinds of health care professionals, but retains overall therapeutic responsibility for the patient. The GMC has never gone further than this in spite of a considerable softening of the medical profession towards complementary medicines (as exemplified by the second BMA report). The GP may be impressed by the results of some complementary treatments, but to take responsibility for the outcomes of treatments which s/he does not understand and whose efficacy has not been demonstrated according to criteria which the medical profession accepts, would still be a highly risky business. As we have seen, there are problems for CPs in the systems of accountability embodied in medical practice and some feel that they could do more for patients if they had more control over the context of treatment. Yet the privileging of bio-medical knowledge and practice which is embedded in the NHS, combined with unchanging legal and professional notions of the relations between doctors and other kinds of practitioner, make it difficult to see how the CPs could be given equal authority with doctors within the NHS.

Second, practitioners of complementary medicines typically come from an institutional background which is different from that of biomedical doctors. Many of the more professionalised forms of complementary medicine have developed practices of record keeping and accounting comparable to those of doctors. That is, they keep confidential notes which record patients' consultations and treatments, and their notion of the ethics of the patient–practitioner relationship is essentially like that which doctors are supposed to observe. However, complementary medicines have grown up in a private health care context where the limiting factor on the possibilities for treatment has been the market. Private biomedicine also operates in a market context;

but it benefits from systems of referral and training as well as material facilities already well-established and financed by the public sector. In private complementary practice the practitioner can treat the patient for as long as they both wish it, provided the patient can pay. The resource limitations on practice in the public sector are quite different. In return for the opportunity to treat patients who could never afford private treatment, CPs have to accept restrictions which have their origins in bureaucratic accounting for time, money, space and expertise. Whilst there is nothing in their knowledge bases which is inherently hostile to practice in a public bureaucratic context, most complementary practitioners have developed their practice and expectations elsewhere. To the extent that integration means integration into the NHS, the process is bound to involve a certain amount of culture shock for CPs. This is not to say that GPs do not also feel that their clinical practice is constrained by resource considerations, nor that doctors in general do not chafe under the increased managerialism of the NHS, only that they have more prior experience of the culture and institutions of bureaucracy.

It is difficult therefore to see how integration into the public sector could be other than asymmetrical. For the effects of 'integration' to be more than local and sporadic, the issue of medical education needs to be addressed. But even then, it is hard to see how integration could be a coming together of equally valued systems of knowledge. Acceptance of the practical effects of the established medical dominance on the part of CPs is the price that must be paid for the wider access to complementary medicine which the NHS could deliver.

Appendix 1 Current ways of delivering CAM

Model	Approach	Pros	Cons
General practice	1 GPs or nursing staff using CAM	Access	Expertise?
	2 Independent CAM practitioners on NHS premises but privately or charitably funded	Access	Cost to patient
GP non-fund-holding practices	3 Referral to specialist CAM centres (see below) (NHS or otherwise funded)		Access Liaison with GP?
	4 Private referral to independent CAM practitioners (Referral by conventional specialists to whom GPs have referred may be reimbursed by private medical insurance for some CAM therapies)		Cost, liaison?
GP fund-holding (GPFH) practices	1 Any of the above can apply in GPFH practices		
	2 CAM practitioners working as part of the multi-professional primary care team	Access Liaison	
	3 Referral to independent CAM practitioners' premises: individually or via block contract	Access Liaison	
GPs and networks	1 Many GPs provide basic CAM treatments, having attended courses	Access	Expertise?
	2 Currently a training model giving GPs in primary care competencies in homeopathy has attracted 10% of Scottish GPs	Access Expertise Integrated	
	A network of specialist homeopathic doctors provides support under agreed terms of service		

Appendix 1 – contd

Model	Approach	Pros	Cons
CAM centres	1 Main homeopathic hospitals in London and Glasgow are national referral centres for homeopathy, acupuncture, manipulative and nutritional therapies Mainly outpatients but also some in-patient provision	Therapy packages	
NHS Acute Trusts	2 Increasing use of osteopaths in physiotherapy departments, but generally haphazard implementation of this and other main CAM therapies in secondary care	Access	
	3 Most palliative care units and hospices (>90%) use some form of touch-based CAM therapies, usually by nursing staff or volunteers	Access	
	4 Pilot projects funded by and implemented on hospital premises: (a) out-patient care, e.g. pain clinic (b) in-patient care, e.g. massage on cardiac ICU (c) dedicated unit, e.g. Lewisham CAM centre, Royal Marsden Rehabilitation Centre (d) nurse-led initiatives, e.g. Oxford Institute of Nursing: aromatherapy Macmillan Practice Development Unit: massage	 QA QA	Stable funding? Integrated/QA? Integrated Liaison with GP Integrated? Integrated? Integrated?
Independent units	Independent provider organisations contracted by District Health Authorities (DHAs) to offer CAM services for specified conditions: e.g. Southampton Centre for Study of Complementary Medicine	GP liaison 'Therapy packages'	
DHA initiatives	1 DHA funding via NHS Community Trust for units based in community, e.g. Liverpool Centre for Health		Stable funding? Liaison with GP
	2 DHA funding to independent CAM practitioners in pilot initiatives, e.g. Calderdale & Kirklees project		Stable funding? QA?
	3 Mental health initiative, e.g. Camden Street project		Integrated?

Charitable projects	Offering subsidised or free treatment, usually to specific client groups, e.g. Bristol Cancer Help Centre, Lighthouse (AIDS), Pathways (drug addiction) (Referrals via GPs, other primary health and community care workers; also self-referral)	Stable funding? Liaison with GP Integrated? Integrated?
CAM training clinics	CAM treatment at low cost by supervised trainees, e.g. British School of Osteopathy, London School of Acupuncture and Trad. Chinese Medicine	Centralised? Liaison with GP Integrated?
Corporate services	1 Via occupational health, e.g. M&S osteopathy service 2 Via occupational counselling services, e.g. massage	Liaison with GP Liaison with GP

Source: Foundation for Integrated Medicine (1997: 38)

Appendix 2 Collaborations discussed in this chapter

Source	Name of centre	Brief description of collaboration
Budd *et al.* 1990	Wells Park General Practice (South London)	Osteopathic and acupuncture services provided by CPs in GP practice premises. Charitable and statutory funding sources. GP referral and some self-referral
Donnelly 1995 and Whelan 1995	Liverpool Centre for Health	Referral centre funded by Health Authority. GP referral from many practices. Separate premises
Emanuel *et al.* 1996	Bolton Complementary Therapies pilot scheme	Seven therapists employed on sessional basis to treat musculo-skeletal problems. GP referral from eight practices. Funded by Bolton FHSA and Wigan and Bolton DHA
Kettle 1993 and Chevallier 1994	Hoxton Health Group (London)	Community- and CP-driven initiative now funded by DHA and other sources. Initiated in out-patients' hospital department. GP referral and some self-referral
Paterson and Peacock 1995	Warwick House Medical Centre, Taunton (Somerset)	Nine CPs rent rooms and share facilities in non-fund-holding GP practice. GP referral and self-referral. Fees paid by patients. Regular meetings between GPs and CPs
Peters 1994 and Reason *et al.* 1992	Marylebone Health Centre (London)	NHS GP practice. GPs refer patients to CPs providing service on-site. CP service funded by grants from various non-statutory bodies
Reason 1995	Phoenix Surgery, Cirencester (Gloucestershire)	Six-partner GP practice provides osteopathy and acupuncture at reduced private rate delivered by CPs on-site. GP referral
Ritchie and Ritchie 1991	Craigmillar Health Project, Edinburgh	Originated as urban and community project. Provides acupuncture, shiatsu, massage and reflexology for local people. Mostly self-referral but GPs have begun to refer patients for acupuncture (more than half new intake). Regular meetings betwen GPs and acupuncturists
Hills and Welford 1998	Glastonbury Health Centre (Somerset)	Five complementary therapies made available on practice premises. Service and CPs funded by Somerset Health Authority. GP referral only

Notes

1 *Kur* is a health regime akin to naturopathy, with a particular emphasis on the value of therapeutic bathing.
2 This is not meant to imply that working-class people will never have had exposure to or knowledge of non-biomedical forms of healing. It is likely that in some areas of the country, working-class people used the services of local herbalists and practitioners of various forms of manipulation which were cheaper than those of the GP in pre-NHS days. However, therapies such as acupuncture, homeopathy or reflexology would not have been available in such communities (see Sharma 1995: 65ff).

References

British Medical Association (1986) *Alternative Therapy: Report of the Board of Science and Education*, London: BMA.
—— (1993) *Complementary Medicine: New Approaches to Good Practice*, Oxford: Oxford University Press.
Budd, C., Fisher, B., Parrinder, D. and Price, L. (1990) 'A model of co-operation between complementary and allopathic medicine in a primary care setting', *British Journal of General Practice* 40: 376–8.
Cant, S. and Sharma, U. (1999) *A New Medical Pluralism? Alternative Medicine, Doctors, Patients and the State*, London: UCL Press.
Chevallier, A. (1994) 'Working within the NHS', *Natural Medicines Society News* no. 31: 3–4.
Christie, V. (1991) 'A dialogue between practitioners of alternative (traditional) medicine and modern (western) medicine in Norway', *Social Science and Medicine* 32 (5): 549–52.
Donnelly, D. (1993) 'Interim report on therapists' experiences', unpublished paper.
—— (1995) 'Integrating complementary medicine within the NHS: a therapist's view of the Liverpool Centre for Health', *Complementary Therapies in Medicine* 3 (2): 84–7.
Eisenberg, D., Kessler, R., Foster, C., Norlock, F., Calkins, M. and Delbanko, T. (1993) 'Unconventional medicine in the United States', *New England Journal of Medicine* 328: 246–52.
Emanuel, J.,Warburton, B., Popay, J. and Siddal, J. (1996) *'A Bit of Manipulation' and 'A Few Needles': An Evaluation of GP Referrals to Complementary Therapists for Musculo-skeletal Problems*, Salford: Public Health Research and Resource Centre.
Foundation for Integrated Medicine (1997) *Integrated Healthcare: A Way Forward for the Next Five Years?*, London: Foundation for Integrated Medicine.
Hernesniemi, A. (1994) 'Co-work between a medical doctor and a traditional healer', in H. Johannessen, L. Launsø, S. Olesen and F. Staugård (eds), *Studies in Alternative Therapy 1: Contributions from the Nordic Countries*, Odense: Odense University Press.
Hills, D. and Welford, R. (1998) *Complementary Therapy in General Practice: An Evaluation of the Glastonbury Health Centre Complementary Medicine Service*, Glastonbury: Somerset Trust for Integrated Health Care.
Hoffman-Dorninger, R. (1995) 'Integrated medicine', in H. Johannessen, S. Olesen and J. Andersen (eds), *Studies in Alternative Therapy 2: Body and Nature*, Odense: Odense University Press.

Kaptchuk,T., Edwards, R. and Eisenberg, D. (1996) 'Complementary medicine: efficacy beyond the placebo effect', in E. Ernst (ed.) *Complementary Medicine: An Objective Appraisal*, Oxford: Butterworth-Heinemann.

Kettle, C. (1993) 'Hoxton health group: a central resource for complementary health care', *Complementary Therapies in Medicine* 1 (3): 148–52.

Larkin, G. (1992) 'Orthodox and osteopathic medicine in the inter-war years', in M. Saks (ed.), *Alternative Medicine in Britain*, Oxford: Clarendon Press.

Launsø, L. (1989) 'Integrated medicine: a challenge to the health-care system', *Acta Sociologica* 32 (3): 237–51.

Maretzki, T. (1987) 'The Kur in West Germany as an interface between naturopathic and allopathic ideologies', *Social Science and Medicine* 24 (12): 1061–8.

May, C. and Sirur, D. (1998) 'Art, science and placebo: incorporating homeopathy in general practice', *Sociology of Health and Illness* 20 (2): 168–90.

Melchart, D. (1996) 'Integration of complementary medicine in research at the University of Munich', in S. Olesen and E. Høg (eds), *Studies in Alternative Therapy 3: Communication in and about Alternative Therapies*, Odense: Odense University Press.

Market and Opinion Research International (MORI) (1989) *Research on Alternative Medicine* (conducted for *The Times* newspaper), London: MORI.

National Association of Health Authorities and Trusts (NAHAT) (1993) *Complementary Therapies in the NHS*, Birmingham: NAHAT.

Paterson, C. and Peacock, W. (1995) 'Complementary practitioners as part of the primary health care team: evaluation of one model', *British Journal of General Practice* 45: 255–8.

Peters, D. (1994) 'Co-operation between doctors and complementary practitioners', in S. Budd and U. Sharma (eds), *The Healing Bond*, London: Routledge.

Pietroni, P. (1992) 'Beyond the boundaries: relationship between general practice and complementary medicine', *British Medical Journal* 305: 564–6.

—— and Chase, H. (1993) 'Partners or partisans? Patient participation at Marylebone Health Centre', *British Journal of General Practice* 43: 341–4.

Reason, P. (1995) 'Complementary practice at Phoenix Surgery: first steps in co-operative inquiry', *Complementary Therapies in Medicine* 3 (1): 37–41.

——, Chase, D., Desser, A., Melhuish, C., Morrison, S., Peters, D., Wallstein, D., Webber, V. and Pietroni, P. (1992) 'Towards a clinical framework for collaboration between general and complementary practitioners: discussion paper', *Journal of the Royal Society of Medicine* 85 (March): 161–4.

Redmond-Pyle, E. (1996) *GPs' Beliefs and Practices vis-à-vis Non-orthodox Medicine: An Anthropological Analysis*, MSc. dissertation in medical social anthropology, University of Keele.

Reilly, D. and Taylor, M. (1993) 'Developing integrated medicine: report of the RCCM fellowship, Glasgow 1987–1990, *Complementary Therapies in Medicine* 1 (1): 3–41.

Resch, K. and Ernst, E. (1996) 'Research methodologies in complementary medicine: making sure it works', in E. Ernst (ed.), *Complementary Medicine: An Objective Appraisal*, Oxford: Butterworth-Heinemann.

Research Surveys of Great Britain (RSGB) (1984) *Omnibus Survey on Alternative Medicine*, London: RSGB.

Ritchie, R. and Ritchie, D. (1991) 'The Craigmillar Health Project: helping people to define their own health needs', *Complementary Medical Research* 5 (3): 160–4.

Sharma, U. (1995) *Complementary Medicine Today*, London: Routledge.

Thomas, K., Fall, K., Parry, J. and Nicholl, J. (1995) *National Survey of Access to Complementary Health Care via General Practice*, Sheffield: Sheffield University Medical Care Research Unit.

Wharton, R. and Lewith, G. (1986) 'Complementary medicine and the general practitioner', *British Medical Journal* 292: 1498–1500.

Whelan, J. (1995) 'Complementary therapies and the changing NHS: a development officer's view', *Complementary Therapies in Medicine* 3 (2): 79–83.

Worth, C. (1995) 'Why and how the NHS is going complementary', *Therapist* 3 (1): 9–12.

13 Medical uncertainty revisited

Renée C. Fox

Introduction

In June 1997, at the invitation of Meg Stacey, I gave several lectures at the University of Warwick, travelling from Oxford where I was spending the academic year as a visiting professor to do so. It was a bracing experience to find myself in the lively intellectual milieu of Warwick's Department of Sociology – an appreciated contrast to the ingrown atmosphere and marginalised status of sociology at the University of Oxford. One of the presentations that I made centred on medical uncertainty, a phenomenon with which I have been preoccupied throughout my career. At the time, I was in the early stages of planning an essay that would re-examine the forms of uncertainty I had previously identified and analysed, in the light of relevant medical, social and cultural developments that had occurred during the 1980s and 1990s. The essay had been solicited by medical sociologist Roy Fitzpatrick for the *Handbook of Social Studies in Health and Medicine* that he was co-editing with Gary Albrecht and Susan Scrimshaw.[1] It seems fitting that, given the 1997 visit to the University of Warwick afforded me the opportunity to discuss some of the underlying concepts and emerging insights, this revised version is included as a tribute to Meg and her contribution to medical sociology.

The colloquy about medical uncertainty should be placed in the larger framework suggested by Ray Porter (1998) in his panoramic 'medical history of humanity', entitled *The Greatest Benefit to Mankind*. Both at the inception of that volume and in its conclusion, he characterises Western medicine, at the close of the twentieth century, as undergoing a 'fundamental crisis' of definition and mandate, orientation and direction. It is a paradoxical crisis, he avers, growing out of medicine's impressive scientific and clinical achievements – especially those that have occurred since the Second World War – and the 'inflated expectations' that 'its triumphs' have brought in their wake. 'Medicine's finest hour is the dawn of its dilemmas', he aphoristically states (ibid.: 3–4, 716–18).

In several regards, I would go further than Roy Porter in interpreting what he portrays as the anomie that currently surrounds our medicine. Surveying

American and British medical literature published during the 1990s as part of my reconsideration of medical uncertainty, I was struck by the fact that it not only contained many indicators of the kind of 'disorientation' that Porter described, but also telling signs of unsureness about basic attributes of medical knowledge and medical thought. Equally notable, in the United States at any rate, is the troubled lack of certainty that many physicians are experiencing and voicing in response to the organisational and financial, as well as the scientific and clinical, changes taking place in medicine: changes, in the words of one middle-aged physician, 'that have been transforming medicine in our lifetime so thoroughly as to make me wonder if this is the same field that I entered in the 1960s'. If, in addition, we turn our attention to the sorts of quandaries around which the field of bioethics has been unfolding since the early 1970s, it appears that the dilemmas medicine faces at this historical juncture reach beyond its boundaries to include questions of value and belief that are more-than-medical and also more-than-ethical.

These are the perturbations in present-day medicine that my re-exploration of medical uncertainty uncovered and on which I should like to focus my discussion. By and large, they have not been extensively described or discussed by social scientists. Therefore, I shall consider them mainly through the medium of scientific and medical literature, and the insights that sociological reflection on that literature yields. But first, some mention of the conditions of uncertainty that seem to be generic to medical knowledge and medical practice in all historical eras will provide grounding for that discussion.

Fundamental forms of medical uncertainty

The problems and kinds of uncertainty identified in the essay on the 'training for uncertainty' of medical students that I published in 1957 (Fox 1957) appear to have persisted over time. In spite of all the changes that have transpired in and around medicine during the past four decades, medical students continue to attest that learning to recognise the abiding presence of uncertainty in medicine and to deal with it are challenging quintessences of becoming a physician (Silver 1964: 127–8). The kinds of uncertainty that mature as well as developing physicians recurrently encounter and with which they grapple are both cognitive and existential in nature. As I have written (Fox 1957, 1959, 1978a, 1980), they include forms of uncertainty that stem from the impossibility of mastering the entire corpus of medicine's knowledge and skills; from the many gaps and limitations in medical knowledge and effectiveness that exist despite medicine's continuous advances; from difficulties associated with distinguishing between personal ignorance and ineptitude; and the lacunae and incapacities of medicine itself. In addition to these intellectual, scientific and technical uncertainties of medicine, physicians must deal with the uncertainties and mysteries of human illness, and its attendant pain and suffering, of life and of death that are inherent to medicine and medical care, and with the questions of meaning that they evoke. Changes that have occurred in medical science, technology and practice and in their social and cultural environs during the past few decades have contributed to the emergence of different expressions of these types of uncertainty. But a number of the themes around which such recent manifestations of uncertainty have crystallised are not new; rather, they are 'updated' and, in some instances, accentuated versions of long-standing propensities and patterns of modern Western medicine.

Uncertainty and the prospect of 'genetic medicine'

This is even true of the medical uncertainty that has been called forth by what is indubitably the most significant and transformative biological discovery of the twentieth century: the identification of the self-complementary, double helix structure of DNA by Francis Crick and James Watson. This discovery, and Crick and Watson's subsequent work showing the way toward analysis of the genetic code and how genetic material directs the synthesis of proteins, ushered in the so-called 'biological revolution' in which the 'new' molecular and cell biology, with its genetic focus, became ascendant. A veritable explosion of information and knowledge has ensued, epitomised by the Human Genome Project, the international scientific effort to identify, map and sequence what are estimated to be the 80,000 genes in the human genetic code.

Even though the Human Genome Project is approaching completion and the attainment of its formidable goal of producing the equivalent of a periodic table of human biology, what the clinical value of all this genetics knowledge will prove to be, what it will contribute to the detection, prevention, delay, 'repair' and cure of human disease, and how and to what extent it will be integrated into the practice of medicine are still indeterminate. The nature of molecular and genetic knowledge is highly reductionistic; it disaggregates biological systems by breaking them into smaller parts; and there is as yet no conceptual framework within which this kind of micro-knowledge can be synthesised, consolidated and made pertinent to the organismic, pathophysiological level of medicine. Furthermore, despite exuberant expectations concerning the prospects of gene therapy and over 300 clinical gene-therapy protocols that have been approved to date, none has as yet succeeded. 'We cannot predict when the benefits of gene therapy will be realised', concluded a US National Institutes of Health committee appointed to assess its current status and promise (Collins and Bochm 1999; Orkin and Moltulsky 1995).

'The relationship between medical knowledge and medical practice is complex' physician-historian Kenneth Ludmerer (1999) points out; and it is not unprecedented for there to be a discrepancy between them. 'Nor is it unusual for an inclusive organic, and holistic way of framing problems, and [a] reductionist and mechanism-oriented' one to coexist in medical thinking. Quite to the contrary, medical historian Charles E. Rosenberg contends, these two 'conflictive' modes of thought have been central to Western medicine throughout its history and, though 'oppositional' and tension-ridden, they are also 'mutually constitutive' in practice (Rosenberg 1998b). However, I would venture to suggest that, in both these regards, the hiatus that presently exists between 'medicine and molecules' is exceptionally large, and that, despite the pregnant conviction that the therapeutic impact of 'the coming integration of genetics into clinical medicine [will be] no less dramatic than the arrival of the antibiotic era more than a half century ago' (Collins and Bochm 1999: 49), this as-yet-unbridged gap is a powerful paradigmatic source of medical uncertainty and limitation. In the United States, a serious decline in the number of physician-scientists, with the consequent possibility that this will diminish a two-way flow of questions, observations and information between laboratory and clinic, may impede or delay closing the gap (Ahrens 1992).

Uncertainty and the 'emergence' and 're-emergence' of infectious diseases

A second change in the cognitive base of contemporary medicine that has opened up new areas of uncertainty, and reopened old ones, is related to what is called in the medical literature 'the emergence and re-emergence of infectious diseases'. These terms refer to the appearance and/or rapid expansion of new infectious diseases in the human population; to the new recognition of those that are already extant and widespread in the population; and to the resurgence of previous plagues, often in new, more severe forms. The pathogenic microbes are frequently viruses, but bacteria and parasites are also involved in these infections. The spectrum of diseases they cause range from HIV/AIDS, Ebola haemorrhagic fever, Legionnaire's disease, Lyme disease, and bovine spongiform encephalopathy ('mad cow' disease), to cholera, dengue, yellow fever, malaria and tuberculosis, among many others.

There is a 'back to the future' dimension to this 'return' of infectious diseases that has occurred at a point in Western medical history when it had become commonplace to suppose that such diseases and their dissemination were not only under control but, in cases like smallpox and poliomyelitis, virtually eradicated. An epidemiological transition was assumed to have taken place 'from an "age of pestilence and famine", in which the mortality pattern was dominated by high rates of infectious disease deaths, especially in the young, to the current "age of degenerative man-made diseases", in which mortality from chronic diseases predominate[d]' (Armstrong *et al.* 1999: 61).

Until recently, this transition was thought to have brought about 'a permanent reduction in infectious disease mortality' in advanced modern societies such as the United Kingdom and the United States. However, the emergence and re-emergence of infectious diseases has undermined the premise that 'gains against infectious diseases [can] be taken for granted'; it has increased awareness of their 'potential volatility' and it has heightened the sense that 'since there is no guarantee the future trends will be stable', vigilance about the 'threats posed by microbes' is called for (ibid.: 66).

The surfacing of a devastating new disease like HIV/AIDS, which progressively brings about the collapse of the body's immune system, for which the only therapy that presently exists is a battery of drugs that temporarily alleviate its symptoms and postpone its fatal outcome, and that has rapidly escalated from a 'clinical oddity' to a global pandemic, constitutes a cultural shock as well as a catastrophic medical and public health happening. As physician Samuel Thier (1986: vii) has pointed out:

> In an era when young physicians have never seen a case of measles or polio and when once life-threatening bacterial infections disappear in two or three days with antibiotic therapy, the AIDS epidemic seems almost unreal. The temptation to believe that a vaccine or a miracle drug is just over the horizon may be overwhelming for both health care providers and the general public.

Furthermore, the phenomenon of emerging and re-emerging infectious diseases has thrown into question the optimistic supposition articulated by physician-essayist Lewis Thomas (1985: 4–5), that there is a relatively 'short, finite list of important disabling, and sometimes fatal illnesses that we are unable to deal with as effectively as we, and our patients hope'; but that 'all the items on the list have changed from blank mysteries to approachable scientific problems'; and that 'ultimately, given the right kind of research and a certain amount of luck, all of them can be solved'.

To a sobering degree, the incidence of infectious diseases and their spread appears to be precipitated by human conditions and behaviour – for example, by changes in patterns of agriculture and irrigation, massive rural-to-urban population movement, increasing population density in cities, global travel and trade, immigration, warfare, refugee migration and internment, economic crises, political upheavals, famine, poverty and homelessness. Even more humbling, historian William McNeill (1993: 5–6) states, is that our human attempts to 'make things the way we want them, and, by skill, organisation and knowledge, to insulate ourselves from local and frequent disasters . . . change natural and ecological relationships'. In turn, this creates 'new situations that become unstable . . . [and] vulnerabili[ties] to some larger disaster'. Such ecosystem disruptions are as true of medical interventions as of other forms of action intended to be ameliorative. An important and threatening example of this phenomenon is the fact that certain strains of microbes have become resistant to a substantial proportion of antibiotic drugs considered first-line treatment, partly because they have been extensively, often excessively, used in humans and also 'in veterinary medicine, animal husbandry, agriculture, and aquaculture' (Tenoyer and Hughes 1996: 303).

In Charles Rosenberg's view, the current 'meta-epidemiological' tendency to make causal connections between unceasing human manipulation and alteration of the environment – including medical manipulation – and the incidence of old and new infectious and chronic diseases is reinforced by a late-twentieth-century iteration of a persistent cultural theme: what he describes as 'change-oriented cultural angst' about 'the risks of civilisation' and 'the pathogenic consequences of progress'. The 'penumbra of social meanings' surrounding this theme, he writes, comprise 'a parable that has been continually reformulated and restated, . . . always with the profound capacity to express questions about the limitations of ambitions no more than human and of progress no more than material' (Rosenberg 1998a: 716, 726, 730).

Uncertainty and prognosis

Another conceptual shift occurring in present-day medicine is the increasing importance that medical prognosis has assumed – a development that has augmented problems of uncertainty faced by physicians when they are called upon to make explicit predictions about the outcome of a patient's illness or condition. Physician-sociologist Nicholas A. Christakis has shown that 'diagnosis and therapy [have always received] more attention than prognosis in patient care, medical research, and medical education'. He attributes this in part to the tendency in medical thinking to make diagnosis the central concern of the clinical encounter, and to view both therapy and prognosis as following directly from it. Once a diagnosis is made and therapy is initiated, a 'relatively fixed, non-individualistic, and standardised' clinical course of a disease is presumed to unfold (Christakis 1999). In the eyes of other physicians – for example, James M. Gilchrist, editor of a volume on prognosis in *Neurology – 'prognosis* has fallen into greater disuse' in recent years. To use a modern term, he writes, it has been 'down-regulated' (Gilchrist 1998; Dalessio 1999). Nicholas Christakis's extensive, in-depth study of physician attitudes and behaviour with regard to prognosis reveals, as he puts it, 'a *dread* of prognostication . . . Physicians would rather not formulate or discuss prognosis', he states. This is because they associate prognosis with the limits of their diagnostic and therapeutic powers and with the grave illnesses and impending deaths of patients. In addition, Christakis has discovered that below the surface of their apprehension about prognosticating – particularly under these circumstances – lies magic-infused clinical thinking: physicians' shared inclination to believe that any negative predictions they make about patients' medical states and their outcomes may have 'self-fulfilling prophecy' effects, whether or not they communicate their sombre expectations to patients. For these reasons, Christakis found, physicians not only have a tendency to skew prognosis-setting in a positive, optimistic direction, but also to play down and, if possible, avoid medical forecasting (Christakis 1999).

Nevertheless, current and pending developments in medical science and technology, and in the social settings in which medicine is practised, are making prognostication more important, and more difficult for physicians to avoid than in the past. The increasing prevalence of chronic disease involves physicians in the ongoing process of anticipating, forestalling and mitigating adverse events associated with the trajectory of the disease or with the cumulative side-effects of its long-term treatment. The invention and deployment of new forms of medical technology, such as genetic testing, prenatal ultrasound and amniocentesis, produce prognostic data about genetically borne disorders, pregnancy and the condition of the foetus that put physicians under greater pressure to provide clinical predictions. In the United States, where a growing number of physicians are now working under the auspices of managed care organisations that review their practice behaviour and emphasise the economic and efficient allocation of scarce resources, doctors are being asked to base clinical decisions such as the timing and duration of hospitalisation and the referral of patients for terminal hospice care on prognostic assessments of the course of the illnesses involved. Intensifying interest in ethical and bioethical aspects of medical care and research and public as well as professional concern about them have also accentuated the significance of prognosis in physicians' relationships and communication with patients. For example, the fact that informed voluntary consent from patients to the diagnostic and therapeutic ministrations they undergo has become an ethical imperative not only obliges physicians to explain to patients what the procedures are, but what they are expected to accomplish, and what risks and untoward effects they may involve.

Uncertainty and the irony of iatrogenesis: side-effects and error

To a striking degree, the medical uncertainty surrounding prognosis, emerging and re-emerging diseases and the advent of molecular biology are all accompanied by another source of uncertainty: perhaps the most ironic of all, because it is a concomitant of actions that physicians take on behalf of their patients. Throughout medical history, the means that physicians have used to diagnose and treat patients' disorders have always had a mixture of beneficent and harmful consequences. Paradoxically, the impressive advances of modern medicine have in certain ways increased its iatrogenically-induced adverse effects on patients, exemplifying what Charles Rosenberg has termed 'pathologies of clinical progress' (Rosenberg 1998a: 726). As the modes of diagnosing and treating disease and illness have become more powerful and effective, they have also grown more dangerous, exposing patients to greater potential risk, suffering and harm through their anticipated and unanticipated negative consequences.

Whole textbooks devoted to this phenomenon are now being written and published. One such text, entitled *Iatrogenic Neurology*, is a volume of 500 pages and 26 chapters, which comprehensively reviews the neurological side-effects of commonly prescribed pharmacological, radiological and surgical treatments of a wide range of medical conditions (Biller 1998). But the complications engendered by the array of therapies available for the treatment of disease are not only neurological in nature. The current armamentarium of cancer treatments, for instance, consists of surgical procedures and radio-therapy and chemotherapy regimens that, however ameliorative or curative, are highly invasive, in some cases mutilating, and can cause physically and psychologically painful symptoms such as fever, infection, anaemia, severe fatigue, hair loss, incontinence, impotence and premature menopause. Or to cite another example, the combinations of anti-retroviral drugs, including protease inhibitors, that have brought about what seems to be a dramatic improvement in the symptoms, daily round and life-span of persons infected with HIV, involve such 'high pill burdens [with] numerous adverse effects . . . [and] myriad drug interactions', that many recipients of these 'drug cocktails' find it difficult to adhere to the regimen necessary for optimal results (Cohen and Fauci 1998: 87).

Whether the drugs are used to treat cancer, HIV/AIDS, neurological disorders or other disease conditions, the incidence of pharmacological iatrogenesis is high. This is partly due to the fact that, in spite of all the pharmacological progress that has been made, no overall therapy of drug action has as yet been developed. Therefore, it is difficult for physicians to foretell how favourable and/or unfavourable an individual patient's responses to particular drugs will be, or to predict how a patient with a chronic disease will react to the cumulative effects of long-term – in some cases, lifelong – treatment with a particular drug or drug combination. Errors that are committed in the practice of medicine are another significant source of iatro-genesis. There is nothing new in medicine about mistakes that cause injurious consequences. However, the increasingly hazardous and intricate character of the instrumentalities that present-day medicine wields enhances the potential gravity of the errors that take place, and the difficulty of ascertaining why they occur and how they can be prevented.

Marc R. de Laval, a paediatric cardiac surgeon affiliated with the Great Ormond Street Hospital for Sick Children in London, has systematically documented and analysed the ways in which errors, accidents and failures occur in the performance of what is known as the arterial switch procedure in cardiac surgery. This operation, designed to correct a congenital heart mal-formation, consists of switching the great arteries around, with transfer of the coronary arteries. The latter, de Laval explains, is 'the most delicate part of the operation [because] it involves the excision of vessels about one milli-metre in diameter from the aorta and their implantation onto the pulmonary artery'. De Laval likens cardiac surgery to a 'complex socio-technical system' that 'shares many similarities with high hazard enterprises, such as the avi-ation industry, nuclear power plants, marine and railroad transportation, [and] chemical plants'. Within what he calls this 'framework of complexity', in collaboration with psychologist James Reason, author of the book *Human Error* (Reason 1990), he conducted a multi-medical centre study of the interactions between individual, team, institutional and organisational human factors and high-technology in the outcomes of 230 arterial switches performed in the United Kingdom over a period of 18 months, focusing special attention on negative outcomes. One of his most striking sets of findings was that in the sort of complex, danger- and risk-fraught system in which cardiac surgery proceeds, 'a tiny difference in initial conditions can be amplified over time to enormous differences' and ' a small event can be just as important for the outcome as a large one'. De Laval illustrated what he termed these 'non-linear interactions of human and technical components' with two scenarios.

In the first scenario, 'a rotation of just a few degrees of the left coronary artery during its implantation to the pulmonary artery results in inadequate myocardial perfusion', with the consequence that the patient spends three weeks in the intensive care unit – rather than 24 hours – and leaves the hospital well, but only after one month. In the second scenario, 'a kink in the arterial line while a patient is on life support [that] remains unnoticed for a few minutes because of a faulty alarm system . . . results in a temporary but profound hypotension from which the patient sustains severe and permanent brain damage' – 'catastrophic consequences' that necessitate lifetime care (de Laval 1996, 1998; de Laval *et al.* 1994).

Uncertainty and individually focused versus collectively oriented medicine

Reconciling and integrating the one-on-one, doctor–patient relationship of clinical medicine with population-based reasoning and action is another long-standing problem in modern medicine, fraught with uncertainty, that physicians constantly face. It is not only a cognitive problem, but one that entails deep role conflicts between what physician-jurist M. Gregg Bloche calls 'clinical fidelity' to patients, their individual wellbeing and welfare and commitment to 'the social purposes of medicine'. In Bloche's view, 'neither medical ethics nor law can resolve this [role] contradiction' that 'vexes' clinical practice. Rather, it must be 'mediated . . . case by case, in myriad clinical circumstances' (Bloche 1999).

The most classic form that the conflict between 'clinical loyalty' and 'social purpose' has taken in medicine is structured around public health concerns – centring on instances when physicians are called upon to take community-wide health considerations into account in ways that may curtail or run counter to patients' individual interests and their autonomy. Vaccination, choosing antibiotics with attention to slowing the development of resistant bacterial strains, reporting contagious diseases to public authorities, and using public health orders to compel persons to be examined for dangerously transmissible disease such as tuberculosis or to be mandatorily detained until they complete full treatment for it – as the Health Code of New York City has permitted since 1993 – are all examples of this kind of action.

The intellectual, clinical and moral tensions and uncertainties that coalesce around the problematic of handling and mediating the individual and collective dimensions of medicine, and of how physicians can adhere to both an 'individual ethic' and a 'distributive ethic' (Kassirer 1998: 197), have been augmented by a number of developments in recent years that have shifted the focus of clinical medicine toward a more aggregate, population-based perspective. These include: the emergence and re-emergence of infectious diseases; the epidemiological tendency of chronic diseases to take their greatest toll on the health and life expectancy of persons in the lowest and poorest strata of advanced modern societies like the United Kingdom and the United States; the growing importance of managed care organisations in the United States; and the burgeoning emphasis on what is termed 'evidence-based medicine'.

Epistemological uncertainty

The uncertainty issues raised by evidence-based medicine are especially important and revelatory. For, although it has been envisioned as a 'new paradigm' that helps to dispel medical uncertainty by providing 'a new set of skills and methods of reasoning that allow physicians to incorporate a growing body of medical evidence into practice' (Tonelli 1998: 1234), evidence-based medicine has brought to the surface fundamental epistemological uncertainty about the nature of good clinical research, good clinical practice, and the relationship between them.

According to what might be called its official definition, 'the practice of evidence-based medicine means integrating individual clinical expertise with the best available external clinical evidence', derived from the basic sciences of medicine and from patient-oriented clinical research, conducted via large, randomised controlled clinical trials or from the systematic review (including meta-analysis) of a number of smaller, more disparate published clinical studies (Sackett *et al.* 1997: 2). Despite medical professional appreciation of the ways in which this approach can improve the quality and quantity of evidence available to physicians and patients, numerous thoughtful British and American physicians have expressed strong reservations and concern about some of its attributes and potential consequences (Grimley-Evans 1995; Hunter 1996; Hurwitz 1997a, b; Naylor 1998). Evidence-based medicine, they contend, is tipped in the direction of a kind of 'biomedical positivism' that defines clinical research in a narrowly scientistic and quantitatively empirical way. It oversimplifies the complexity of the clinical situation, they say, especially of clinical decision making – thereby 'spurious[ly] claim[ing] to provide certainty in a world of clinical uncertainty' (Hunter 1998: 6). It downplays the importance of 'non-evidentiary' aspects of medicine, they maintain, of clinical experience, expertise and judgement; pathophysiological knowledge; first-hand clinical observation; and responsiveness to patients' wishes, preferences and values. Partly as a consequence of its focus on measurable outcomes in the populations of patients enrolled in clinical trials, they opine, evidence-based medicine pays insufficient attention to the individual particularities of individual patients – to the physiological, psychological, social and cultural differences between them. In all these regards, and on a more 'philosophical' level, physician Mark R. Tonelli writes, 'there is an intrinsic gap' between clinical research and clinical practice. The existence of this gap, he states, 'means that evidence can never directly dictate care; the evidence cannot tell us when it is best to ignore the evidence' (Tonelli 1998: 1238–9).

The at once basic and far-reaching sort of epistemological uncertainty that evidence-based medicine and the ongoing discussion of its assets and limitations have brought forth is notable. To begin with, evidence-based medicine rests on the disquieting assumption that a great deal that advanced modern medicine professes to know is neither strongly supported by reliable and valid scientific findings nor clinically efficacious and efficient. Evidence-based medicine is seen by its proponents as a way of significantly improving this state of affairs. But in the challenges to what critics of evidence-based medicine regard as its excessive claims, two other sorts of epistemological uncertainty are voiced: questions about whether there is any 'simple accepted definition [of] what constitutes valid and useful research' (Taylor and Buterakos 1998); and statements about the need to develop a better understanding of the knowledge base and mode of reasoning of clinical medicine and practice (Tonelli 1998: 1239).

Uncertainty regarding the nature of medical knowledge and way of thought is not confined to debate about evidence-based medicine. This was one of the most striking and, for me, surprising patterns that my perusal of the medical literature for this chapter made apparent. Whether they deal with phenomena associated with HIV/AIDS, cancer or inflammatory bowel disease, for example, infectious or chronic syndromes, processes of diagnosis, prevention, treatment, care or prognosis, or methods of collecting and analysing medical data, many recent journal articles express concern about current problems of epistemological uncertainty. Here are some illustrative excerpts from the literature I surveyed:

> Big gaps remain in our knowledge of HIV, and it may be that we need a more complex response in terms of therapeutic approaches . . . Similarly, prevention has focused largely on fairly simple psychological approaches . . . The gaps are even bigger in determining how to prevent a million people from becoming infected with AIDS this year . . . and at the same time care for nearly 30 million people with HIV living in developing countries.
>
> (Piot 1998: 1844–5)

> In a recent commentary of AIDS therapy, the phrase 'Failure isn't what is used to be . . . but neither is success' was coined (Cohen, 1998). Failure has generally been defined in virological terms; the inability to achieve complete suppression of viral replication. However, treatment failure is

not only viral resistance. In fact, definition of failure or success of treatment is a far more complex phenomenon.

(Perrin and Telenti 1998: 1871)

Renal cell carcinoma continues to fool internists and noninternists alike ... One source of error [is] the clinicians' overreliance on the use of patterns ... Pattern recognition greatly simplifies problem solving ... Occasionally, however, we rely on pattern recognition to a fault, trying to fit square pegs into round holes.

(Saint *et al.* 1998: 381)

Diseases like inflammatory bowel disease that have systemic manifestations can pose daunting diagnostic challenges ... The focus and training that physicians bring to a clinical case typically create cognitive expectations that determine their attention to and interpretation of events ... [T]hese elements can be important to reasoning in the presence of uncertainty while also being a source of error in diagnostic interpretation.

(Berkwits and Gluckman 1997: 1683–4)

The National Institutes of Health convened a consensus conference in January 1997 to examine new evidence of the effectiveness of mammographic screening for breast cancer for women ages 40 to 49 years ... Critics of the panel stated resoundingly that it had reached the 'wrong' conclusion, understating the effectiveness of mammography, exaggerating the potential harms of false-positive results, and raising unnecessary fears about the safety of mammography. The implication that the panel should not have had these concerns or expressed them perpetuates the notion that there is only one correct way to interpret evidence. Who can say when evidence is 'good' enough?

(Woolf and Lawrence 1997: 2105–6)

Two articles in this issue reach apparently conflicting conclusions regarding the safety of the short postpartum hospital stays that are now 'standard for apparently well mothers and newborns ... Science does not and probably can not supply airtight evidence that longer stays are more effective ... In the absence of an adequate base of scientific knowledge about [how] to achieve the best health outcomes, it appears rational and ethical to be guided by a combination of good judgement, caution, and compassion in weighing the best evidence available'.

(Braverman *et al.* 1997: 334–6)

It is impossible to say, on the basis of recent evidence alone, whether the results of a large randomized, controlled trial or those of a meta-analysis of many smaller studies are more likely to be close to the truth ... We never know as much as we think we know.

(Ballar 1997: 559–60)

Embedded in such journal passages are a series of epistemological questions; how much of what medical scientists and physicians think they know is real knowledge – certain enough, or based on sufficiently good grounds for this claim to be made? What are the connections between medical knowledge, judgement and belief? How can errors of cognition, perception, judgement and belief be recognised, analysed and reduced, if not eliminated? What kinds of relationships exist between scientific and non-scientific aspects of medicine? Between simplicity and complexity in medical accuracy, understanding and effectiveness? And between the scientific basis of medicine, its clinical application to diagnosis, therapy, prognosis and prevention, and to the formulation and implementation of health policy? These articles also consider the way in which what physician-scientist Ludwik Fleck termed the characteristic 'thought-style' of medicine (Löwy 1990) contributes to the pattern-recognition and critical problem-solving capacities of physicians and to the built-in biases that result from their internalised conceptions and misconceptions; with problems of achieving consensus between medical professionals when they disagree in clinical and policy contexts; and with how to better join, and more fruitfully integrate patient-, population- and globally oriented medicine, and attention to the disparate health, illness and medicine conditions and needs in the 'two worlds' of developed and developing countries.

The foregoing suggests that the current 'disorientation' of modern Western medicine invoked by Roy Porter not only involves its clinical accomplishments and crisis of success, its limitation and liabilities, but also its underlying cognitive framework, its concepts, means of gathering and evaluating data and of establishing facts, and its modes of analysis and interpretation.

Vocational uncertainty

Along with multiple forms of uncertainty, which I have identified, in the United States physicians are also facing uncertainty in their professional status and roles. The main precipitants of this vocational uncertainty are the nation-wide restructuring of health insurance and reorganisation of health care delivery that are taking place as the country moves rapidly towards a predominantly managed care system. What consequences this will have for the employment of physicians; the fields within medicine that they select and deselect; their conditions of work; their incomes; the scope, continuity and quality of care they offer to patients, and the relationships they establish with them; the sorts of professional decision making and autonomy they will and will not be able to exercise; and for the meaning, fulfilment and frustration they will experience in their chosen careers, are among the serious vocational questions that doctors, medical students and 'pre-med' students are facing.

A somewhat anomalous situation exists in the United States in this regard. Many physicians in practice are feeling dispirited by the changing conditions of medical practice. Even if they acknowledge that the degree of professional autonomy they previously enjoyed was excessively paternalistic and self-interested, the diminution of independence that physicians experienced during the 1990s confronted them with unresolved conflicts over the leeway they would like to have in determining the medical actions they take on behalf of their patients, and the organisational, financial and time constraints that are now imposed on them by managed-care gatekeepers. Although young persons interested in becoming physicians are keenly aware of these uncertainties and conflicts (*Pulse* 1997, 1998), an unprecedentedly large number of US college and university students were seeking admission to medical schools throughout the 1990s. We need more knowledge and understanding of the young women and men opting for medical careers at this time of transition and indeterminacy in the profession: their conceptions of being a physician, what motivates them to become doctors, and how they aspire to practise medicine under the emerging new conditions.

'Bioethical' uncertainty

Finally, medicine is the epicentre of the uncertainty that underlies the development of what has come to be known as bioethics. Ostensibly, this area of reflection, inquiry and action that surfaced at the beginning of the 1970s and has grown more prominent ever since is concerned with problematic ethical concomitants of medical research, and of particular advances in biomedicine and medical technology. Its conceptual framework and discourse have been strongly influenced by the logico-rational positivism and principalism of Anglo-American analytic philosophy. But whether the concrete issues raised are related to abortion or euthanasia, for example, to assisted means of reproduction, organ transplantation or cloning; irrespective of what specific quandaries are under discussion and regardless of what moral principle is invoked – be it autonomy, beneficence, non-maleficence or justice; larger, uncertainty-pervaded meta-questions of value, belief and meaning underlie bioethical deliberation. These thematic questions are as religious and metaphysical as they are medical and moral.

What is life? What is death? When does life begin? When does it end? What is a person? What is a child? A parent? A family? What does it mean to be human? Who are my brothers and my sisters, my neighbours and my strangers? Is it better not to have been born at all than to have been born with a severe genetic defect? How vigorously should we intervene in the human condition to repair and improve ourselves? And when should we cease to desist? This at once elemental and transcendental questioning coded into the deep structure of bioethics suggests, as I have written, that 'bioethics is not just bioethics', and that it pertains to more than medicine and more than ethics. It also seems to be a metaphorical language and a symbolic medium through which social uncertainty about our modem Western cultural tradition and world-view is being publicly articulated and pondered.

Conclusion

The modalities of uncertainty I have discussed are closely connected with a variety of changes that are occurring both within and around medicine at this historical juncture. The gamut of these changes is broad: they are scientific and technological, cognitive and ethical, conceptual and empirical, methodological and procedural, and social and cultural in nature. And they have ramifying implications for the way of thought, the value system and the practice of medicine that affect how it is delivered and experienced by health professionals, patients and their families. As the grounding of medicine shifts in multidimensional ways, long-standing sources and manifestations of uncertainty have been reactivated, accentuated or modified, and new ones have formed. It is with extensive uncertainty about its state of knowledge and accomplishments, its value-commitments and its future directions, and with a mixture of confidence and insecurity, that modern Western medicine faces the twenty-first century. Because medicine is so integrally associated with the most profound questions about our individual and collective origins and identity, our sense of purpose and meaning, our shared human condition and our ultimate mortality, its relationship to uncertainty is also an indicator of how sure and unsure we are of where we have come from and where we are going, societally and culturally, as we enter the new millennium.

Note

1 We are grateful to Sage Publications for permission to reprint this revised version of the essay written for Gary L. Albrecht, Ray Fitzpatrick and Susan C. Scrimshaw (eds), *Handbook of Social Studies in Health and Medicine*, London: Sage 1999.

References

Ahrens, Edward A. (1992) *The Crisis in Clinical Research*, New York: Oxford University Press.

Armstrong, Gregory L., Conn, Laura A. and Pinner, Robert W. (1999) 'Trends in infectious disease mortality in the United States during the 20th century', *Journal of the American Medical Association* 281 (1): 61–6.

Atkinson, Paul (1984) 'Training for certainty', *Social Science and Medicine* 19 (9): 949–56.

Bach, F.H., Fishman, J.A., Daniels, N., Promios, L., Anderson, B., Carpenter, C.B., Forrow, L., Robson, S.C. and Fineberg, H. (1998) 'Uncertainty in xenotransplantation: individual benefit versus collective risk', *Nature Medicine* 4 (2): 141–4.

Ballar, John C. III (1997) 'The promise and problems of meta-analysis', *New England Journal of Medicine* 337 (8): 559–61.

Berkwitz, Michael and Gluckman, Stephen J. (1997) 'Seeking an expert interpretation', *New England Journal of Medicine* 337 (23): 1682–4.

Biller, José (ed.) (1998) *Iatrogenic Neurology*, Woburn, MA: Butterworth-Heinemann.

Bloche, M. Gregg (1999) 'Clinical loyalties and the social purposes of medicine', *Journal of the American Medical Association* 281 (3): 268–74.

Blumberg, Baruch and Fox, Renée C. (1985) 'The Daedalus effect: changes in ethical questions relating to hepatitis B virus', *Annals of Internal Medicine* 102 (3): 390–4.

Braverman, Paula, Kessel, Woodie, Egerter, Susan and Richmond, Julius (1997) 'Early discharge and evidence-based practice: good science and good judgement', *Journal of the American Medical Association* 278 (4): 334–6.

Christakis, Nicholas A. (1995) *Prognostication and Death in Medical Thought and Practice*, PhD dissertation, University of Pennsylvania, Philadelphia.

——(1999) *Death Foretold: Prophecy and Prognosis in Medical Care*, Chicago: University of Chicago Press.

Cohen, Jon (1998) 'Failure isn't what it used to be . . . but neither is success', *Science* 279 (5354): 1133–4.

Cohen, Oren J. and Fauci, Anthony S. (1998) 'HIV/AIDS in 1998: gaining the upper hand?', *Journal of the American Medical Association*, 280 (1): 87–8.

Collins, Francis S. and Bochm, Karina (1999) 'Avoiding casualties in the genetic revolution: the urgent need to educate physicians about genetics', *Academic Medicine* 74 (1): 46–9.

Cournand, André (1977) 'The code of the scientist and its relationship to ethics', *Science* 198 (4318): 699–705.

Dalessio, Donald J. (1999) Review of James M. Gilchrist (ed.), *Prognosis in Neurology, Journal of the American Medical Association* 281 (2): 191.

De Laval, Marc R. (1996) The Edgar Mannheim Lecture (manuscript).

——(1998) 'Thinking beyond the third dimension', inaugural lecture on appointment as Professor of Cardiothoracic Surgery at the University of London (manuscript).

——, François, Katrien, Bull, Catherine, Brawn, William and Spiegehalter, David (1994) 'Analysis of a cluster of surgical failures: application to a series of neonatal switch operations', *Journal of Thoracic and Cardiovascular Surgery* 107 (3): 914–24.

Evans, J. Grimley (1995) 'Evidence-based and evidence-biased medicine', *Age and Ageing*, 24: 461–3.

Fox, Renée C. (1957) 'Training for uncertainty', in Robert K. Merton, George Reader and Patricia L. Kendall (eds), *The Student-Physician: Introductory Studies in the Sociology of Medical Education*, Cambridge, MA: Harvard University Press.

——(1959) *Experiment Perilous: Physicians and Patients Facing the Unknown*, Glencoe, IL: Free Press. (Reissued with a new epilogue, New Brunswick, NJ: Transaction Publishers, 1997.)

——(1962) 'Medical scientists in a chateau', *Science* 136 (3515): 476–83.

——(1964) 'An American sociologist in the land of Belgian medical research', in Phillip E. Hammond (ed.), *Sociologists at Work*, New York: Harper and Row.

——(1976) 'The sociology of medical research', in Charles Leslie (ed.), *Asian Medical Systems: A Comparative Study*, Berkeley, CA: University of California Press.

——(1978a) 'The autopsy: its place in the attitude-learning of second-year medical students', in Renée C. Fox, *Essays in Medical Sociology: Journeys into the Field*, New Brunswick, NJ, and Oxford: Transaction Books.

——(1978b) 'Is there a new medical student?', *Transactions and Studies* 45 (4): 206–12.

——(1980) 'The evolution of medical uncertainty' *Millbank Memorial Fund Quarterly/Health and Society* 58: 1–49.

Gilchrist, J. (ed.) (1998) *Prognosis in Neurology*, Boston, MA: Butterworth-Heinemann.

Grimley-Evans, J. (1995) 'Evidence-based and evidence-biased medicine', *Age and Aging* 24: 461–3.

Hunter, D.J. (1996) 'Rationing and evidence-based medicine', *Journal of Evaluation in Clinical Practice* 2: 5–8.

Hurwitz, B. (1997a) Personal communication, 17 June.

—— (1997b) 'Clinical guidelines: philosophical, legal, emotional and political considerations', draft paper commissioned by *British Medical Journal*.

Light, Donald (1979) 'Uncertainty and control in professional training', *Journal of Health and Social Behavior* 20 (4): 310–22.

Löwy, Ilana (1990) *The Polish School of Philosophy of Medicine: From Tytus Chalubinski (1820–1889) to Ludwik Fleck (1896–1961)*, Dordrecht, Boston, MA, and London: Kluwer Academic Publishers.

Ludmerer, Kenneth M. (1999) *Time to Heal: American Medical Education in the Twentieth Century*, New York: Oxford University Press.

Martensen, Robert L. and Jones, David S. (1997) 'Searching for medical certainty: medical chemistry to molecular medicine', *Journal of the American Medical Association* 278 (8): 609.

McNeill, William H. (1993) 'Patterns of disease emergence in history', in Stephen S. Morse (ed.), *Emerging Viruses*, New York: Oxford University Press.

Morse, Stephen S. (1993) 'Examining the origins of emerging viruses', in Stephen S. Morse (ed.), *Emerging Viruses*, New York: Oxford University Press.

Naylor, C. David (1998) 'What is appropriate care?', *New England Journal of Medicine* 338 (26): 1918–20.

Orkin, Stuart H. and Motulsky, Amo G. (1995) 'Report and recommendations of the panel to assess the NIH [National Institutes of Health] investment in research on gene therapy', unpublished, non-paginated text.

Parsons, Talcott (1951) 'Social structure and dynamic process: the case of modern medical practice' in Talcott Parsons, *The Social System*, Glencoe, IL: Free Press.

Perrin, Luc and Telenti, Amalio (1998) 'HIV treatment failure: testing for HIV resistance in clinical practice', *Science* 280 (5371): 1971–3.

Piot, Peter (1998) 'The science of AIDS: a tale of two worlds', *Science* 280 (5371): 1844–5.

Porter, Roy (1998) *The Greatest Benefit to Mankind: A Medical History of Humanity*, New York: W.W. Norton (first American edition).

Public Health Service USA (1996) 'Guidelines on infectious disease issues in xenotransplantation', draft.

Pulse (medical student section of the *Journal of the American Medical Association*) (1997) 'An uncertain future: physician jobs in the balance', 277 (1), 68–73.

—— (1998) 'Making a living: alternative careers for physicians', 279 (17): 1398–1403.

Reason, James (1990) *Human Error*, Cambridge: Cambridge University Press.

Rosenberg, Charles E. (1998a) 'Pathologies of progress: the idea of civilisation as risk', *Bulletin of the History of Medicine* 72: 714–30.

—— (1998b) 'Holism in twentieth-century medicine', in Chris Lawrence and George Weisz (eds), *Greater Than its Parts: Holism in Biomedicine, 1920–1950*, New York: Oxford University Press.

Sackett, D.L., Richardson, W.S., Rosenberg, W. and Haynes, R.B. (1997) *Evidence-based Medicine: How to Practise and Teach EBM*, New York and London: Churchill-Livingstone.

Saint, S., Saha, S. and Tierney, L.M. Jr (1998) 'A square peg in a round hole', *New England Journal of Medicine* 338: 379–83.

Silver, M.T. (1964) 'The student experience', in D.C. Tosteson, A.J. Adelstein and S.T.

Canter (eds), *New Pathways to Medical Education: Learning to Learn at Harvard Medical School*, Cambridge, MA: Harvard University Press.

Taylor, D. Kay and Buterakos, James (1998) 'Evidence-based medicine: not as simple as it seems', *Academic Medicine* 73 (12): 1221–2.

Tenoyer, F.C. and Hughes, J.M. (1996) 'The challenge of emerging infectious diseases: development and spread of multiple resistant bacterial pathogens', *Journal of the American Medical Association* 275: 300–4.

Thier, Samuel O. (1986) 'Preface', in *Mobilizing Against AIDS: The Unfinished Story of a Virus*, Cambridge, MA: Harvard University Press.

Thomas, Lewis (1979) *The Medusa and the Snail*, New York: Viking Press.

—— (1985) From an unpublished talk delivered at the University of Cincinnati Medical Center, 18 October (manuscript).

Tonelli, Mark R. (1998) 'Philosophical limits of evidence-based medicine', *Academic Medicine* 73 (12): 1234–40.

Tosteson, Daniel C. and Goldman, David C. (1994) 'Lessons for the future', in Daniel C. Tosteson, S. James Adelstein and Susan T. Carver (eds), *New Pathways in Medical Education: Learning to Learn at Harvard Medical School*, Cambridge, MA: Harvard University Press.

Ubel, Peter A., Arnold, Robert N. and Caplan, Arthur L. (1993) 'Rationing failure: the ethical lessons of the retransplantation of scarce organs', *Journal of the American Medical Association* 270 (20): 2469–74.

Woolf, Steven H. and Lawrence, Robert S. (1997) 'Preserving scientific debate and patient choice: lessons from the consensus panel of mammography screening', *Journal of the American Medical Association* 278 (23): 205–7.

14 Resisting 'fatal unclutteredness'

Conceptualising the sociology of health and illness into the millennium

Virginia Olesen

Introduction

Because it is well-nigh impossible in a single essay to consider, never mind do justice to, the implications of Meg Stacey's extensive and powerful work in the sociology of health and illness, I here focus on several critical concepts and their implications and then the quality and character of her conceptualisations. Economic, intellectual and social developments buffet scholars, researchers and thinkers in the sociology of health and illness. At the same time we shape the field with our thinking, research and concepts. Conceptualisation *is* the coin of the realm. As context for my observations, I briefly review the history of the sociology of health and illness, highlighting complexities which did not characterise earlier thinking and trends which impinge on the field.

Sociology of health and illness in perspective

The sociology of health and illness is a relatively young field characterised by increasing complexity. We have borrowed freely from other conceptual realms in sociology and other social sciences, but we have also generated knowledge which has deepened and enriched conceptual, theoretical and methodological realms within the larger discipline of sociology. Chief among the emergent complexities has been the recognition emergent from a wide range of empirical work that patients in health care contexts are far from passive beings in whatever context they find themselves. Rather, they are active and engaged with others in that context and literally create outcomes, new relationships and new structures. Awareness of the complexities and characteristics of patients and their contexts in which larger social, material and cultural issues are at play now seems somewhat commonplace, but was a marked departure from the homogeneous medical perspective of the 1950s, which carried considerable implications for conceptual and empirical work in our field (Annandale 1998: 26–7; Williams and Calnan 1996).

Patient as worker

Meg Stacey's concerns with the division of labour in health care were and are a critical part of that departure. Posing the critical question, Who are the health workers?, she called for sociological incisiveness with her admonition: 'Sociologically we need to be clear about who is doing what and why' (Stacey 1984: 193). Building on that call, she took Everett Hughes's (1971) idea of the patient as work object far beyond his original insight to conceptualise the patient as a worker in the health care division of labour. She argued powerfully that patient as worker also produced health alongside the providers, though she was careful not to elevate these workers to the level of partners.

Consider the shift from a view in which the passive patient was locked into the doctor's all-knowing interventions to one in which the patient actively negotiates with a physician or other provider, inside or outside scientific medicine. Those early structural views of the care context, valuable though they were in opening the previously unexamined topic of medical care to the sociological gaze, nevertheless severely limited understanding and the possibilites for research (Charmaz and Olesen 1997: 456; Annandale 1998: 264; Bury 1997). The patient was not a passive dope, but an actor capable of collaborating and negotiating with or resisting providers, even bossing or overturning providers. Here are glimpses of the important insights which feminist scholars brought to the sociology of health and illness regarding women's place and action in care systems.

The patient is both worker and work object in interaction with others in the system. The elegant simplicity of this idea opened vistas not thought of before and questioned a number of well-established but shop worn concepts and then-fashionable views of what was going on in health care.

Among the outworn fashionable perspectives which the concept of the patient as worker upended was a limited conceptualisation of the doctor–patient relationship as the only significant interaction. That view had overlooked patient contacts with other providers. Her insight that the patient is also an actor and a worker opened the way to consider these other interactants, for instance, nurses, physical therapists and informal providers such as family, with whom the patient interacts and who care for the patient (Annandale 1998: 264; Atkinson 1995: 34; James 1994). We've also come to see, as Annandale (1998: 248) has cogently observed, splits and diversities within and among these providers. All doctors are not alike; all nurses are not alike. As Strauss and Bucher (1961) theorised several decades ago, being dynamic entities, the professions are subject to divisiveness, splits and regroupings. Recognising the multiple players and their shifting professional situations substantially altered the scope of our analysis and expanded our interpretative strengths. What had been thought to be homogeneous became recognised as variegated. What had been seen as simple and linear came to be viewed as complex and multi-levelled. The upshot: a more dynamic sociology of health and illness.

That more dynamic sociology of health and illness offered the analytic capacity to interpret alterations of all sorts and in situations where earlier formulations did not open insight or understanding and, indeed, evoked misunderstanding and sometimes a dehumanised view of the patient. Parallel research elsewhere demonstrated the work of hospitalised patients and the implications of that work for rethinking organisational structure (Strauss *et al.* 1982). I think it could be also argued that conceptualising the patient as worker created an intellectual ambience in which conceptualising the social construction of illness became possible and, indeed, necessary.

Meg's formulation of patient as worker also casts the 'problem' of patient compliance in an entirely new light and denudes the term compliance of its invidious and undifferentiated views of patients. As work by anthropologists has shown, 'non-compliant' patients often have their own good reasons, grounded in their realities and the work of being patients (Hunt *et al.* 1989).

Patient as economic actor

Looking just at the US but recognising the push in Britain, Canada and elsewhere to make health care more efficient, these efforts date back at least to the 1920s but have been stepped up in the 1980s and 1990s with a shift from fee for service to managed care. Rising costs of technology in all forms (equipment, drugs, treatments), costs of care not covered by co-payments, increasing demands for care by an ageing population fuelled these pressures. In the US these changes have left few, if any, care contexts untouched. Fee-for-service contexts, health maintenance organisations, general hospital care and the new for-profit hospital chains run by corporations are all affected. The changes impinge on those working within them who enact the meanings of these strictures. The impact, of course, may differ for different participants: a provider who has to determine how long a patient can stay in hospital and still be reimbursed for care faces a different situation than nurses who must deal with increased patient loads, shortened hospital stays for all but the sickest patients and burgeoning regulations regarding appropriate performance (Olesen and Bone 1998; Olesen 2000).

In this era of the bottom line and downsizing, with economic and material considerations writ large, it is now more tempting than ever to think of the patient as an economic actor, a consumer or client. Meg Stacey's (1976) incisive critique of the idea of patient as consumer was ahead of its time. She later argued that the term consumer 'devalued the potential of the patient status' (1984: 161). As noted, it overlooked the patient's part as worker and, equally important, erased the factor of suffering in patienthood, eradicating the interrelations between illness and culture (Morris 1998: 15). Moreover, it seemed to lodge suffering in the realm of discourse; but suffering is not simply a matter of discourses, it is grounded, it is a part of patient work and being (Bury 1997: 14). As she reminds us in a beautifully written passage on the utility of the terms, client, consumer and patient: 'Patient will do since it derives from the Latin *pati*, to suffer' (Stacey 1976: 200).

Conceptualising the patient as sufferer does not exclude thinking of the patient simultaneously as an economic actor with material interests in the health care system. The concept of patient as sufferer refuses a simple-minded binary in which patient is *either* patient *or* economic actor. Patient is both.

Informal caregiving

Standing alongside her reconceptualisation of the patient as a worker are Meg's early and influential insights about unpaid, informal caregiving. In the 1980s she called for recognition that care takes place simultaneously in the private domain and in the public domain, that rewards and sanctions differ in the two domains, and emphasised the necessity of understanding how they interlock and are interdependent (Stacey 1984: 168). This move highlighted the gender, race and class issues in health care work of all kinds and shifted thinking away from an impoverished reliance on marketplace concepts back to fundamental social relations in the work of caring. This framed a much wider, more relevant view of health care work and all health workers, and in so doing elevated our thinking in the sociology of health and illness to more complex and more productive ways than had previously been the case.

We've slowly come to recognise, even if we don't always conceptualise productively in our theories and research, the unpaid providers who nurture and care for the acute or chronically ill adult or child. In part this recognition has emerged from a growing awareness of the place of chronic illness. Chronic illness, once not at all conceptualised, has been recognised as a central experience for many, if not most, people, both elderly and young and for their caregivers. As Charmaz (2000: 277) has written:

> Chronic illness poses more social, interactional and existential problems than acute illness because it lasts . . . Experiencing chronic illness means much more than feeling physical distress, acknowledging symptoms and needing care. It includes metaphor and meaning, moral judgements and ethical dilemmas, identity questions and reconstruction of self, daily struggles and persistent troubles.

The biologically disruptive experience of chronic illness, as Bury (1982) has pointed out, also presents a different time frame and social ethic: matters may drag on and there may be no clearly marked end, no defined period such as the postoperative recovery from surgery, but continual grappling with limited abilities, growing disabilities and the eventual descent into death.

Even as framing illness as an acute, discrete, dominant event gave way to the more processual and dynamic views seen in chronicity, so have our conceptualisations of providers blurred and shifted, inspired in part by Meg's conceptualisation of informal caregivers (Stacey 1984). The technological work done at home by family caregivers and the support rendered by non-professional others overlap and impinge on what used to be solely contained in the institutional setting (Olesen 1997: 405). In this connection Gallagher (1994: 74) has also recently warned against 'drawing too tight a circle of exclusion around the elements of the treatment process' in which treatment, particularly long-range treatment such as dialysis, is seen as separate and distinct from the rest of the patient's life.

What had been overlooked was foregrounded; what formerly was absent became integral and critical to a full analysis of health care work. A more rounded picture of the health care contexts emerged: the dialysis patient cared for at home (Gerhardt and Brieskorn-Zinke 1986), the labours of women caring for elderly parents or relatives (Abel 1990), the work of mothering ill and healthy family members (Graham 1985).

This formulation, however, reaches well beyond the sociology of health and illness and speaks to more general sociological issues. More precisely, the division of labour, that stalwart of sociological thinking, could no longer be seen in traditional ways. A different and considerably more complex picture emerged. Moreover, this formulation had other implications. In analysing the work of unpaid labourers, it is possible 'to explicate the creation and recreation of gender in the continually changing contours of a class of workers who are unpaid but critical to care' (Olesen 1989: 6). Examination of unpaid care in its gendered, raced and classed attributes affords glimpses of the workings of stratification systems and of the structure of society itself.

In the recognition of the patient as a worker and as a suffering being, albeit also an economic one, and in expanding and altering the long-ossified views of the division of labour to revise ideas of the public and the private and the place of unpaid labour we see some of Meg Stacey's most elegant concepts and formulations.

The aesthetics of conceptualisation

Thoroughly sociological, Meg's concepts nevertheless are elegant. I could have described them as 'robust', that overworked term with muscular overtones, but I prefer the desciptor elegant, for it points to an aesthetic in her conceptual work that gives her many contributions, these and others not discussed here, a very long shelf life. Graceful and elegant, they are also vigorous, an attribute which centres them in the history and shaping of the sociology of health and illness.

Particularly important is the issue of voice. As Cohen and Rogers (1994: 304) have argued, 'narrative voice influences theoretical work'. They ask how theorists employ voice to establish intellectual autonomy and how the use of voice establishes credibility with readers. Meg Stacey's narrative voice is strongly informed by, but never subservient to, sociological and feminist theory, is always original and creative, invoking a refreshing intellectual autonomy. At the same time her passionate common sense in her narrative voice invites credibility. Her narrative voice couples first-rate, innovative sociological theorising with a deep recognition of human elements familiar to us all. Thus she realises originality and credibility, those qualities we all hope for in our work.

In the work briefly reviewed here she was disruptive, overturned taken-for-grantednesses, excavated unexamined ideas and in so doing opened new spaces for exploration, argumentation, research and even practice. These formulations were well ahead of the curve and helped shape a contemporary, vital sociology of health and illness with new complexities fit for uncertain times and altering care scenarios. The work exemplified what the Indian novelist Bhatari Mukerjee (1994: 6) has felicitously termed 'resisting a fatal unclutteredness'.

Resisting a fatal unclutteredness: sociology of health and illness for the millennium

I turn to three ideas deriving from Meg's contributions where I find considerable potential for reconceptualising in our field. First, questioning the place and nature of emotions in rationalising care systems. Second, extending the concept of suffering. Third, thinking of how we frame problems in the sociology of health and illness.

Emotions in rationalising health care systems

Meg anticipated the problem and importance of conceptualising emotions in rationalising health care systems when she commented: 'the emotional component of human service has been ignored by classical theories, but is critical to them' (Stacey 1981: 174). If the patient is a passive blob in the health care scenario, conceptualising emotions is not possible or even desirable. Though the whole question of the emotions, like that of the body to which it is closely related, was neglected for decades within sociology and in the sociology of medicine and the sociology of health and illness, recent attention has shown this topic to be of critical significance.

Excellent collections (James and Gabe 1996; Bendelow and Williams 1998; Fineman 1994) have established an intellectual footing for the consideration of emotions in social life and health care which has opened new arenas for research, analysis and theory to understand in a more nuanced and rounded way issues and problems in health care systems.

Simultaneously, there has been a burst of informative empirical work on doctors' emotions (deCoster 1997); nurses' emotional management (Lawler 1991; Burfoot 1994; Bone 1997); emotional socialisation of nursing and medical students (Smith 1992; Mills and Kleinman 1988); emotional climates of wards and units (Kotarba *et al.* 1997; Aiken *et al.* 1997a, 1997b); nursing homes (Diamond 1992; Foner 1994); emotional experiences of families with terminally ill family members (Timmermans 1994; Mamo 1999); emotional management between physicians and nurses (James 1994); and among members and workers in a psychodrama-based encounter group (Thoits 1996), to name but a few excellent studies.

What remains as a task for conceptualisation is the interplay of emotions in health care organisations and contexts undergoing the processes of rationalisation noted earlier. It is not useful to assume that because these contexts are being rationalised, emotional issues drop out. That oversimplified view both empirically and theoretically inhibits nuanced understanding of these complex changes. Emotions are implicated in reason, rationality and rationalisation. We already have at hand a useful repertoire of conceptualisations with which to understand this issue: Hochschild's (1983) emotional labour and feeling rules; James's (1994) 'status shields'; Olesen's (1990) 'emotional lag'; Couch's (1992) 'evocative transformations'; Jaggar's (1989) 'outlaw emotions'; Thoits's (1996) 'deviant emotions' are but a few of these.

We can add to this useful roster, being aware of certain caveats which will facilitate conceptualisation. It is critical, as Radley (1988) has warned, to avoid individualising and to keep firmly in mind the intertwined and reciprocal nature of the individual and the social. Social here means social contexts and their interactants as well as features of the organisations of which they are a part and which they help transform. Emotional interactions occur socially and resonate among the participants who may or may not alter their expections, behaviours, ideas of themselves and even the rationalising rules. This calls to mind again Meg's conceptualisations of the workers in health care.

Beyond this recognition, it is important that our conceptualisations have the capacity to capture the fluidity of multiple selves and situations. All participants in health care bring a multiplicity of selves emergent from and influenced by the multiple realities which characterise their lives (Schutz 1962: 207–9). Thus, these interactants possess shifting, unstable emergent 'mobile subjectivities' (Ferguson 1993) which move along the complex trajectories of race, gender, sexual orientation, social class position and internalised views of being a provider/patient/caregiver. These contribute to layered complexities of emotional experience in rationalised contexts, as research in nursing homes by Diamond (1992) and Foner (1994) demonstrates.

Conceptualisation of emotions in rationalising contexts should also recognise the emotional and social order which emerges from emotion-laden interactions in care contexts (Strauss *et al.* 1963, 1982). The dynamics of an emergent social order, always in play, always in flux, are propelled by emotional matters which fuel these dynamics and bring to a temporarily stabile level understandings, norms, forms which come out of a wide range of encounters. Emotional interactions, as Collins (1981) and others have pointed out, are structure-building interactions, but the forms and structures which are created and emerge themselves are subject to the flux of further emotion-laden interactions. Selves, interaction and social organisation are intertwined, impinge on one another and emerge from one another. Bury (1997) has sounded an important caution to medical sociologists not to become caught in management scenarios and thereby lose our critical edge. Astute, critical conceptualisation of emotions in these many settings steers us away from becoming lost in the accountants' spreadsheets.

In sum, with regard to conceptualising emotions within these rationalising contexts, we must be alive to the dynamics and complexities – no settling for easy stasis here – and to recognition that structures, selves and interactions – all emotionally saturated – are continually emergent and impinging. Selves and social contexts are creating and being created.

Suffering

As Meg has astutely reminded us, suffering is ever-present in health care contexts. There is, of course, a great deal to be said about suffering and the emotional complexities of that in the rationalising scenarios just discussed. Who will comfort the dialysis patient at home? What of the overworked physician who has little time for yet another patient in pain? How do nurses distribute their emotional capital in situations where more is demanded but less is possible? All of these and more are crucial questions, but I wish to take the issue in a different direction.

Though Meg quite properly was critical of conceptualising the patient as consumer, nevertheless the patient and his/her family are players in health care economic scenarios. Even as the administration of comfort and support are crucial for the suffering – physical – patient, so are issues of the participation in health care economics for the patient and his/her family. Therein lie, at least in the United States and elsewhere where health care is not available to all who need it, elements of suffering related to economic matters that have been overlooked or at least under-conceptualised in the literature on health care inequality and in our thinking about the sociology of health and illness. I refer here to the question of the anxiety, fear, depression, guilt, in situations where insurance policies fail, buckle, are non-existent or where access to care of whatever type, medical and/or complementary, is limited or non-existent.

Mary Zimmerman's (1999) cross-national studies in Finland and the US of cases where insurance policies have failed families with children diagnosed with serious cancer and who need considerable help investigate this critical issue. Her interviews reveal from the US respondents the anguish, anxiety, fear and more when the insurance or health care coverage will no longer take care of the expensive cancer treatments needed for the ill child. One of Zimmerman's crucial points is that these worries and anxieties enter the definition and construction of what is health? what is illness? what is health care? The emotions are in play and intertwined with the economics. This adds a new dimension which demands our conceptual energies if we are to understand fully emotional complexities in care situations and the part they play. It calls for new sensibilities, new awarenesses, new dynamics in empirical work.

Framing problems in our field

As the editors of an early edition of the *Handbook of Medical Sociology* noted:

> There is no point here in trying to unravel the mystique that surrounds why different conceptual and theoretical frameworks achieve popularity at one point in time and not at another within sociology. Undoubtedly, in part, this depends upon the recognition given works of particular men [they used the term men: women were not mentioned] at a particular time. In part, in all sociology, it is related to the social and political forces that influence the directions of scientific and intellectual thought.
>
> (Freeman *et al.* 1972: 501)

However, these observations do not really comprehend why certain issues become conceptualised and others do not.

The terrain of our field is now quite different from even a decade ago, a point Scambler makes in comparing the collection of theoretical essays he edited in 1987 and a more recent collection done with Higgs (1998). Issues had emerged, become conceptualised and endured or faded. The dynamics of change in the sociology of sociological knowledge in our field were not clear. However, some vital conceptualisations, such as Meg's framing of the patient and unpaid persons as health care workers and her underscoring of the place of suffering, seem to be born out of passion for the topic. This was also true of the long-neglected question of gendered issues in health care, especially regarding women – one of my own early essays in that field was entitled, 'Rage is not enough: scholarly feminism and research in women's health' (Olesen 1989).

In addition to our intellectual, theoretical, political and disciplinary preferences, there is an issue of how we view our work and concepts emotionally. Issues are more than just interesting in the abstract, they are passion laden. Beyond the question of our own feelings about our work, the emotional discourses which surround and suffuse issues in the sociology of health and illness are themselves indicators of which issues do or do not become foregrounded and merit our attention. Here I am indebted to the thinking of Donilene Loseke (1999), who is examining the issue of emotions discourse and how social problems come to be constructed.

There are innumerable issues in the sociology of health and illness which could compete for our attention: what are the emotional discourses around these issues and how do those discourses create us and our work? It is instructive to think about AIDS, where emotional discourses, and other factors in the issue, helped bring it to the fore and into our purview, and to contrast that with the long-standing scandalous rates in the US of high infant mortality, where emotional discourses do not seem to construct the problem in a way which compels our field to conceptualise and worry about this issue.

Do emotional discourses sustain the viability of the issue or health problem and, if so, how? Hilgartner and Bosk (1988) more than a decade ago argued that there was a tip point for the emergence and fading of social problems in the American public. Are there are emotional discourses surrounding the tip point for issues in our field and what are their characteristics? The emotional discourses which bring health care issues to our attention also carry boundaries and baggage which may capture us, but, if we are alive to complexities, may keep our conceptualisations subtle, supple, useful and free and help us avoid 'blinders and blinkers' in our field (Murcott 1977).

In sum, I have tried to examine three issues among many issues deriving from Meg's work which I think present opportunities for reconceptualising in our field: first, the nature of emotional care in rationalising care systems; second, extending the concept of suffering to include emotions generated by patients' financial concerns; third, analysing our own emotions and the emotional discourses that surround and create emergent issues in our field. Such reconceptualisation and attentiveness to new complexities resist a 'fatal unclutteredness' which would ossify the humane, meliorative and theoretical aspects of our work. The troubling and complicating of once-taken-for-granted concepts, as Meg Stacey's rich legacy shows, lead to new resonances more fully compatible with this uncertain epoch and more promising to take into the new millennium (Olesen 1998: 4). The pursuit of a humane, just and empirically astute sociology of health and illness, the animating spirit of Meg's long and productive career, requires no less.

References

Abel, E.K. (1990) 'Family care of the frail elderly', in E.K. Abel and M.K. Nelson (eds), *Circles of Care: Work and Identity in Women's Lives*, Albany, NY: State University of New York Press.

Aiken, L.H., Lake, E.T., Sochalski, J. and Sloane, D.M. (1997a) 'Design of an outcomes study of the organization of hospital AIDS care', *Research in the Sociology of Health Care* 14: 3–26.

—— Sloane, D.M. and Lake, E.T. (1997b) 'Satisfaction with inpatient acquired immunodeficiency, a national comparison of dedicated and scattered bed units', *Medical Care* 35: 948–62.

Annandale, E. (1998) *The Sociology of Health and Medicine*, Cambridge: Polity Press.

Atkinson, P. (1995) *Medical Talk and Medical Work*, London: Sage.

Bendelow, G. and Williams, S.J. (eds) (1998) *Emotions in Social Life: Critical Themes Contemporary Issues*, New York: Routledge.

Bone, D. (1997) 'Feeling squeezed: dimensions of emotion work in nursing under managed care', unpublished doctoral dissertation, Department of Social and Behavioral Sciences, School of Nursing, University of California, San Francisco.

Burfoot, J. (1994) 'Outlaw emotions and the sensual dynamics of compassion: the case of emotion as an instigator of social change', unpublished paper, Middlebury, VT: Department of Sociology, Middlebury College.

Bury, M. (1982) 'Chronic illness as disruption', *Sociology of Health and Illness* 4: 167–82.

—— (1997) *Health and Illness in a Changing Society*, New York: Routledge.

Charmaz, K. (2000) 'Experiencing chronic illness', in G.L. Albrecht, R. Fitzpatrick and S. Scrimshaw (eds), *Handbook of Social Studies in Health and Medicine*, London: Sage.

—— and Olesen, V. (1997) 'Ethnographic research in medical sociology: its foci and distinctive contributions', *Sociological Methods and Research* 25: 452–94.

Cohen, I.J. and Rogers, M.F. (1994) 'Autonomy and credibility: voice as method', *Sociological Theory* 12: 304–18.

Collins, R. (1981) 'On the microfoundations of macrosociology', *American Journal of Sociology* 86: 984–1014.

Couch, C.J. (1992) 'Evocative transformations and social relationships', in N.K. Denzin (ed.), *Studies in Symbolic Interaction*, vol. 13, Greenwich, CT: JAI Press.

deCoster, A.V. (1997) 'Physician emotion management', unpublished paper, Baton Rouge, LA: Department of Sociology, Louisiana State University.

Diamond, T. (1992) *Making Grey Gold: Narratives of Nursing Home Care*, Chicago: University of Chicago Press.

Ferguson, K. (1993) *The Man Question: Visions of Subjectivity in Feminist Theory*, Berkeley, CA: University of California Press.

Fineman, S. (1994) *Emotions in Organizations*, Newbury Park, CA: Sage.

Foner, N. (1994) *The Caregiving Dilemma: Work in an American Nursing Home*, Berkeley, CA: University of California Press.

Freeman, H., Levine, S. and Reeder, L.G. (1972) 'The present status of medical sociology', in Howard E. Freeman, Sol Levine and Leo G. Reeder (eds), *Handbook of Medical Sociology*, Englewood Cliffs, NJ: Prentice-Hall.

Gallagher, E.B. (1994) 'Quality of life issues and the dialectic of medical progress: illustrated by end-stage renal disease patients', *Advances in Medical Sociology* 5: 67–90.

Gerhardt, U. and Brieskorn-Zinke, M. (1986) 'The normalization of hemodialysis at home', in J.R. Roth and S.B. Ruzek (eds), *Research in the Sociology of Health Care*, vol. 4, Greenwich, CT: JAI Press.

Graham, H. (1985) 'Providers, negotiators, mediators: women as the hidden carers', in E. Lewin and V. Olesen (eds), *Women, Health and Healing: Toward a New Perspective*, London: Tavistock Methuen.

Hilgartner, S. and Bosk, C. (1988) 'The rise and fall of social problems: a public arenas model', *American Journal of Sociology* 94: 53–78.

Hochschild, A.R. (1983) *The Managed Heart: The Commercialization of Human Feeling*, Berkeley, CA: University of California Press.

Hughes, E.C. (1971) *The Sociological Eye*, Chicago: University of Chicago Press.

Hunt, L.M., Jordan, B. and Browner, C.H. (1989) 'Compliance and the patient's perspective: controlling symptoms in everyday life', *Culture, Medicine and Psychiatry* 13: 315–34.

Jaggar, A.M. (1989) 'Love and knowledge: emotion in feminist epistemology', in A.M. Jaggar and S.R. Bordo (eds), *Gender/Body/Knowledge: Feminist Reconstructions of Being and Knowing*, New Brunswick, NJ: Rutgers University Press.

James, N. (1994) 'Divisions of emotional labour: disclosure and cancer', in S. Fineman (ed.), *Emotion in Organizations*, Thousand Oaks, CA: Sage.

James, V. and Gabe, J. (1996) *Health and the Sociology of the Emotions*, Oxford: Blackwell.

Kotarba, J.A., Ragsdale, D. and Morrow, J.R. Jr (1997) 'Everyday culture in a dedicated HIV/AIDS Hospital Unit', in J.J. Kronenfeld (ed.), *Research in the Sociology of Health Care*, vol. 14: *The Evolving Health Care System: Necessary Changes for Providers of Care, Consumers and Patients*, Greenwich, CT: JAI Press.

Lawler, J. (1991) *Behind the Screens: Nursing, Somology and the Problem of the Body*, London: Churchill Livingstone.

Loseke, D. (1999) 'Emotions discourse and the construction of social problems', unpublished paper presented to the Midwest Sociological Association.

Mamo, L. (1999) 'Death and dying: confluences of emotion and awareness', *Sociology of Health and Illness* 21: 13–36.

Mills, T. and Kleinman, S. (1988) 'Emotions, reflexivity and action: an interactionist analysis', *Social Forces* 66: 1009–27.

Morris, D.B. (1998) *Illness and Culture in the Postmodern Age*, Berkeley, CA: University of California Press.

Mukherjee, B. (1994) *The Holder of the Word*, London: Virago.

Murcott, A. (1977) 'Blind alleys and blinkers: the scope of medical sociology', *Scottish Journal of Sociology* 1: 2–5.

Olesen, V.L. (1989) 'Caregiving, ethical and informal: emergent challenges in the sociology of health and illness', *Journal of Health and Social Behavior* 30: 1–10.

—— (1990) 'The neglected emotions: a challenge to medical sociology', *Medical Sociology News* 16: 11–15.

—— (1997) 'Who cares? Formal and informal providers', in S.B. Ruzek, V.L. Olesen and A.E. Clarke (eds), *Women's Health, Diversities and Complexities*, Columbus, OH: Ohio State University Press.

—— (1998) 'Resisting fatal unclutteredness: reflections on the history of the sociology of health and medicine', unpublished paper presented at the ASA Medical Sociology Plenary, August.

—— (2000) 'Emotions and gender in US health care contexts: implications for change and stasis in the division of labor', in S.J. Williams, M. Calnan and M. Bury (eds), *Health, Medicine and Society: Key Theories, Future Agendas*, Newbury Park, CA: Sage.

—— and Bone, D. (1998) 'Emotions in rationalizing organizations: conceptual notes from professional nursing in the US', in S.J. Williams and G. Bendelow (eds), *Emotions in Social Life: Critical Themes and Contemporary Issues*, New York: Routledge.

Radley, A. (1988) 'The social form of feeling', *British Journal of Social Psychology* 27: 5–18.

Scambler, G. (ed.) (1987) *Sociological Theory and Medical Sociology*, London: Tavistock.

—— and Higgs, P. (1998) *Modernity, Medicine and Health: Medical Sociology towards 2000*, London: Routledge.

Schutz, A. (1962). 'On multiple realities', in M. Natanson (ed.), *Alfred Schutz, Collected Papers: The Problem of Social Reality*, vol. i, The Hague: Martinus Nijhoff.

Smith, P. (1992) *The Emotional Labour of Nursing*, London: Macmillan.

Stacey, M. (1976) *The Health Service Consumer: A Sociological Misconception*, Sociology of the National Health Service, Sociological Review Monograph no. 22, Keele: University of Keele.

—— (1981) 'The division of labour revisited, or overcoming the two Adams', in P. Abrams, R. Deem, J. Finch and P. Rock (eds), *Practice and Progress: British Sociology 1950–1980*, London: Allen and Unwin.

—— (1984) 'Who are the health workers? Patients and other unpaid workers in health care', *Economics and Industrial Democracy* 5: 157–84.

—— (1988) *The Sociology of Health and Healing*, London: Unwin Hyman.

Strauss, A.L. and Bucher, R. (1961) 'Professions in process', *American Journal of Sociology* 66: 325–34.

——, Schatzman, L., Bucher, R., Erlich, D. and Sabshin, M. (1963) 'The hospital and its negotiated order', in E. Freidson (ed.), *The Hospital in Modern Society*, New York: Free Press.

——, Fagerhaugh, S., Suzcek, B. and Wiener, C.L. (1982) 'Sentimental work in the technological hospital', *Sociology of Health and Illness* 12: 254–78.

Thoits, P. (1996) 'Managing the emotions of others', *Symbolic Interaction* 19: 85–109.

Timmermans, S. (1994) 'Dying of awareness: the theory of awareness contexts revisited', *Sociology of Health and Illness* 16: 322–39.

Williams, S.J. and Calnan, M. (1996) *Modern Medicine: Lay Perspectives and Experience*, London: UCL Press.

Zimmerman, M. (1999) 'TLC or CFO? Conflicted caregivers in the health care market', unpublished paper presented to the Midwest Sociological Society.

Concluding comments

Meg Stacey

My reaction to this collection of essays is to rejoice. Reading it has given me much pleasure and reminded me what a wonderful conference it was – so many smiling faces! The essays are remarkably diverse, yet they constitute a unity. The contributors, who include a biologist, anthropologists and soci-ologists, range in age and experience from young new authors to the inter-nationally acclaimed. The strong representation from abroad is welcome. Especially wonderful for me – sitting in a world that sometimes seems increas-ingly alienating – is to see so many people working in areas important to me, developing new areas and ways of working whose importance I can heartily commend. This brings a sense of relief: the world is not so alien after all.

Suffering

The question of suffering has underpinned much of the work I have tried to do over the years, particularly the suffering which we human beings inflict on one another, individually or collectively. The treatment of children in hospital was one such striking example in the 1960s. How was it, how does it still happen, that in trying to improve health more pain is inflicted? One can accept with Parsons that treatment may involve inflicting pain. The unneces-sary and unintended suffering in the hospital treatment of children struck me so forcibly: unintended and *unrecognised* suffering. In looking for *why*, so much in so many areas has had to be attended to: work organisation; profes-sional organisation; the private/public divide; the gender order; the division of labour; the legacies of history – my colleagues have discussed aspects of all of these and more, both directly and indirectly.

Suffering was not always an acceptable word. A colleague on the second children-in-hospital study (Hall and Stacey 1979), having read the section headed 'Illness, treatment and suffering' in my concluding chapter, advised against using the word 'suffering'. I suppose the fear was that it would be seen as 'unscientific'; it spoke out loud of the messiness of human happenings that reductivist science ignores. Our work would be seen as 'tainted' if emotion were expressed. I ignored the advice. I am not sorry. Was the following the most unacceptable passage in the whole section?

It is the business of medicine to identify disease and to ameliorate or cure it. Ultimately the purpose of this is that suffering shall be reduced, but attention is directed to the disease rather than to the suffering or the person who is suffering. The concentration on disease seems to have the effect of distracting attention from what cannot be defined as disease, and therefore (unintentionally no doubt), to distract attention from, or to refuse to accept the evidence of, suffering which cannot be put down to an identifiable disease entity ... the failure to recognize or treat pain which is not physical pain.

(Ibid.: 185–6)

Our systematic studies, using a variety of methods, had shown that some children undoubtedly suffered during hospitalisation. Why not say so bluntly?

There is nothing scientistic about the chapters in the present book. Happily the scientism that threatened to overwhelm sociology did not succeed as it has in some parts of psychology (see Rose and Rose 2000). Our authors are all aware that emotions and values imbue the lived experiences of patients and their carers as well as those of us who research and teach. Lynda Birke's criticism of social constructionism (Chapter 2) is, at least in part, impelled by her personal experiences of menstrual pain derived from her own internal gynaecological 'bits and pieces' as she calls them – these are not *simply* socially constructed. Virginia Olesen refers to the 'passion for the subject' that has impelled much creative research. In that context Olesen refers to her own early feminist essay 'Rage in not enough: scholarly feminism and research in women's health'. I suspect Joan Haran's passion for women's right to chose is what gave her the energy to pursue her complex analysis (Chapter 4). An integral part of Hilary Rose's analysis of reactions to clinical genetics is the 'personal distress' which parents feel when prenatal diagnostic testing leads to a necessary decision to abort or not to abort (Chapter 3).

Not only do these contributors have no embarrassment in talking about suffering, the importance of including and understanding emotions is made plain. Gillian Bendelow notes how emotions lie at the juncture of fundamental dualisms, mind/body, nature/culture, public/private. The child-centred methodologies she developed reflect this understanding. Simon Williams's approach is more academically theoretical, but not without feeling; he refers, for example, to moving beyond such sub-specialisms as the sociology *of* emotions or the sociology *of* the body towards a more 'passionate sociology' (Game and Metcalfe 1996). The contributors include some who have done – and do – just that. Williams's reflections on the relations between the social sciences and biology are part of the growing tide of scholarly opinion that has found reductive analysis an unsatisfactory route to the proper understanding of human beings and their social life, a life integrally involving feelings and emotions.

Priscilla Alderson's chapter on the consent of children and their parents to surgery shows clearly the importance of including feelings and perceptions in the equation (Chapter 11). Giving informed consent for medical treatment cannot be entirely reduced to rational procedures. For example, cutting out 'voluntariness' from consent, as has been suggested (Faden and Beauchamp 1986: 257), tidies it up, but '[c]onsent then dwindles into a polite formality which tolerates patients' idiosyncratic preferences *abstracted from those issues in their daily lives which make their hopes and fears significant*' (my emphasis). As her research showed, parents' consent to complex treatment plans is a *process*, not an event: people need time to acquire knowledge as deeply absorbed and experienced awareness of the personal implications; 'factual information' is not enough. The moral considerations involved throughout are not separated from everyday life. Priscilla Alderson's work illustrates well the 'fatal unclutteredness' that would 'ossify the humane, meliorative and theoretical aspects of our work', to which Virginia Olesen draws attention (Chapter 14).

The dam bursts

In recent years the dam which held back the collective expression of patients' sorrow and anger has burst. Doctors have increasingly been called to account and in the process the extent of that anger and sorrow has become plain. As those of us who listened to patients over the past 30 or 40 years have been aware, there was a great deal of underground distress ranging from a feeling of not having been treated as a full human being, to other more serious complaints: parents who were not listened to when they tried to convey their conviction that a particular medical treatment was not working, but on the contrary was doing their child harm; parents who were not properly told about the full nature of a child's illness and the manner of his/her death – or with whom the doctor did not share her/his doubts and uncertainties (see Power 1998); parents who have carried this pain with them for decades. Parents who, like those in Bristol, had accepted operative treatment for their babies; babies who were returned to them seriously damaged or dead. Such heart surgery is inherently and unavoidably risky, but these parents found that their children had been operated on by surgeons whose rates of death and damage were above average; also that a medical whistle-blower had been so unsupported that he emigrated. A parents' movement developed. The General Medical Council's (GMC) disciplinary action and the subsequent public inquiry are now on record (GMC 2001; Bristol Royal Infirmary Inquiry 2001).

Twenty, possibly even ten, years ago, most medical practitioners were unaware of the force of pent-up sorrow and anger that had found no satisfactory route for expression, or of the resultant determination to 'find the truth' and 'see justice done'. Practitioners, with honourable exceptions, were not even aware of their role in this. One of my most used transparencies when talking about the old GMC was one that simply said:

Meaning Well

Doing Badly

There was a tendency among too many doctors to see the complainants and protesters as 'unbalanced', unable to accept their bereavement because of individual pathology, rather than recognising their own failures of information and communication or their own technical incompetence. In the past, routes to express complaints were all too often blocked; the attitudes and behaviour of the GMC was, as its President Sir Donald Irvine has said, part of the problem (Irvine 2001: 8). The Patients' Charter and attempts to improve the complaints machinery raised expectations; the public was far less subservient than it had been at the start of the NHS. The faltering nature of the procedures, however, increased frustration.

The uncovering of the widespread practice of removing organs from children's corpses without first telling the parents, let alone gaining their fully informed consent, has added to the pain, fury and despair of individuals and groups of patients. In an apparently secular society there is a sense in which the human body remains sacred – and it seems especially so in death. The dead body requires respectful treatment in honour of, and affection for, the recently living and vibrant being that it was. Respectful treatment is also an important component of the healing of the bereaved. The body 'belongs' to the relatives, parents, children, partners; it is in some sense part of their very being. For the bereaved to find they have only laid to rest part of their loved one stirs emotions of great depth – especially when added to suspicions of incompetent or unsympathetic treatment. Theirs is the sorrow and the mourning.

Divisions of work, occupations and specialisms

Remarkable changes have taken place in the division of labour and the nature of specialisation since I read sociology in the 1940s and even since I came to study health care in the 1960s. Some have been liberating; all have brought their own difficulties. Four sets of changes are particularly striking – the first three being closely connected with the shifting division between the public and private domains:

- the changing gender and generational orders;
- the changing relationships between patient and professional;
- third-party involvement in formerly intimate domestic matters;
- the re-emergence of alternative and complementary healing modalities.

Changing gender and generational orders

Women have penetrated the public worlds of work and play. Still not always fully accepted and certainly not yet receiving equal pay for equal worth; still at risk of being seen as sex objects rather than persons in our own right; constantly exploited in advertisements, nevertheless women are in there, in the public domain and in sufficient numbers to help and support each other. What a change is there! Children's position in the division of labour has also changed, more respected as persons and in some ways given more space, but also more surveillance, by caring parents and by the state.

The division of health care labour reflects these changes. In the mid nineteenth century all medical practitioners were men – one woman slipped through, but that gap in the hedge was soon blocked. By the outset of the twentieth century male-dominated medicine worked alongside midwives, independent but able only to deal with 'normal' deliveries and thus subject to medical authority. Nurses worked to doctors who had ultimate authority *de jure* if not always *de facto*. By mid century little had changed, but change was on the way. The beginning of the twenty-first century sees male and medical domination no longer unchallenged; gender biases in medical specialties continue and some new ones emerge. Nursing has a completely new look.

Celia Davies has brought the 'gender agenda' (Chapter 5), as she calls it, up to date with regard to professional self-regulation, juxtaposing the gendered nature of the GMC with that of the United Kingdom Central Council (UKCC). 'We cannot', she says, 'understand masculinities apart from femininities or the gendered work of nurses apart from the gendered health work of doctors. Medicine and nursing are locked together in a binary relation, a relation that affirms the one and denies the other . . . '. She argues further that '[i]f health work is characterised by "binary othering", the institutions set up by those differently positioned by the binary divide *can have the appearance but never the reality of equivalence*' (my emphasis). The strategies of the Council of a subordinated occupation are gendered: not because of any essential difference between women and men, but because gender was crucial to its social formation. How right Celia is to conclude: 'If current regulatory practice is to be reformed and perhaps . . . unified across the professions, then it needs to confront and transcend the gender legacies at the heart of its present institutional structures.' In Irvine's Royal Society of Medicine lecture (Irvine 2001) I noted sadly that neither sex nor gender was mentioned.

Changing relationships between patients and professionals

In 1948, patients who yesterday were charity patients today became patients with a right to be there, a right deriving from their contributions to the state through insurance payments and taxes. Many found it hard to claim the new status, could not even believe it. After a while, however, the old subservience began to be shed. Medical knowledge gradually became more available –

although to my knowledge one medical officer tried to block *The Lancet* and the *British Medical Journal* being ordered for the university library. Gradually organisations of patients and carers got underway, some working closely with interested doctors. The 'active patient', as Hilary Rose puts it (Chapter 3), is now taking over. Despite warnings, doctors have been slow to understand that they can no longer get away with the old secretive, paternalistic attitudes, as the Bristol and Alder Hey protests show.

In January 2001 the President of the GMC gave an address to the Royal Society of Medicine, 'The public and the medical profession: a changing relationship', aimed at rallying his colleagues in face of necessary reforms (Irvine 2001). By no means all of the audience shared his conviction that doctors and patients should henceforth work in partnership.

Gillian Lewando Hundt's chapter demonstrates again, but in a totally different context – among the Bedouin Arabs of the Negev – that before, during and after childbirth the women actively chose among the many relevant services the Israeli state made available (Chapter 6). The women are guided by their culture, their religion and their social and economic circumstances.

Third-party involvement in formerly intimate affairs

A striking change was third-party involvement entering the moment of conception – heralded by the birth of the first test-tube baby in 1978. Public involvement in private matters had taken a leap even larger than the near-universal hospitalisation of childbirth a decade before. The 'new genetics' takes this further forward again.

On the one hand, information about the very constitution of our bodies can fall into the hands of governmental authorities – note the mapping of the genes of the entire Icelandic population. (I await Hilary Rose's research report on this, currently in the hands of the Wellcome Trust.) But not everything can or will fall to governments, consultants or pharmaceutical companies. It is not and will not be just a matter for medical scientists and practitioners. New sets of relations are developing, driven by the exigencies of applying the new genetics in real-life situations: interpenetrations of new kinds between the private and the public domains and changes in professional client–patient relationships. The patient as producer as well as consumer of health care emerges in new ways. 'Genetic knowledge', as Rose says, 'has to be situated in an intimate context.'

The dangers of exploitation of patients and corruption of the new knowledge on the part of medical professionals and commercial interests, notably pharmaceutical corporations, remain ever present. Rose recognises that critical comment is 'almost drowned out by the deluge of Gene-talk'. However, in some areas at least, *genethics* will be built from below. She argues that women and their partners – picking their way through their reproductive choices, dealing with the knowledge of pathology for which no therapy is presently available – are *central* to the application of genetic knowledge.

Furthermore, this is the only way to avoid consumer eugenics and state eugenics. New institutions are needed which are both more transparently democratic and have greater legitimacy and power than present advisory bodies. They have to work in the face of 'immense industrial and financial forces'.

The re-emergence of complementary and alternative healing modalities

When allopathic medicine gained state recognition with the Medical Regulation Act in 1858, the knell started tolling for all other kinds of healers. Not banned (they simply could not call themselves 'registered medical practitioners'), they were not allowed in state employ in the armed forces or elsewhere. As the state influence over health grew, so did the effect of this restriction, first with National Health Insurance and then when the NHS was established. Everyone was now able to get health care free at the point of delivery. Medicine, by now biomedicine, had achieved effective domination over all other types of practitioner (see, for example, Larkin 1983, 1995; Power 1984; Saks 1992; Stacey 1988).

However, in the last 30 or more years increasing numbers of people have turned to alternative and complementary practitioners (CPs for short), notwithstanding the fees. Biomedical and the formerly banished practitioners are now beginning to work together. Questions arise, which Ursula Sharma examines in Chapter 12: is 'integration' of all the varied types of healing happening? could it happen? or does medicine still dominate? The short answers to this seem to be: 'no' to the first; 'not under present circumstances' to the second; and 'yes', biomedicine does.

A number of difficulties come between CPs and GPs in achieving co-operation, let alone integration, in practice. The first obstacle is the organisation of therapeutic responsibility, controlled by the GMC and permeating the entire NHS, which continues to restrict CPs' independence: the GP must retain ultimate responsibility for the patient. Second, the wide differences in education and training between GPs and most CPs are an impediment. Not surprisingly, co-operation is better and more effective when considerable mutual education has taken place, but frequently this is done outside paid CP sessions. The third comes from 'market forces': a great advantage of the CPs working with GPs is that many people who could not afford to pay for CPs then have access to their healing skills. Over against this CPs have to submit to NHS bureaucratic accounting for time, money, space and expertise, and lose the freedom which private practice accords. Attitudes exacerbate – or even create – difficulties. Some GPs say they treat CPs as equals (although the latter do not always think so); others would like to have CPs as subordinate allies, as practice nurses and physiotherapists are: a status CPs resist. They each have their own knowledge base and trained practice skills.

Sharma concludes somewhat pessimistically that 'it is hard to see how integration could be a coming together of equally valued systems of know-ledge'. In practice, accepting 'established medical dominance on the part of CPs is the price that must be paid for wider access to complementary medi-cine' delivered by the NHS. Are there no alternative solutions open to gov-ernment? Types of knowledge and understanding – especially when linked with power and/or profit – seem to be crucial to so many of the concerns of this book.

Theory, method and knowledge

Irvine (2001: 3) reminded us how great was the professional and public enthusiasm for the new science and technology of medicine around the time of the foundation of the NHS in 1948. A hierarchical division of labour with hospital consultants at its apex was established: '[S]cience and scientific research became embedded at the top of the profession's values and incentive systems, with the so-called "soft parts" of medicine – notably communication with patients and relatives, and teaching – apparently much less valued' (Irvine 2001: 2). Medical attention, following the scientific mode, looked ever more deeply and ever more minutely 'down into the cells'.

The kind of science that was espoused

Classical science rested on a 'conviction of fundamental simplicity [which] was . . . seen as essential for rationality itself . . . and has had a specially strong influence on ideas about the nature of science. Being "scientific" appeared to involve above all an unconquerable faith in this ultimate sim-plicity' (Midgley 1992: 35, discussing Prigogine and Stengers 1984). Discover-ies of the complexity and continual movement and instability of matter may have led contemporary scientists to dismiss this view, but this was the science which medicine espoused and which led it to develop into biomedicine. From this have arisen some of our greatest blessings but also very great hazards. Faith in simple uncluttered propositions has also led scientists to undertake some extraordinary myth-making, as Midgley reveals, taking apart such giants as Barrow and Tipler, Dyson, Monod (Midgley 1992, 1994). Her chap-ter in *Alas, Poor Darwin* (Rose and Rose 2000) shows the inutility, as well as the absurdity, of 'memology' (a fashion set off by Dawkins): the attempt to apply to culture the atomising approach, so successful in relation to matter of all kinds.

The image of a deterministic gene is another such: 'we are shaped by our genes', this argument runs. We are no longer offered 'a straightforward old-fashioned deity [rational science did a good deal to trash that idea] but, more creepy still, a kind of plotting ego at the heart of our own body cells. We emerge as the pawns of our own tissues, pawns deluded into thinking that they are the players' (Midgley 1994: 87). But, Midgley reminds us, we are, in truth, conscious subjects and active agents (ibid.: 90).

Despite the many wonderful medical treatment successes that have flowed from the scientific approach – without microsurgery and laser beams I would not be typing this chapter – by end-century the early hopes of a conquest of disease had faded. The thalidomide tragedy was perhaps the first seriously to shake public faith in the new medicine, including in that case the pharmaceuticals. New diseases emerged and old ones re-emerged, as Renée Fox reminds us (Chapter 13); doubt and uncertainties abound. 'Nature' refuses to be controlled, let alone beaten. Ever more complex technologies and treatments demanded ever more training, skill and devotion to the tasks in hand. Yet, as Midgley (1992, 1994) demonstrates, the scientific method leaves out much that we need to understand about the world and our lives: other conceptual frameworks and other methods are also needed.

This thinking bears closely on the central point of Virginia Olesen's chapter (14), 'Resisting fatal uncluttteredness', a wonderful phrase she has drawn from Bharati Mukherjee (1994). Priscilla Alderson's research, discussed above, is a particularly relevant example. However, the whole array of essays in this book illustrates the points about different methods being needed for different understandings.

Methodology and epistemology

The range of methodologies encompassed in this book excites me: it's great seeing people going about things in new ways. There was a time, perhaps 50 years ago, when sociology looked on contemporary social relations and theorised them without reference to their historical origins. Times have changed. Just how important history is to understanding the present scene comes out clearly in Celia Davies's analysis of the regulation of health care professions (Chapter 5), in Joan Busfield's account of how ideas about mental illness have changed over the last 200 years, including the relationship of particular labels to sex and gender (Chapter 7) and in Anne Murcott's account of the disposal of dead bodies – which moved from the private, or at least neighbourhood, domain to the public, but is now being brought back again by a few radical folk (Chapter 6).

Gillian Bendelow and Geraldine Brady draw out the varied ways in which research on or about children has changed in historical time and also differs between disciplines. These changes are traced from the early quantitative approach of psychologists to child behaviour, through the tardy recognition by sociologists that children are social beings and associated research in the mid twentieth century, to a more child-centred research and one that brings children firmly into the division of labour as active agents. Through the 'draw and label' technique Bendelow and her colleagues (and now others) have come to appreciate children's understanding about their illness and medication – views that turn out to be quite different from what their parents had imagined (Chapter 9). Priscilla Alderson has used methods that have demonstrated that children have much greater competence to decide about their own treatment options than former assumptions and methods had suggested. Children are competent social actors, they have agency, as Bendelow puts it, but they are also in a structured position in which adults have the power and authority. Adults also are in structured positions, of course. Lesley Doyal reminds us of this (Chapter 10).

Renée Fox's methodology is at once historical and contemporary. On re-entering the field of *medical uncertainty* that she researched in the 1950s (Fox 1957, 1959) she used 1990s' British and American medical and scientific literature. These were her primary sources to assess the extent and nature of change and continuity from the 1950s to the 1990s. This comparison reveals that some old uncertainties persist, albeit sometimes in new manifestations, as in the case of genetics, which starkly reveals the gap between the highly reductionist genetic science and potential 'genetic medicine'. As yet there is 'no conceptual framework within which the [reductionist] micro-knowledge can be synthesised, consolidated and made pertinent to the organismic, pathophysiological level of medicine'. But this is a new form of a long-existing co-existence in medicine.

Uncertainties are 'both cognitive and existential'. Just as genetics reveals more starkly old problems, so 'evidence-based medicine' raises profound issues: uncertainty regarding the nature of medical knowledge; gaps in knowledge; and questions of evidence – about what? for what? for whom? Medicine's cognitive framework is called into question. There is epistemological uncertainty.

In different mode, Lesley Doyal's excellent discussion of policy and gender equity rests importantly on quantitative research, but demonstrates the importance of conceptualisation in addressing her problem. Her wish is for methods and theories that will help to show how to improve human wellbeing – a concern I share. She complains that some work on 'the body' is unhelpful, being overly theorised and abstract, tending to lead to paralysis. I do empathise with that. So she starts her analysis of 'gender' by looking at the biological and social domains separately, indicating how some knotty problems have drawn researchers from both domains nearer together – a notable example being HIV/AIDS. Gillian Lewando Hundt's chapter relies on analysis of clinical and health delivery statistics as to the treatment received in, around and after childbirth by Bedouin Arab women. Its richness and credibility rests on in-depth interviews of selected samples of women.

I have long thought that sensitive and well-written novels can convey a greater understanding of the social world and its culture than can 'the analytically distinct categories of abstract social theory' (Haran: Chapter 4) and also, I have thought, than the survey-based analyses that too often lead to a 'so what?' response. Social anthropology apart, there was in my younger days a dearth of narrative accounts of subjective experience. I was thinking then largely about novels set in the 'real world'.

Joan Haran's comparative analysis of a piece of science fiction and a ghosted autobiography takes a further step. She points to how 'common senses' are both produced and mediated by such novels and to how they can play a critical role in the development of social theory. These interests chime with those of Virginia Olesen, who asks whether emotional discourses sustain the viability of an issue or health problem and, if so, how? Comparing them, Haran fears the dystopic sci-fi account may well predict the future for American women better than the biographical account of the woman doctor who provides abortions; women's freedom to chose may be by no means secure. The pro-life utterances President Bush made with almost his first breath in office suggest she may be right. Virginia Olesen has challenged researchers to investigate when and what part emotional discourses play in future events. This terrain might be an interesting example.

The problems with specialising

Lynda Birke's chapter fascinated me. She, the only biologist among the authors, describes how public understanding of our insides is distorted by the scientists' use of graphics leading us, for example, to imagine that we have lots of empty spaces inside, where in reality there is little. The *biological* reduction to abstractions had not really penetrated my mind – it seems not so obvious as those of physics. 'Modern scientific illustrations', she says, 'are highly stylised: organs appear taken out of context of a body . . . [s]ometimes they are so abstracted they no longer bear much relationship to the living organism.' Female sex organs relevant to reproduction but not to pleasure (no clitoris) are shown, for example: 'The body . . . becomes a set of replaceable parts – as indeed it is within the rhetoric of biomedicine.' Transplant surgery is the outstanding example, but this replaceability, as Birke says, does not fit with the way people live their lives or how they *experience* transplant surgery.

What I found most fascinating, however, was Birke's revelation that the bodies *sociology* has dealt with generally have surfaces but no insides – not in this case a distortion, but an absence. This suggests (if true, and I'm no expert on the sociology of the body) that as sociologists we are still more bound by the Cartesian split than I had realised. Thinking of the mind/body divide, I recalled the great stress laid on connecting the mind and the body in Buddhism, that so-ancient body of thought (like 2,500 + years). Some meditation practices, for example, not only propose conscious breathing to link body and mind, but also reflecting on the state of one's body, including a check on all the major *internal* organs.

Lynda Birke is so right to say that in the West today 'we rarely think in terms of how living the body within society (the subject of so much recent theorising) impacts on the body's internal processes'. We know in quantitative terms about correlations with characteristics of populations and the presence of disease, but not the processes. OK, so we know it's a virus or a pollutant, but we do not know why it strikes these persons and not those similar ones: the individual/society problems again. As Linda Birke concludes, we seriously need dialogue across the disciplinary divide. Those biologists who are talking about agency seem good ones to start with.

A trouble is the inbuilt tendency for each specialism to believe it has the blueprint that will save the world – or more modestly, a blueprint without which the world cannot be saved. This derives partly from the excitement and commitment people feel for their own discipline and the way it (or their bit of it) selects problems for study and goes about studying them. My (unsystematic) observation over the years is that cries for multidisciplinary research or interdisciplinary research (much harder) come from outside rather than from within the discipline – from funders who need to see relevance for the 'real' world. Out there people, societies, cultures are not chopped in bits and 'anyone' can see that all sorts of ways of looking are needed to get a proper grip.

As Virginia Olesen points out, this applies to 'rational management'. I use inverted commas advisedly. Current notions of good management flow from a particular interpretation of what is reasonable. They have a strong scientistic, rather than scientific, flavour – they descend from *Voltaire's Bastards*, as John Rawlston Saul (1993) proposes. (Unfortunately his chapter on health is not the strongest, but the general argument is interesting.) Virginia Olesen draws particular attention to the emotional dilemmas that rationalising environments produce – indicating that sociologists of health and healing and of the emotions need to look at these issues. Her plea is fuelled by the consequences in the US's health care non-system: when insurance runs out on a seriously ill patient treatment, no longer funded, ceases. Crises in the UK do not happen quite like that: we still cling to treatment free at the point of delivery. However, some health authorities do not make available certain treatments and may refuse expensive but unproven treatments in some chronic cases. Restrictions thus have their origin in policy decisions rather than in the insurance exclusiveness or the limits of what the insurance covers. When governed by policy decisions the economics lie at a further remove from the patient; but choices still have to be made. As Lesley Doyal points out in her chapter, policy choices have to be made as to how much priority to give to achieving gender equity over against other necessary social goals such as checking racism or reducing poverty.

Death in peace and war

Anne Murcott has pointed out that I did not deal with death and the disposal of the dead in either Banbury study. I am delighted Anne is herself taking up the subject. Lynda Birke (Chapter 2), as well as mentioning her own physical suffering, remarked upon the suffering war brings – the only reference to war in this book up to now. Yet war (often state sanctioned) is a cause of death, disability and disease and is associated with disturbed states of mind. Medical sociology has not generally taken this on board; I offered no leads in my earlier work.

As critics have remarked to me, the Second World War was not discussed in

Tradition and Change (Stacey 1960). Why? The war was too recent: indeed, when I first went to Banbury it was still happening. 'Everyone' knew about it; its specific effects in Banbury were referred to, such as the town being 'closed' because of the numbers of people who had moved there. My sense is that it was too soon for analysis. The reality of participant observation reflects the omissions as well as the inclusions of those whose lives one is sharing and observing. The First World War is the one to which reference is made in *Tradition and Change*, as an historical marker after which things had changed significantly.

Time passes, new life experiences change perceptions. The NATO war against Serbia had just begun when the conference, the origin of this book, was held. (Yes, I know they said it was not a war; but so it was, and illegal at that.) Our government's action upset me. My own experience of living in a repeatedly bombed city made me acutely aware of what was happening to the Serbs and later also to the Kosovars – and 1940's missiles were not tipped with depleted uranium. I became aware of this omission in the sociology of health and illness in a way that I had not in all the many previous wars. I commented on it in my concluding address. The whole history of the twentieth century provides empirical evidence that violence solves nothing: rather, violence breeds violence. Predictably this would happen in the Balkans – as all too soon it did.

Why has medical sociology not taken the health consequences of war on board? Maybe the analytical methods of modern science and of logic as practised, leading us to fragment and divide our disciplines, make it easier for us to evade some painful, difficult and dangerous topics. Wars, after all, come under military studies or peace studies, not under the provision of health care or the sociology of medical knowledge.

There is something uncannily similar between aspects of modern medicine and modern war: both involve high-precision instruments, application of the latest techno-science and the separation of one problem from all others. Since the Gulf war we hear of 'clinical war'. We now know that the precision bombing may be less than precise, killing many civilians – just as we now know about medical iatrogenesis. It is 9 years since the Gulf war was allegedly over, but bombing raids continue – their wisdom at last being questioned. Sanctions still imposed on Iraq – by US and British governments – have so damaged the health of the population, and particularly of Iraqi children, that one UN official after another has resigned, no longer able to support the policies in face of these health consequences: Denis Halliday, co-ordinator of humanitarian relief in Iraq and at the time Assistant Secretary-General of the UN, resigned in 1998; on 13 February 2000, his successor Hans von Sponeck also resigned, followed two days later by Jutta Burgahlt, head of the World Food Programme in Iraq (Pilger 2000: 29). Unicef reports that more than 4000 children under 5 die each month than would have died before sanctions (ibid.: 26). Anupama Rao Singh, Unicef's senior representative in Iraq, is reported as saying that in 10 years Iraqi child mortality has gone from one of the lowest in the world to the highest (ibid.). The wisdom of sanctions was at last being questioned when Baghdad was suddenly bombed; again civilians were injured and killed.

Returned members of the armed forces repeatedly report 'mystery' illnesses. Depleted uranium is thought to be one cause. Later we hear that peacekeeping forces in Kosovo report illness: skilled investigators have found evidence of depleted uranium both on abandoned military equipment and in civilian areas. For long the talk was exclusively of health consequences for armed forces personnel; only much later was anxiety about the health of those the action was designed to protect added to the discussion – and then not by official sources. We do not know the health consequences of the attacks on Serbia, what contamination their land and people have suffered. Pollution of the Danube must affect its whole course through Europe.

My search for peace workers at the time of the NATO war led me to Cynthia Cockburn's work and a network called Women in Black (WIB for short). In her book *The Space Between Us: Negotiating Gender and National Identities in Conflict* (1998), Cynthia focused on groups where women have come together across deep divisions of nationality, religion and ethnicity, sometimes all of those at once, to work for peace from the grass roots and together to ameliorate the suffering that armed conflict imposes, particularly on women and their children, offering health aid to raped and wounded women. Cockburn's empirical studies, based on participation with the groups, describe and analyse women's activism in Northern Ireland, in Israel/ Palestine, in Bosnia/Herzegovina.

In October 1999 I attended the WIB conference in Montenegro, Federal Republic of Yugoslavia. About 250 women from all over the world gathered: from Italy, the Balkan states, Israel, Belgium, Holland, Germany, France, UK, Norway, North America, Latin America and Russia. They ranged from Eastern Orthodox or Muslim 'traditional' mothers through every shade of feminism to radical lesbians. This motley array contained widely differing views, for example those who supported the NATO action and the majority who regretted it. A thread running through the conference was 'Not "either . . . or", but "neither . . . nor"'. All of us experienced pressure at home to support *either* NATO *or* Milosevic; all of us wanted *neither* Milosevic *nor* NATO's action. (Do those dualities remind you of other similar litanies such as nature/nurture, micro/macro, biomedical/alternative?)

Cockburn reports that, working together, the women's peace groups become increasingly aware of, and articulate about, the masculinism that underlies armed conflict. The women are also aware that rape is not just an individual act but is used as a weapon of war. When armed violence breaks out the women's groups that cross divides find it harder to keep together. The violence increases the pull of nationalities and religious affiliations. As they did in Northern Ireland, currently in the Middle East the groups work hard to stay together, at considerable personal risk. WIB members from many parts of the world are going (January/February 2001) to Israel/Palestine to support their sisters as the tension increases.

There are, of course, many peace groups, mediators, women and men, who do valiant work to reduce violence (see, for example, Curle 1995). My imagination was caught, however, by women working together across the many divides, learning to understand and respect each other, to become strong together. They speak out and write and protest non-violently, seeking to change the political scene. These women seem to point to one way out of a dark world, so detrimental to health: conscious, small-scale interactions that buck the trend of the dominant consciousness; which offer practical demonstrations of co-operative possibilities and which should be linked in to any peace-making effort. I would like to see sociologists and anthropologists in my successor generations taking up the challenge of examining the health aspects of the causes and consequences of violent conflicts and working also on health promotion in those areas.

Renée Fox is right to suggest that the medical uncertainties are not unconnected with more general uncertainties at the start of this new century: 'the dilemmas that medicine faces at this historical juncture reach beyond its boundaries to include questions of value and belief that are more-than-medical and also more-than-ethical'. She concludes (p. 250, above) that:

> It is with extensive uncertainty about its state of knowledge and accomplishments, its value-commitments and its future directions, and with a mixture of confidence and insecurity, that modern Western medicine faces the twenty-first century . . . its relationship to uncertainty is also an indicator of how sure and unsure we are of where we have come from and where we are going, societally and culturally, as we enter the new millennium.

The way we study, the way we create understanding of ourselves and the world is crucial to finding a vision by which we can go forward constructively – in which unnecessary and unintended suffering is reduced. Breaking away from the fractured accounts of traditional science to a more contextualised and inclusive view is liberating, providing a more humane vision. The task is urgent: our globe and all of us living beings within it are in trouble. Wonderful though many of the feats of science and technology are, rely on them though we do in our daily lives, the downside of concentrating on highly specialised segments, of going ever deeper down into the cells, and thus losing our view not only of the whole but of the contexts of the fragments of cells, is threatening planetary disaster. Of course there is a sense in which we have to look carefully at parts, at smaller sections of some kind. The trick must be never to forget about the whole to which our part relates – probably in multiple ways. This is where Hilary and Steven Rose's (2000) book, for example, is so important, bringing together as it does so many different takes on the gene question.

It is crucial, too, that we – and I mean all of us, biologists, humanists, social scientists, the lot – constantly remember that maxim of well-conducted science: always to be willing and open to being proved wrong. This is a main reason why science has been able to proceed so far. Forgetting that maxim, yielding to a desire to gain or retain power or authority or to a desire for more profits – or just being obstinate and ego-centred – not only distorts science, it could spell disaster for the globe. To that maxim I would add: always remember the wider context in which any one aspect is located and the interactions therewith.

Dear friends, thank you all for that wonderful conference and for putting this book together. I didn't know I'd done all those things and I'm still not sure I did. However, if it has helped, I'm glad. If anything I have said in my concluding remarks has caused unwitting offence, please forgive. It's wonderful to see you all doing such great things. May your work flourish!

References

Bristol Royal Infirmary Inquiry (2001) *The Inquiry into the Management and Case of Children Receiving Complex Heart Surgery at the Bristol Royal Infirmary*, <http://www.bristol-inquiry.org.uk> (accessed May 2001).

Cockburn, C. (1998) *The Space Between Us: Negotiating Gender and National Identities in Conflict*, London and New York: Zed Books.

Curle, A. (1995) *Another Way: Positive Response to Contemporary Violence*, Oxford: Jon Carpenter.

Faden, B. and Beauchamp, T. (1986) *A History and Theory of Informed Consent*, New York: Oxford University Press.

Fox, R. (1957) 'Training for uncertainty', in R.K. Merton, G. Reader and P.L. Kendall (eds), *The Student-Physician: Introductory Studies in the Sociology of Medical Education*, Cambridge, MA: Harvard University Press.

—— (1959) *Experiment Perilous: Physicians and Patients Facing the Unknown*, Glencoe, IL: Free Press.

Game, A. and Metcalfe, A. (1996) *Passionate Sociology*, London: Sage.

General Medical Council (2001) Bristol disciplinary cases, <http://www.gmc-uk.org> (accessed May 2001).

Hall, D. and Stacey, M. (1979) *Beyond Separation: Further Studies of Children in Hospital*, London: Routledge and Kegan Paul.

Irvine, Sir Donald (2001) *The Public and the Medical Profession: A Changing Relationship*, The Lloyd Roberts Lecture, Royal Society of Medicine, London: General Medical Council.

Larkin, G.V. (1983) *Occupational Monopoly and Modern Medicine*, London: Tavistock.

—— (1995) 'State control and the health professions in the United Kingdom', in T. Johnson, G. Larkin and M. Saks, *Health Professions and the State in Europe*, London: Routledge.

Midgley, M. (1992) *Science as Salvation: A Modern Myth and its Meanings*, London and New York: Routledge.

—— (1994) *The Ethical Primate: Humans, Freedom and Morality*, London and New York: Routledge.

Mukherjee, B. (1994) *Holder of the World*, London: Virago.

Pilger, J. (2000) 'Squeezed to death', *Guardian Weekend* 4 March: 26–32.

Power, C. (1998) 'When things go wrong what should be said?', *Bulletin of Medical Ethics* 141: 13–21.

Power, R. (1984) *A Natural Profession? Issues in the Professionalism of British Nature Cure 1930–1950*, MSc thesis, Polytechnic of the South Bank, London.

Prigogine, I. and Stengers, I. (1984) *Order Out of Chaos: Man's New Dialogue with Nature*, London: Collins Fontana.

Rose, H. and Rose, S. (2000) *Alas, Poor Darwin: Arguments Against Evolutionary Psychology*, New York: Harmony.

Saks, M. (ed.) (1992) *Alternative Medicine in Britain*, Oxford: Clarendon Press.

Saul, J.R. (1993) *Voltaire's Bastards: The Dictatorship of Reason in the West*, Toronto and Harmondsworth, Middx: Penguin.

Stacey, M. (1960) *Tradition and Change: A Study of Banbury*, London: Oxford University Press.

—— (1988) *The Sociology of Health and Healing: A Textbook*, London: Unwin Hyman.

Index